T0176526

Antiplatelet Therapy in
Cardiovascular Disease

Antiplatelet Therapy in Cardiovascular Disease

EDITED BY

Ron Waksman, MD, FACC
Associate Chief of Cardiology
Director of Cardiovascular Research and Advanced Education
MedStar Heart Institute at MedStar Washington Hospital Center
Washington, DC, USA

Paul A. Gurbel, MD, FACC, FAHA
Director, Sinai Center for Thrombosis Research
Associate Chief for Research
Department of Medicine
Sinai Hospital of Baltimore;
Professor of Medicine
Johns Hopkins University School of Medicine
Baltimore, MD;
Adjunct Professor of Medicine
Duke University School of Medicine
Durham, NC, USA

Michael A. Gaglia, Jr., MD, MSc
Assistant Professor of Medicine
Division of Cardiovascular Medicine
University of Southern California Keck School of Medicine
Los Angeles, CA, USA

WILEY Blackwell

Contents

List of Contributors

Yousif Ahmad, BMedSci, BMBS, MRCP
Cardiology SpR and Honorary Research Fellow
National Heart and Lung Institute
Imperial College London
London;
University of Birmingham Centre for Cardiovascular Sciences
City Hospital
Birmingham, UK

Dominick J. Angiolillo, MD, PhD
Associate Professor of Medicine
Director, Cardiovascular Research
University of Florida College of Medicine
Jacksonville, FL, USA

Nachiket Apte, MBBS
Resident
Sinai Center for Thrombosis Research
Sinai Hospital of Baltimore;
Johns Hopkins University School of Medicine
Baltimore, MD, USA

Deborah E. Aronson, PhD
Medical Publication Editor
The Zena and Michael A. Wiener Cardiovascular Institute
The Icahn School of Medicine at Mount Sinai
New York, NY, USA

Nevin C. Baker, DO
Fellow, Interventional Cardiology
MedStar Washington Hospital Center
Washington, DC, USA

Sameer Bansilal, MD, MS
Assistant Professor
The Zena and Michael A. Wiener Cardiovascular Institute
The Icahn School of Medicine at Mount Sinai
New York, NY, USA

Eric R. Bates, MD
Professor of Internal Medicine
Division of Cardiovascular Diseases
Department of Internal Medicine
University of Michigan
Ann Arbor, MI, USA

Kevin P. Bliden, BS, MBA
Program Manager
Sinai Center for Thrombosis Research
Sinai Hospital of Baltimore
Baltimore, MD, USA

Laurent Bonello, MD, PhD
Medical Doctor (Cardiology)
Département de Cardiologie
Hôpital Nord
Chemin des Bourrely
Marseille, France

Nicoline J. Breet, MD, PhD
Cardiologist in Training
Department of Cardiology
St Antonius Hospital
Nieuwegein, The Netherlands

Andrzej Budaj, MD, PhD, FESC
Professor of Medicine
Director
Department of Cardiology
Postgraduate Medical School
Grochowski Hospital
Warsaw, Poland

Marco Cattaneo, MD
Professor of Internal Medicine
Dipartimento di Scienze della Salute
Unità di Medicina 3
Ospedale San Paolo
Università degli Studi di Milano
Milano, Italy

Matthew J. Chung, MD
Adjunct Assistant Professor of Medicine
Duke University Medical Center;
Hospitalist Physician
Durham Veterans Affairs Medical Center
Durham, NC, USA

Lidija Covic, PhD
Co-Director
Hemostasis and Thrombosis Laboratory
Molecular Oncology Research Institute
Division of Hematology/Oncology
Tufts Medical Center;
Assistant Professor of Medicine and Biochemistry
Tufts University School of Medicine
Boston, MA, USA

Flávio de Souza Brito, MD
Clinical Research Fellow
Division of Cardiology
Duke University Medical Center
Duke Clinical Research Institute
Durham, NC, USA

Germano di Sciascio, MD, FACC, FESC, FSCAI
Professor and Chairman of Cardiology
Department of Cardiovascular Sciences
Campus Bio-Medico University of Rome
Rome, Italy

Vijay A. Doraiswamy, MD, FACP
Fellow
Cardiovascular Medicine
University of Arizona
Tucson, AZ, USA

J. Emilio Exaire, MD
Assistant Professor of Medicine
The University of Oklahoma Health Sciences Center
Oklahoma City, OK, USA

Pierre Fontana, MD, PhD
Associate Professor
Co-director
Geneva Platelet Group
University of Geneva;
Division of Angiology and Haemostasis
Geneva University Hospitals and Faculty of Medicine
(Geneva Platelet Group)
Geneva, Switzerland

Francesco Franchi, MD
Postdoctoral Research Associate
University of Florida College of Medicine
Jacksonville, FL, USA

Michael A. Gaglia, Jr., MD, MSc
Assistant Professor of Medicine
Division of Cardiovascular Medicine
University of Southern California Keck School of Medicine
Los Angeles, CA, USA

Martin Gesheff, BS
Research Study Coordinator
Sinai Center for Thrombosis Research
Sinai Hospital of Baltimore
Baltimore, MD, USA

Paul A. Gurbel, MD, FACC, FAHA
Director, Sinai Center for Thrombosis Research
Associate Chief for Research
Department of Medicine
Sinai Hospital of Baltimore;
Professor of Medicine
Johns Hopkins University School of Medicine
Baltimore, MD;
Adjunct Professor of Medicine
Duke University School of Medicine
Durham, NC, USA

Christian Hamm, MD
Professor of Internal Medicine and Cardiology
Department of Internal Medicine and Cardiology
Kerckhoff Heart and Thorax Center
Bad Nauheim, Germany

Arnoud W.J. van't Hof, MD, PhD
Interventional Cardiologist
Head
Department of Research
Isala Academy
Isala Klinieken
Zwolle, The Netherlands

Thomas Hohlfeld, MD
Professor of Pharmacology
Associate Director
Institute of Pharmacology and Clinical Pharmacology
UniversitätsKlinikum
Heinrich-Heine Universität Düsseldorf
Düsseldorf, Germany

Stefan James, MD, PhD
Director
Cardiac Catheterization Laboratory
Associate Professor of Cardiology
Uppsala Clinical Research Center;
Uppsala University Hospital
Uppsala, Sweden

Young-Hoon Jeong, MD, PhD
Associate Professor of Medicine
Division of Cardiology
Department of Internal Medicine
Gyeongsang National University Hospital
Jinju-si, South Korea

Jacek Kubica, MD, PhD
Professor of Medicine
Department of Cardiology and Internal Medicine
Ludwik Rydygier Collegium Medicum
Nicolaus Copernicus University
Bydgoszcz, Poland;
Systematic Investigation and Research on Interventions
and Outcomes (SIRIO)-MEDICINE Research Network

Athan Kuliopulos, MD, PhD
Director
Hemostasis and Thrombosis Laboratory
Molecular Oncology Research Institute
Tufts Medical Center;
Professor of Medicine and Biochemistry
Tufts University School of Medicine
Boston, MA, USA

Marc Laine, MD
Medical Doctor (Cardiology)
Département de Cardiologie
Hôpital Nord
Chemin des Bourrely
Marseille, France

Ana Laynez, MD
Attending Physician
Division of Cardiology
Department of Internal Medicine
MedStar Washington Hospital Center
Washington, DC, USA

Seung-Whan Lee, MD
Associate Professor
Division of Cardiology
University of Ulsan College of Medicine
Asan Medical Center
Seoul, Republic of Korea

Eli I. Lev, MD
Associate Professor of Medicine and Cardiology
Department of Cardiology
Rabin Medical Center
Petah-Tikva;
Tel-Aviv University
Tel-Aviv, Israel

Joshua P. Loh, MBBS
Fellow
Interventional Cardiology
MedStar Washington Hospital Center
Washington, DC, USA

Fabio Mangiacapra, MD, PhD
Attending Cardiologist
Department of Cardiovascular Sciences
Campus Bio-Medico University of Rome
Rome, Italy

Ray V. Matthews, MD
Professor of Medicine
Director of Interventional Cardiology
Division of Cardiovascular Medicine
University of Southern California Keck School of Medicine
Los Angeles, CA, USA

Talha Meeran, MBBS
Resident
Sinai Center for Thrombosis Research
Sinai Hospital of Baltimore;
Johns Hopkins University School of Medicine
Baltimore, MD, USA

Roxana Mehran, MD, FACC
Professor of Medicine (Cardiology)
Director of Interventional Cardiovascular Research and
Clinical Trials
The Zena and Michael A. Wiener Cardiovascular Institute
The Icahn School of Medicine at Mount Sinai;
Cardiovascular Research Foundation
New York, NY, USA

Rosetta Melfi, MD
Attending Cardiologist
Department of Cardiovascular Sciences
Campus Bio-Medico University of Rome
Rome, Italy

Sa'ar Minha, MD
Fellow
Interventional Cardiology
MedStar Washington Hospital Center
Washington, DC, USA

Ana Muñiz-Lozano, MD
Post-doctoral Research Associate
University of Florida College of Medicine
Jacksonville, FL, USA

Aung Myat, BSc(Hons), MB, BS, MRCP
SpR Cardiology & BHF Clinical Research Training Fellow
Cardiovascular Division
King's College London BHF Centre of Research Excellence
The Rayne Institute
St Thomas' Hospital
London, UK

Eliano Pio Navarese, MD, PhD
Interventional Cardiologist and Assistant Professor
Department of Cardiology and Internal Medicine
Ludwik Rydygier Collegium Medicum
Nicolaus Copernicus University
Bydgoszcz, Poland
President of Systematic Investigation and Research
on Interventions and Outcomes (SIRIO)-MEDICINE
Research Network

Annunziata Nusca, MD
Attending Cardiologist
Department of Cardiovascular Sciences
Campus Bio-Medico University of Rome
Rome, Italy

Martin Orban, MD
Cardiologist
Department of Cardiology
Medizinische Klinik und Poliklinik I
Klinikum der Universität München
Ludwig-Maximilians-Universität München
Munich, Germany

Anna Oskarsson, MSc
Research Fellow
Department of Medical Sciences, Cardiology
Uppsala Clinical Research Center
Uppsala, Sweden

Franck Paganelli, MD, PhD
Professor of Cardiology
Département de Cardiologie
Hôpital Nord
Chemin des Bourrely
Marseille, France

Duk-Woo Park, MD
Assistant Professor
Division of Cardiology
University of Ulsan College of Medicine
Asan Medical Center
Seoul, Republic of Korea

Seung-Jung Park, MD, PhD, FACC
Professor of Medicine
Division of Cardiology
University of Ulsan College of Medicine
Chairman, Cardiovascular Center
Asan Medical Center
Seoul, Republic of Korea

Matthew J. Price, MD, FACC, FSCAI
Director
Cardiac Catheterization Laboratory
Division of Cardiovascular Diseases
Scripps Clinic;
Assistant Professor
Scripps Translational Science Institute
La Jolla, CA, USA

Sunil V. Rao, MD
Associate Professor of Medicine
Duke University Medical Center
Duke Clinical Research Institute;
Director
Cardiac Catheterization Laboratories
Durham Veterans Affairs Medical Center
Durham, NC, USA

Simon R. Redwood, MD, FRCP, FACC, FSCAI
Professor of Interventional Cardiology and Honorary
Consultant Cardiologist
Cardiovascular Division
King's College London BHF Centre of Research Excellence
The Rayne Institute
St Thomas' Hospital
London, UK

Jean-Luc Reny, MD, PhD
Associate Professor of Medicine
Co-director
Geneva Platelet Group
University of Geneva;
Director
Division of Internal Medicine, and
Rehabilitation
Trois-Chêne Hospital;
Geneva University Hospitals and Faculty of Medicine
(Geneva Platelet Group)
Geneva, Switzerland

Fabiana Rollini, MD
Postdoctoral Research Associate
University of Florida College of Medicine
Jacksonville, FL, USA

Jorge F. Saucedo, MD
Clinical Professor, Cardiology
NorthShore Medical Group
Evanston, IL, USA

Karsten Schrör, MD
Professor of Pharmacology
Retired, Director of Institute of Pharmacoloy and
Clinical Pharmacology
UniversitätsKlinikum
Heinrich-Heine Universität Düsseldorf
Düsseldorf, Germany

Dirk Sibbing, MD
Interventional Cardiologist and
Clinical Researcher
Department of Cardiology
Medizinische Klinik und Poliklinik I
Klinikum der Universität München
Ludwig-Maximilians-Universität München
Munich, Germany

Marvin J. Slepian, MD
Professor of Medicine
Director
Interventional Cardiology
University of Arizona
Tucson, AZ, USA

Glenn Stokken, MD
Resident
Department of Medicine
University of Arizona
Tucson, AZ, USA

Udaya S. Tantry, PhD
Laboratory Director
Sinai Center for Thrombosis Research
Sinai Hospital of Baltimore
Baltimore, MD, USA

Jurriën M. ten Berg, MD, PhD, FESC, FACC
Interventional Cardiologist
Department of Cardiology
St Antonius Hospital
Nieuwegein, The Netherlands

Pierluigi Tricoci, MD, MHS, PhD
Assistant Professor of Medicine
Division of Cardiology
Duke University Medical Center
Duke Clinical Research Institute
Durham, NC, USA

Muthiah Vaduganathan, MD, MPH
Internal Medicine Resident Physician
Department of Medicine
Massachusetts General Hospital
Harvard Medical School
Boston, MA, USA

Marco Valgimigli, MD, PhD, FESC
Senior Interventional Cardiologist
Associate Professor of Cardiology
Thoraxcenter
Erasmus Medical Center
Rotterdam, The Netherlands

Christoph Varenhorst, MD, PhD
Cardiologist and Hospital Physician
Department of Medical Sciences, Cardiology
Uppsala Clinical Research Center;
Uppsala University Hospital
Uppsala, Sweden

Ron Waksman, MD, FACC
Associate Chief of Cardiology
Director of Cardiovascular Research and Advanced Education
MedStar Heart Institute at MedStar Washington Hospital Center
Washington, DC, USA

Ping Zhang, MD, PhD
Instructor of Medicine
Hemostasis and Thrombosis Laboratory
Molecular Oncology Research Institute
Tufts Medical Center;
Departments of Medicine
Tufts University School of Medicine
Boston, MA, USA

Foreword

We have long known that platelets are pivotal in preventing bleeding and in the clot-formation response to arterial disruption, be it spontaneous or man-made. But only in the recent past, beginning in the 1990s, have we learned more about the complex biology of platelets and the hundreds of agonists by which they can be activated. Aspirin, while a very important platelet inhibitor, works only on the particular thromboxane pathway. When parenterally administered IIb/IIIa glycoprotein inhibitors were developed, we had the misconception that "the final common pathway" to platelet aggregation was being addressed. While these agents had an incremental effect beyond aspirin, the orally active P2Y12 receptor blocking drugs proved to have a level of efficacy simulating the IIb/IIIa inhibitors. And we further learned there was marked heterogeneity of response to the prototypic P2Y12 antiplatelet, clopidogrel, which is partially accounted for by genomic variants in the cytochrome required for its metabolism to an active drug. Newer P2Y12 agents have been developed that circumvent this issue, but they again emphasize the difficult and delicate trade-off of preventing a clot versus promoting a bleeding complication. To add to the complexity, there are now a variety of ways that platelet function can be assessed, even at point-of-care, but there is still considerable controversy as to how and whether these assays should be used in clinical practice.

Now, Drs. Ron Waksman, Paul A. Gurbel and Michael A. Gaglia, Jr., who are highly regarded researchers in the field, have put together a book that dissects the complex antiplatelet story. The book first gets into the underpinning of platelet biology, then delves into the various platelet function tests. Following this background, there is a systematic review of each of the major antiplatelet agents that have undergone extensive clinical trial evaluation. The last two sections deal with use of these agents with percutaneous coronary intervention, other clinical indications, and lack of their responsiveness.

This comprehensive monograph spans the gamut from the platelet cellular biology to the results of the most recent, large-scale clinical trials. All tolled, there have been well over 250,000 patients who have been enrolled in worldwide clinical trials of antiplatelet agents for vascular disease. Accordingly, there is an enormous body of knowledge to synthesize and learn from. This book certainly fulfills an unmet need, bringing together experts if the field from around the world to provide insights and useful perspective. *Antiplatelet Therapy in Cardiovascular Disease* will undoubtedly be a useful resource for cardiologists and physicians who care for patients requiring antiplatelet therapy.

Eric J. Topol, MD
Scripps Clinic and The Scripps Research Institute
La Jolla, CA, USA

Preface

Platelets play pivotal roles in the pathogenesis of cardiovascular disease, a leading cause of mortality worldwide. Inhibition of platelet function is now a key therapeutic strategy for cardiovascular disease, and novel strategies are rapidly emerging. *Antiplatelet Therapy in Cardiovascular Disease* provides a comprehensive and up-to-date overview that spans basic biology, translational research, and clinical treatment. The book is divided into five sections. In Section I, we review major discoveries in platelet physiology and receptor function that have advanced the development of new antiplatelet agents. Section II provides a comprehensive analysis of the major methods being employed clinically to assess platelet function and the pharmacodynamic effects of antiplatelet therapy. The pharmacology of established and novel antiplatelet agents is extensively reviewed in Section III. A specific group of patients who have benefitted from antiplatelet therapy are those with coronary and peripheral arterial disease treated with percutaneous interventions. Section IV is dedicated to the latter group and reviews the controversial areas of pre-PCI antiplatelet therapy and the duration required for dual antiplatelet therapy after coronary stent implantation. In addition to the role of antiplatelet therapy in reducing thrombotic complications, we also review the emerging evidence demonstrating the clinical importance of antiplatelet therapy-related bleeding. Section V is focused on the very controversial and rapidly evolving topics of antiplatelet responsiveness and personalized antiplatelet therapy. In this section, we comprehensively address persistent ischemic event occurrence in the era of potent antiplatelet therapy, an unmet need that is particularly high in specific subgroups. Personalized antiplatelet therapy holds the promise of optimal avoidance of ischemic event occurrence and bleeding.

International experts in basic science, interventional and noninterventional cardiology, and translational medicine have come together to produce the state-of the-art chapters contained in this book. *Antiplatelet Therapy in Cardiovascular Disease* targets a broad audience, including clinical and basic scientists, practicing clinicians, medical students, and allied healthcare professionals who seek concise and in-depth knowledge of antiplatelet therapy.

We are grateful to our medical editor Kathryn Coons and to the publishing staff for their assistance in bringing this book to print. We hope that you will find the book useful in widening your knowledge of the field of antiplatelet therapy in cardiovascular disease.

Ron Waksman, Paul A. Gurbel, and Michael A. Gaglia, Jr.

Section I

Platelet Biology and Pathophysiology

1 Platelet Pathophysiology and its Role in Thrombosis

Paul A. Gurbel[1,2,3] and Udaya S. Tantry[1]
[1] Sinai Hospital of Baltimore, Baltimore, MD, USA
[2] Johns Hopkins University School of Medicine, Baltimore, MD, USA
[3] Duke University School of Medicine Durham, NC, USA

Platelets were first described as disklike structures by Osler in 1873 [1]. Seven years later, their anatomical structure and role in hemostasis and experimental thrombosis were described by Bizzozero [2]. An *in vitro* method to quantify platelet aggregation was reported by Born in 1962. Born stated that "If it can be shown that adenosine diphosphate (ADP) takes part in the aggregation of platelets in blood vessels, it is conceivable that adenosine monophosphate (AMP) or some other substance could be used to inhibit or reverse platelet aggregation in thrombosis" [3]. The observations of Born provided the fundamental basis for *ex vivo* measurement of platelet aggregation in patients with coronary artery disease (CAD) and for the development of antiplatelet agents. Antiplatelet agents that block these targets were either identified (aspirin) or developed (P2Y$_{12}$ and GPIIb/IIIa receptor blockers) during the past four decades. Currently, the latter agents constitute a major part of the pharmacological strategy to prevent thrombosis, an important cause of myocardial infarction and death [4].

Under normal circumstances, platelets circulate in an inactive form and don't significantly interact with the vessel wall. In the setting of endothelial disease or a breach in the endothelial lining, platelets will attach to the vessel wall. Healthy vascular endothelium prevents platelet adhesion and subsequent activation by producing factors such as ectoADPase (CD39), prostaglandin I$_2$, and nitric oxide. Injury to the endothelium results in exposure of the subendothelial matrix resulting in adhesion, activation, and aggregation of platelets. The latter processes play important roles in coagulation and clot generation at the site of vascular injury ultimately preventing blood loss (hemostasis) and promoting healing [5].

Role of platelets during initiation of atherosclerosis and plaque formation

The normal endothelium loses its antithrombotic properties in the setting of hyperlipidemia, hypertension, smoking, obesity, insulin resistance, and inflammation. Dysfunctional endothelium is characterized by decreased expression of antithrombotic factors. There is enhanced expression of von Willebrand factor (vWF), selectins, tissue factor, fibronectin, integrin $\alpha_v\beta_3$, and plasminogen activator inhibitor and other proinflammatory cytokines, chemokines, and adhesion molecules. An activated but intact endothelium facilitates the adhesion and activation of circulating platelets. Activated platelets on the surface of the endothelium express proinflammatory cytokines and adhesion molecules that further facilitate the binding and internalization of leukocytes into the subendothelial space where they transform into macrophages. Moreover, changes in endothelial permeability and the composition of the subendothelial matrix facilitate the entry and retention of cholesterol-rich low-density lipoprotein (LDL) particles. The macrophages avidly engulf LDL cholesterol and transform into foam cells, leading to fatty streak and plaque formation. Activated platelets further enhance inflammation by expressing platelet factor 4, CD40 ligand, and interleukin-1β [5, 6].

Role of platelets in thrombosis

Occlusive thrombus generation at the site of plaque rupture is influenced by the thrombogenicity of the exposed plaque material (plaque vulnerability), local flow disturbances (vessel vulnerability), and, most importantly, systemic thrombotic propensity involving platelet hyperreactivity, hypercoagulability, inflammation, and depressed fibrinolysis (blood vulnerability). Spontaneous atherosclerotic plaque rupture during acute coronary syndromes and vascular injury during coronary interventions result in the exposure of subendothelial matrix facilitating platelet adhesion and activation. Under the high shear conditions present in arterial blood vessels, initial platelet adhesion is facilitated by binding of the glycoprotein (GP) Ib/IX/V receptor to vWF immobilized on collagen and binding of the platelet GPVI receptor directly to the exposed collagen [4, 5].

Following adhesion, platelets form a monolayer at the site of vessel wall injury (primary hemostasis) and undergo activation resulting in morphologic changes coupled with intracellular calcium ion mobilization. The subsequent intracellular events, particularly downstream from GPVI, lead to the release of two important secondary agonists, thromboxane A_2 (TxA_2) and adenosine diphosphate (ADP). TxA_2 is produced from membrane phospholipids through cyclooxygenase/thromboxane synthase activity, and ADP is released from dense granules. These two locally generated agonists through autocrine and paracrine mechanisms play a critical role in the sustained platelet activation in response to other stimuli and in the final activation of GPIIb/IIIa receptors (final common pathway). The binding of activated GPIIb/IIIa receptors between adjacent platelets through soluble fibrinogen results in stable thrombus generation. It has been proposed that sustained platelet activation of the GPIIb/IIIa receptor and platelet procoagulant activity are critically dependent on continuous downstream signaling from the $P2Y_{12}$ receptor, an important ADP receptor [4, 5].

Plaque rupture also results in tissue factor exposure at the site of vascular injury and the generation of femtomolar amounts of thrombin. Thrombin further promotes platelet activation and the formation of a procoagulant platelet surface where larger amounts of thrombin are generated. Finally, thrombin converts fibrinogen to fibrin, leading to the formation of an extensive fibrin network and a stable occlusive platelet–fibrin clot. In addition to the prothrombotic properties resulting from heightened platelet reactivity, a procoagulant and antifibrinolytic environment in the presence of dysfunctional endothelium markedly enhances clot formation and stability (Figure 1.1) [4, 5, 6, 7].

The clinical manifestations of thrombus generation at the site of plaque rupture depend on the extent and duration of thrombotic occlusion. Mural platelet-rich "white" thrombi often incompletely block coronary blood flow and are present during unstable angina (UA) and non-ST-segment elevation myocardial infarction (NSTEMI). STEMI is often characterized by complete coronary arterial obstruction by thrombi composed of "red thrombi" that are more rich in red blood cells and fibrin. Spontaneous or iatrogenic embolization may occur during percutaneous coronary intervention (PCI). Microemboli of plaque material and thrombus washed downstream from the culprit lesion may lead to distal microvascular occlusion. Thus, distal embolization from either source may cause myocardial ischemia and infarction despite in the presence of a revascularized infarct-related epicardial coronary artery. In addition to thrombus generation at the culprit plaque rupture site, synchronous plaque rupture and luminal thrombosis may occur in ACS patients [7].

Multiple lines of evidence support the important role of platelets in thrombosis and subsequent clinical manifestations. Indirect evidence from congenital platelet disorders and animal models highlighted the role-specific platelet receptors in hemostasis [7]. Using real-time visualization of thrombus formation following vessel wall injury in the microcirculation of living mouse, Furie *et al.* demonstrated the important role of platelet physiology during the clot formation [8]. In patients who died suddenly of ischemic heart disease, Davies found intramyocardial platelet aggregates [9]. Atherectomy specimens taken from the culprit plaques of patients with UA have shown platelet-rich thrombi [10]. Angioscopy has demonstrated the white thrombi on the surface of ruptured plaques. Further evidence for the primary role of platelets during thrombus generation came from studies where arterial thrombus formation was induced by human atherosclerotic plaque substances [11, 12].

Furthermore, platelet activation and high platelet reactivity have been demonstrated in patients with CAD. High platelet reactivity (defined as >230

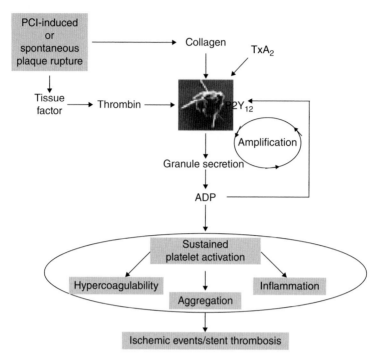

Figure 1.1 Central role of adenosine diphosphate (ADP) $P2Y_{12}$ receptor interaction in platelet activation and aggregation during the occurrence of ischemic events and stent thrombosis. After plaque rupture, tissue factor and collagen are exposed, leading to platelet activation. Three important pathways (thrombin–protease-activated receptor-1, thromboxane [Tx] A2-thromboxane receptor, and between ADP and $P2Y_{12}$ receptor) amplify the response. The ADP–$P2Y_{12}$ interaction plays a central role. PCI indicates percutaneous coronary intervention. (Source: Bonello et al. Working Group on High On-Treatment Platelet Reactivity. Consensus and future directions on the definition of high on-treatment platelet reactivity to adenosine diphosphate. *J Am Coll Cardiol.* 2010; **56**: 919–933. Reproduced with permission of Elsevier.)

platelet reactivity units by VerifyNow P2Y12 assay) during clopidogrel therapy was independently associated with greater coronary artery atherosclerotic burden and plaque calcification as measured by intravascular ultrasound (IVUS) imaging [13]. In the ADAPT-DES study, the largest platelet function study conducted in patients treated with drug-eluting stents and dual antiplatelet therapy, 30-day stent thrombosis occurrence was greatest in patients with high platelet reactivity by the VerifyNow assay [14]. A close association between platelet reactivity, systemic inflammation, and procoagulant marker elevation has also been described in patients with CAD [15, 16, 17].

References

1 Osler, W. (1874) An account of certain organisms occurring in the liquor sanguinis. *Proceedings of the Royal Society of London*, **22**, 391–398.
2 Bizzozero, G. (1881) Su di un nuovo elemento morfologico del sangue dei mammiferi e della sua importanza nellatrombosie nella coagulazione. *L'Osservatore*, **17**, 785–787.

3 Born, G.V. (1962) Aggregation of blood platelets by adenosine diphosphate and its reversal. *Nature*, **194**, 927–929.

4 Gurbel, P.A. and Tantry, U.S. (2010) Combination antithrombotic therapies. *Circulation*, **121**, 569–583.

5 Gurbel, P.A. and Tantry, U.S. (2012) Do platelet function testing and genotyping improve outcome in patients treated with antithrombotic agents? Platelet function testing and genotyping improve outcome in patients treated with antithrombotic agents. *Circulation*, **125**, 1276–1287 discussion 1287.

6 Mann, K.G., Butenas, S., and Brummel, K. (2003) The dynamics of thrombin formation. *Arteriosclerosis, Thrombosis, and Vascular Biology*, **23**, 17–25.

7 Gurbel, P.A., Bliden, K.P., Hayes, K.M., and Tantry, U. (2004) Platelet activation in myocardial ischemic syndromes. *Expert Review of Cardiovascular Therapy*, **2**, 535–545.

8 Furie, B. and Furie, B.C. (2005) Thrombus formation in vivo. *The Journal of Clinical Investigation*, **115**, 3355–3362.

9 Davies, M.J., Thomas, A.C., Knapman, P.A., and Hangartner, J.R. (1986) Intramyocardial platelet aggregation in patients with unstable angina suffering sudden ischemic cardiac death. *Circulation*, **73**, 418–427.

10 Glover, C. and O'Brien, E.R. (2000) Pathophysiological insights from studies of retrieved coronary atherectomy tissue. *Seminars in Interventional Cardiology*, **5**, 167–173.

11 Reininger, A.J., Bernlochner, I., Penz, S.M. *et al.* (2010) A 2-step mechanism of arterial thrombus formation induced by human atherosclerotic plaques. *Journal of the American College of Cardiology*, **55**, 1147–1158.

12 Fernández-Ortiz, A., Badimon, J.J., Falk, E. *et al.* (1994) Characterization of the relative thrombogenicity of atherosclerotic plaque components: implications for consequences of plaque rupture. *Journal of the American College of Cardiology*, **23**, 1562–1569.

13 Chirumamilla, A.P., Maehara, A., Mintz, G.S. *et al.* (2012) High platelet reactivity on clopidogrel therapy correlates with increased coronary atherosclerosis and calcification: a volumetric intravascular ultrasound study. *JACC. Cardiovascular Imaging*, **5**, 540–549.

14 Stone, G.W., Witzenbichler, B., Weisz, G. *et al.* (2013) Platelet reactivity and clinical outcomes after coronary artery implantation of drug-eluting stents (ADAPT-DES): a prospective multicentre registry study. *Lancet*, **382**, 614–623.

15 Tantry, U.S., Bliden, K.P., Suarez, T.A. *et al.* (2010) Hypercoagulability, platelet function, inflammation and coronary artery disease acuity: results of the Thrombotic RIsk Progression (TRIP) study. *Platelets*, **21**, 360–367.

16 Gori, A.M., Cesari, F., Marcucci, R. *et al.* (2009) The balance between pro- and anti-inflammatory cytokines is associated with platelet aggregability in acute coronary syndrome patients. *Atherosclerosis*, **202**, 255–262.

17 Park, D.W., Lee, S.W., Yun, S.C. *et al.* (2011) A point-of-care platelet function assay and C-reactive protein for prediction of major cardiovascular events after drug-eluting stent implantation. *Journal of the American College of Cardiology*, **58**, 2630–2639.

2 Platelet Receptors and Drug Targets: COX-1

Thomas Hohlfeld and Karsten Schrör

Universitätsklinikum, Heinrich-Heine Universität Düsseldorf, Düsseldorf, Germany

Cyclooxygenases (COX, PGH synthases) are key enzymes in the biosynthesis of prostaglandins and thromboxane. Two isoenzymes exist with a 61% of sequence identity, which are products of different genes. COX-1, considered as a constitutive version of the enzyme, is mainly responsible for housekeeping functions [1]. COX-2, the second isoform, is inducible in most tissues and associated with cellular stress (e.g., shear stress in vascular tissue), inflammatory processes, and cell proliferation. Platelets largely express the COX-1 isoform.

Structure, expression, and catalytic activity of platelet COX-1

Both COX isoforms consist of two identical heme-containing subunits inserted in the endoplasmic membrane. The substrate arachidonic acid is bound in a channel extending into the interior of the protein where it is converted by two sequential reactions into prostaglandin G_2 (PGG_2) and prostaglandin H_2 (PGH_2). The first reaction (at the COX site) inserts two oxygen molecules into the substrate fatty acid and catalyzes a cyclization of the carbon backbone. The product, PGG_2, is transformed at a different site (peroxidase site) to PGH_2, which involves the reduction of the 15-hydroperoxide group of PGG_2. In platelets, PGH_2 is further converted by thromboxane synthase into thromboxane A_2 (TXA_2).

The preferred substrate of COX-1 and COX-2 is arachidonic acid, which is released by phospholipase A_2 (PLA_2) from the glycerophospholipids of cell membranes. Ceramide kinase and ceramide-1-phosphate contribute by bioactivation of cytosolic PLA_2. Alternative sources of arachidonic acid are arachidonylethanolamine (anandamide) and 2-arachidonylglycerol [2].

COX activity requires an activating hydroperoxide to generate a tyrosyl radical at Tyr385, which is essential to initiate catalytic activity. Thus, platelet TXA_2 formation also depends on the concentration of

Antiplatelet Therapy in Cardiovascular Disease, First Edition. Edited by Ron Waksman, Paul A. Gurbel, and Michael A. Gaglia, Jr.
© 2014 John Wiley & Sons, Ltd. Published 2014 by John Wiley & Sons, Ltd.

COX-activating lipid peroxides. The local activity of peroxides is particularly high in platelets, allowing for an extensive burst of PGH_2 and TXA_2 synthesis when platelets are activated [3]. A possible consequence in the intact vasculature may be that vascular PG formation (e.g., PGI_2) is more completely suppressed by NSAIDs than platelet TXA_2 synthesis.

Functional role of platelet COX-1

COX-1-deficient mice have reduced arachidonic acid-induced platelet aggregation [4], confirming a wealth of experimental data demonstrating that COX-1 is critical for platelet activation. In addition, nonplatelet COX activity in vascular tissues also regulates vascular function and thrombosis. Hence, cardiovascular effects of NSAIDs depend on the inhibition of platelet TXA_2 via platelet COX-1 and on inhibition of vascular PG formation by extraplatelet COX-1 and COX-2. Their products (e.g., PGI_2 and TXA_2) have opposing biological effects on vasculature (vascular tone, thrombogenicity, growth) and platelets (aggregation, secretion).

Genetic polymorphisms of COX-1 and COX-2 expression in platelets

Sequence analysis of COX-1 has identified genetic variations that alter COX-1 activity (K185T, G230S, L237M) and change COX-1 sensitivity to indomethacin (P17L, G230S) [5]. Another COX-1 variant (G-1006A) has been associated with an elevated risk of ischemic stroke [6]. However, data on the importance of COX polymorphisms for platelet function and platelet sensitivity to aspirin are inconsistent [7].

Several years ago, our laboratory has demonstrated that platelets may also contain the inducible COX isoform COX-2 [8]. Subsequent work from others showed that COX-2 is required for megakaryocyte differentiation [9]. Thus, it is conceivable that COX-2 message and protein are carried over into the mature platelets. Some authors suggested that platelet COX-2 may bypass COX-1 and result in an impairment of the antiplatelet action of aspirin due to the lower sensitivity of COX-2 toward aspirin [10], while others did not detect COX-2-dependent TXA_2 formation by human platelets at all [11]. Further work identified COX-2 mRNA in platelets as a COX-2 variant (COX-2a) with a loss of about 100 bp in exon 5 [12]. The deduced protein was metabolically inactive [13].

Platelet COX-1 as a target for antithrombotic therapy

The usefulness of aspirin for first-line antiplatelet therapy to prevent atherothrombotic complications in vascular disease is well established. This is covered by Chapter 13.

Unlike aspirin, the naNSAID-induced inhibition of platelet COX-1 depends on the half-life in plasma, which is relatively short (few hours) for most compounds. NaNSAIDs also act competitively, allowing the local concentration of arachidonic acid to displace the compounds from their binding sites within the COX-1 substrate channel. Due to a nonlinear relationship between platelet TXA_2 generation and function [14], decreasing naNSAID plasma levels result in rapid and full recovery of platelet function (Figure 2.1A). Thus, naNSAIDs are not appropriate for circadian platelet inhibition.

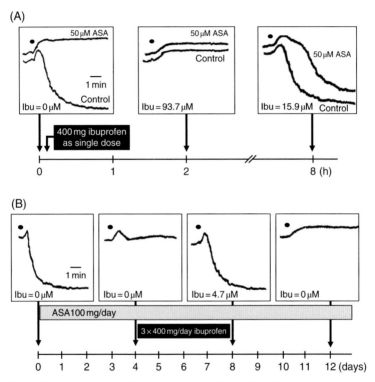

Figure 2.1 Interaction of oral ibuprofen with aspirin in a healthy subject, as demonstrated by arachidonic acid-induced light transmission aggregometry in two settings. (A) Aggregation before (left) and 2 h (middle) and 8 h (right) after an oral dose of 400 mg ibuprofen. Before ibuprofen, *in vitro* addition of 50 μM aspirin completely inhibits aggregation. Two hours after ibuprofen, platelets are inhibited by the high plasma concentration of ibuprofen. Eight hours after ibuprofen, the concentration of ibuprofen has fallen and aggregation has recovered. Remarkably, residual ibuprofen still interferes with the *in vitro* antiplatelet action of aspirin (see text), as shown by the failure of aspirin to prevent aggregation at this time. (B) Continuous oral administration of 100 mg/day aspirin achieves complete platelet aggregation within 4 days. Subsequent cotherapy with ibuprofen (3 × 400 mg over 4 days) abolishes inhibition by aspirin due to pharmacodynamic interaction. Four days after discontinuation of ibuprofen, platelet inhibition by aspirin is restored. Black dots mark the addition of 1 mM arachidonic acid. Actual ibuprofen plasma concentrations (HPLC) are also indicated.

Interaction between aspirin and naNSAIDs at the level of platelet COX-1

Low-dose aspirin cumulatively inactivates platelet COX-1 by acetylation of Ser530 within the substrate channel [15]. Since naNSAIDs are attracted by overlapping binding sites in the COX substrate channel [16], one might expect that COX-1 inhibition by aspirin will be synergistically amplified. This, however, may not be true. Since the initial binding affinity of aspirin in the COX-1 substrate channel is relatively weak compared with naNSAIDs [17], the latter may prevent the access of aspirin by steric hindrance and protect platelet COX-1 from permanent inactivation by aspirin. Since the half-life of aspirin in blood is only approximately 15 min, aspirin will no more be present when the actual naNSAID concentrations have fallen and COX activity is restored.

Another concept of naNSAID/aspirin interaction has been developed from the observation that the two COX subunits are structurally identical but functionally different [1]. There is some evidence that one COX monomer is inactive but controls the activity of the partner monomer, which is catalytically active. This cross talk may be mediated by amino acids at the interface between the two monomers, causing a conformational change of the catalytic subunit. Some NSAIDs appear to bind to the regulatory subunit and exert a noncompetitive inhibition of the catalytic subunit, while others may directly interact with the catalytic subunit. This may modulate the interaction of aspirin with COX-1. A crystallographic analysis and animal experimentation suggested that this mechanism may account for the interaction between aspirin and celecoxib at platelet COX-1 [18].

In vitro and *in vivo* evidence for aspirin/naNSAID interaction

Preexposure of COX-1 enzyme with different COX inhibitors at nanomolar concentrations attenuated COX-1 inhibition by aspirin [19], although the compounds did not inhibit COX-1 activity when applied alone. Studies with healthy subjects have confirmed this *in vitro* interaction. For example, Catella-Lawson *et al.* demonstrated that ibuprofen interferes with aspirin in terms of platelet aggregation and TXA_2 formation with ibuprofen, as long as ibuprofen was applied prior to aspirin [20, 21]. These studies noted that subinhibitory doses of naNSAIDs were still sufficient for preventing inhibition by aspirin. An example that demonstrates the interaction between aspirin and naNSAIDs *in vitro* and *in vivo* is given in Figure 2.1.

Clinical data also support this interaction. For example, a small trial with 18 patients receiving aspirin for stroke prevention and comedication with ibuprofen or naproxen showed at 27 months' follow-up largely unchanged platelet activity upon stimulation by arachidonic acid and collagen, suggesting failure of aspirin treatment [22]. Discontinuation of naNSAIDs or a modified dosing scheme restored platelet inhibition by aspirin. Another, larger study examined 1055 patients with nonfatal myocardial infarction and 4153 controls in a case–control design and showed that the reduction of cardiovascular events by aspirin was abolished when combined with frequent naNSAIDs (mainly ibuprofen) [23].

Concluding remarks

While the central role of COX-1 as key enzyme of platelet TXA_2 formation and target of low-dose aspirin is acknowledged since decades, platelet COX-1 remains subject to relevant and innovative research. All other inhibitors of platelet function, including GPIIb/IIIa inhibitors and ADP receptor antagonists, have been developed on the background of antiplatelet therapy with aspirin. Basic pharmacological as well as clinical properties of this enzyme, such as naNSAID/aspirin interactions, are important for the present and future concepts of antiplatelet therapy.

References

1 Smith, W.L., Urade, Y., and Jakobsson, P.J. (2011) Enzymes of the cyclooxygenase pathways of prostanoid biosynthesis. *Chemical Reviews*, **111**, 5821–5865.

2 Gkini, E., Anagnostopoulos, D., Mavri-Vavayianni, M., and Siafaka-Kapadai, A. (2009) Metabolism of 2-acylglycerol in rabbit and human platelets. Involvement of monoacylglycerol lipase and fatty acid amide hydrolase. *Platelets*, **20**, 376–385.

3 Boutaud, O., Aronoff, D.M., Richardson, J.H., Marnett, L.J., and Oates, J.A. (2002) Determinants of the cellular specificity of acetaminophen as an inhibitor of prostaglandin H(2) synthases. *Proceedings of the National Academy of Sciences of the United States of America*, **99**, 7130–7135.

4 Langenbach, R., Morham, S.G., Tiano, H.F. *et al.* (1995) Prostaglandin synthase 1 gene disruption in mice reduces arachidonic acid-induced inflammation and indomethacin-induced gastric ulceration. *Cell*, **83**, 483–492.

5 Lee, C.R., Bottone, F.G., Jr, Krahn, J.M. *et al.* (2007) Identification and functional characterization of polymorphisms in human cyclooxygenase-1 (PTGS1). *Pharmacogenetics and Genomics*, **17**, 145–160.

6 Lee, C.R., North, K.E., Bray, M.S., Couper, D.J., Heiss, G., and Zeldin, D.C. (2008) Cyclooxygenase polymorphisms and risk of cardiovascular events: the Atherosclerosis Risk in Communities (ARIC) study. *Clinical Pharmacology and Therapeutics*, **83**, 52–60.

7 Goodman, T., Ferro, A., and Sharma, P. (2008) Pharmacogenetics of aspirin resistance: a comprehensive systematic review. *British Journal of Clinical Pharmacology*, **66**, 222–232.

8 Weber, A.-A., Zimmermann, K., Meyer-Kirchrath, J., and Schrör, K. (1999) Cyclooxygenase-2 in human platelets as a possible factor in aspirin resistance. *Lancet*, **353**, 900.

9 Tanaka, N., Sato, T., Fujita, H., and Morita, I. (2004) Constitutive expression and involvement of cyclooxygenase-2 in human megakaryocytopoiesis. *Arteriosclerosis, Thrombosis, and Vascular Biology*, **24**, 607–612.

10 Guthikonda, S., Lev, E.I., Patel, R. *et al.* (2007) Reticulated platelets and uninhibited COX-1 and COX-2 decrease the antiplatelet effects of aspirin. *Journal of Thrombosis and Haemostasis,* **5,** 490–496.

11 Patrignani, P., Sciulli, M.G., Manarini, S., Santini, G., Cerletti, C., and Evangelista, V. (1999) COX-2 is not involved in thromboxane biosynthesis by activated human platelets. *Journal of Physiology and Pharmacology,* **50,** 661–667.

12 Censarek, P., Freidel, K., Udelhoven, M. *et al.* (2004) Cyclooxygenase COX-2a, a novel COX-2 mRNA variant, in platelets from patients after coronary artery bypass grafting. *Thrombosis and Haemostasis,* **92,** 925–928.

13 Censarek, P., Steger, G., Paolini, C. *et al.* (2007) Alternative splicing of platelet cyclooxygenase-2 mRNA in patients after coronary artery bypass grafting. *Thrombosis and Haemostasis,* **98,** 1309–1315.

14 Reilly, I.A. and FitzGerald, G.A. (1987) Inhibition of thromboxane formation in vivo and ex vivo: implications for therapy with platelet inhibitory drugs. *Blood,* **69,** 180–186.

15 Loll, P.J., Picot, D., and Garavito, R.M. (1995) The structural basis of aspirin activity inferred from the crystal structure of inactivated prostaglandin H2 synthase. *Natural Structural Biology,* **2,** 637–643.

16 Selinsky, B.S., Gupta, K., Sharkey, C.T. and Loll, P.J. (2001) Structural analysis of NSAID binding by prostaglandin H2 synthase: time-dependent and time-independent inhibitors elicit identical enzyme conformations. *Biochemistry,* **40,** 5172–5180.

17 Ouellet, M., Riendeau, D., and Percival, M.D. (2001) A high level of cyclooxygenase-2 inhibitor selectivity is associated with a reduced interference of platelet cyclooxygenase-1 inactivation by aspirin. *Proceedings of the National Academy of Sciences of the United States of America,* **98,** 14583–14588.

18 Rimon, G., Sidhu, R.S., Lauver, D.A. *et al.* (2009) Coxibs interfere with the action of aspirin by binding tightly to one monomer of cyclooxygenase-1. *Proceedings of the National Academy of Sciences of the United States of America,* **107,** 28–33.

19 Rosenstock, M., Danon, A., Rubin, M., and Rimon, G. (2001) Prostaglandin H synthase-2 inhibitors interfere with prostaglandin H sythase-1 inhibition by nonsteroidal anti-inflammatory drugs. *European Journal of Pharmacology,* **412,** 101–108.

20 Catella-Lawson, F., Reilly, M.P., Kapoor, S.C. *et al.* (2001) Cyclooxygenase inhibitors and the antiplatelet effects of aspirin. *New England Journal of Medicine,* **345,** 1809–1817.

21 Gladding, P.A., Webster, M.W., Farrell, H.B., Zeng, I.S., Park, R. and Ruijne, N. (2008) The antiplatelet effect of six non-steroidal anti-inflammatory drugs and their pharmacodynamic interaction with aspirin in healthy volunteers. *The American Journal of Cardiology,* **101,** 1060–1063.

22 Gengo, F.M., Rubin, L., Robson, M. *et al.* (2008) Effects of ibuprofen on the magnitude and duration of aspirin's inhibition of platelet aggregation: clinical consequences in stroke prophylaxis. *Journal of Clinical Pharmacology,* **48,** 117–122.

23 Kimmel, S.E., Berlin, J.A., Reilly, M. *et al.* (2004) The effects of nonselective non-aspirin non-steroidal anti-inflammatory medications on the risk of nonfatal myocardial infarction and their interaction with aspirin. *Journal of the American College of Cardiology,* **43,** 985–990.

3 Platelet Receptors and Drug Targets: P2Y$_{12}$

Marco Cattaneo

Ospedale San Paolo, Università degli Studi di Milano, Milano, Italy

P2 receptors

Purine and pyrimidine nucleotides are extracellular signaling molecules that regulate the function of virtually every cell in the body. They interact with P2 receptors, which are divided into two subfamilies: P2Y receptors, seven-membrane spanning proteins coupled to G proteins, and P2X receptors, ligand-gated ion channels [1]. Eight P2Y receptors have been identified so far: P2Y$_1$, P2Y$_2$, P2Y$_4$, P2Y$_6$, P2Y$_{11}$, P2Y$_{12}$, P2Y$_{13}$, and P2Y$_{14}$. They can be subdivided into adenine nucleotide- and uracil nucleotide-preferring receptors: the former (P2Y$_1$, P2Y$_{11}$, P2Y$_{12}$, and P2Y$_{13}$) mainly respond to adenosine diphosphate (ADP) and adenosine triphosphate (ATP). From a phylogenetic and structural point of view, two distinct P2Y receptor subgroups have been identified: the G$_q$-coupled subtypes (P2Y$_1$, P2Y$_2$, P2Y$_4$, P2Y$_6$, and P2Y$_{11}$) and the G$_i$-coupled subtypes (P2Y$_{12}$, P2Y$_{13}$, and P2Y$_{14}$) [1]. Seven P2X receptors have been identified, P2X$_1$–P2X$_7$, which are primarily ATP receptors [1].

Human platelets express three distinct P2 receptors (Figure 3.1): P2Y$_1$ and P2Y$_{12}$, which interact with ADP, and P2X$_1$, which interacts with ATP, with the following order of expression – P2Y$_{12}$ >> P2X$_1$ > P2Y$_1$ [2].

Roles of adenine nucleotides in platelet function

ADP is a weak platelet agonist. As such, it only induces shape change and reversible aggregation in human platelets, while the secretion of platelet δ-granules constituents and the ensuing secondary aggregation that are observed following stimulation with ADP of normal platelet-rich plasma (PRP) are triggered by thromboxane (TX)A$_2$, whose synthesis is stimulated by platelet aggregation [3]. This phenomenon is greatly enhanced when the concentration of plasma Ca^{2+} is artifactually decreased, such as in citrate PRP. ADP plays a key role in platelet function because, when it is secreted

---

Antiplatelet Therapy in Cardiovascular Disease, First Edition. Edited by Ron Waksman, Paul A. Gurbel, and Michael A. Gaglia, Jr.
© 2014 John Wiley & Sons, Ltd. Published 2014 by John Wiley & Sons, Ltd.

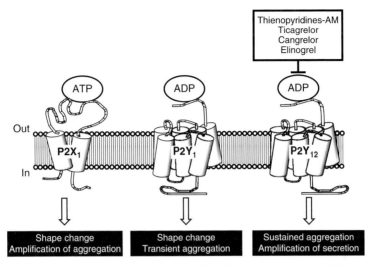

Figure 3.1 Simplified schematic representation of the effects of the interaction of ATP and ADP with platelet P2 receptors (P2X$_1$, P2Y$_1$, P2Y$_{12}$) in platelet function. Inhibitors have been developed for each receptor, but only the P2Y$_{12}$ receptor inhibitors are shown, because they are already used in clinical practice, or are in development, as antithrombotic drugs: the AM of thienopyridines, ticagrelor, cangrelor, and elinogrel.

from δ-granules, it amplifies the platelet responses induced by other platelet agonists and stabilizes platelet aggregates (Figure 3.2) [3, 4]. Transduction of the ADP-induced signal involves inhibition of adenylyl cyclase (AC) and a concomitant transient rise in the concentration of cytoplasmic Ca^{2+}.

Upon platelet exposure to ADP, the G$_q$-coupled P2Y$_1$ receptor mediates a transient rise in cytoplasmic Ca^{2+}, platelet shape change, and rapidly reversible aggregation, and the G$_i$-coupled P2Y$_{12}$ receptor mediates inhibition of AC and amplifies the platelet aggregation response [3, 4]. Concomitant activation of both the G$_q$ and G$_i$ pathways by ADP is necessary to elicit normal aggregation (Figure 3.1) [5]. The importance of concurrent activation of the G$_q$ and G$_i$ pathways for full platelet aggregation is highlighted by the observations that normal aggregation responses to ADP can be restored by epinephrine, which is coupled to an inhibitory G protein, G$_z$, in P2Y$_{12}$-deficient platelets, and by serotonin, which is coupled to G$_q$, in P2Y$_1$ knockout (KO) platelets [3].

ATP, through its interaction with P2X$_1$, activates platelets by inducing a very rapid influx of extracellular Ca^{2+}, which is associated with platelet shape change and amplification of platelet aggregation, especially under high shear stress conditions (Figure 3.1) [6].

P2Y$_{12}$

The human P2Y$_{12}$ receptor was cloned in 2001 [7]: it contains 342 amino acid residues, has a classical structure of a G protein-coupled receptor and, although it was initially demonstrated to be expressed in platelets and the

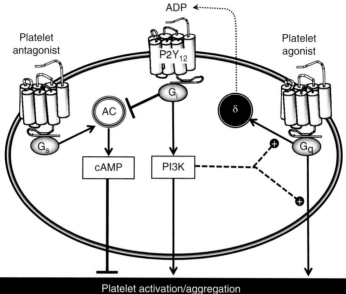

Figure 3.2 Central role of P2Y$_{12}$ in platelet activation and aggregation. ADP, by interacting with P2Y$_{12}$, a seven-transmembrane receptor that is coupled to the inhibitory G protein G$_i$, induces platelet aggregation and amplifies the aggregation response that is induced by other agonists (but also by ADP itself, which interacts also with its other platelet receptor, P2Y$_1$, not shown in this cartoon). In addition, P2Y$_{12}$ stabilizes the platelet aggregates (not shown in this cartoon) and amplifies the secretion of platelet dense granules (δ) stimulated by secretion-inducing agonists (which are coupled to G$_q$). Although P2Y$_{12}$ is coupled to inhibition of AC through G$_i$, this function is not directly related to P2Y$_{12}$-mediated platelet activation. However, it could have important implications *in vivo*, where platelets are exposed to the natural platelet antagonists, such as prostacyclin or adenosine, which inhibit platelet activation/aggregation by increasing platelet cAMP through activation of AC mediated by G$_s$; inhibition of AC by P2Y$_{12}$ counteracts the inhibitory effect of these platelet antagonists, thereby favoring platelet activation and the formation of platelet aggregates *in vivo*. solid line+arrow, activation; truncated solid line, inhibition; dashed line ending with a (+), amplification; dotted line+arrow, secretion.

central nervous system only, its mRNA has recently been detected also in other tissues [4]. Studies of a patient with dysfunctional P2Y$_{12}$ revealed that the integrity of the highly conserved H-X-X-R/K motif in TM6 and of EL3 is important for receptor function [4]. P2Y$_{12}$ has four extracellular cysteines, some of which play an essential role in receptor expression and interact with the active metabolite (AM) of clopidogrel to form a disulfide bond, which irreversibly inactivates the receptor [4]. P2Y$_{12}$ plays a central role in platelet function (Figure 3.2).

Role of P2Y$_{12}$ in ADP-induced platelet activation/aggregation

ADP stimulates P2Y$_{12}$-mediated inhibition of AC through activation of a G$_{\alpha i2}$ G protein subtype [4]. Activation of G$_{\alpha i2}$ by ADP is critical for integrin αIIbβ3 activation and platelet aggregation and has a critical requirement for lipid rafts [4]. It must be noted however that, although inhibition of AC via G$_{\alpha i2}$ is a key feature of platelet activation by ADP, it bears no causal relationship to platelet aggregation [4]. Several studies suggested a crucial role for phosphoinositide 3-kinase (PI3-K) in ADP-dependent, P2Y$_{12}$ receptor-mediated platelet activation, which is likely triggered by the γ,β-subunits of G$_i$ [4]. In addition, it has been shown that ADP induces slow and sustained PI3-K platelet aggregation, which is not preceded by platelet shape change. Some studies demonstrated that pharmacological blockade of P2Y$_{12}$ receptors reduces the ability of platelets to produce TXA$_2$; however, the platelet TXA$_2$ production is normal in patients with P2Y$_{12}$ deficiency [4]. P2Y$_{12}$ amplifies the mobilization of cytoplasmic Ca^{2+} mediated by P2Y$_1$ and other receptors and regulates diacylglycerol-mediated signaling [4].

Role of P2Y$_{12}$ in plateletresp onses to agonists other than ADP

The interaction of ADP with P2Y$_{12}$ amplifies platelet secretion and aggregation and stabilizes platelet aggregates induced by other agonists, such as collagen, TXA$_2$, and thrombin (Figure 3.2). Early studies demonstrated the important role of P2Y$_{12}$ in shear-induced platelet aggregation long before its molecular identification, by using platelets from individuals treated with the antithrombotic drug ticlopidine or from a patient with congenital P2Y$_{12}$ deficiency [4].

Role of P2Y$_{12}$ in thrombin generation

P2Y$_{12}$ shares with P2Y$_1$ the ability to contribute to collagen-induced exposure of tissue factor (TF) and platelet microparticle formation in whole blood and to contribute to the formation of platelet–leukocyte conjugates mediated by platelet surface P-selectin exposure, which results in TF exposure at the surface of leukocytes [4]. However, only the P2Y$_{12}$ receptor was found to be involved in the exposure of phosphatidylserine by thrombin or other platelet agonists and in TF-induced thrombin formation in PRP [4].

Role of P2Y$_{12}$ in inhibition of AC

As mentioned earlier, although inhibition of AC via Gα_{i2} is a key feature of platelet activation by ADP/P2Y$_{12}$, it bears no causal relationship to platelet aggregation, because inhibition of AC by alternative agents that do not stimulate G$_i$ does not induce platelet aggregation. However, inhibition of AC by ADP/P2Y$_{12}$ may play a very important, albeit indirect, role in platelet aggregation *in vivo*, because it negatively modulates the antiplatelet effect of prostacyclin and other platelet antagonists that increase the platelet cyclic adenosine monophosphate (cAMP) levels (Figure 3.2) [8]. This effect, which is not shared by P2Y$_1$, may at least partly explain why the *in vivo* bleeding time is more severely prolonged in P2Y$_{12}$ KO mice compared to P2Y$_1$ KO mice, despite the fact that they display similar impairment of platelet aggregation *in vitro*. Moreover, this function of

ADP/P2Y$_{12}$ may increase the antithrombotic potential of P2Y$_{12}$ inhibitors and may be blunted by the coadministration of high doses of aspirin, which may interfere with prostacyclin production by endothelial cells [8]. The demonstration that high doses of aspirin blunted the antithrombotic effects of the P2Y$_{12}$ inhibitor ticagrelor in the PLATO trial [9] is consistent with this hypothesis.

Role of P2Y$_{12}$ in platelet thrombus formation *in vitro* and *in vivo*

Several studies reported the important role of the P2Y$_{12}$ receptor in platelet thrombus formation and stabilization on collagen-coated surfaces or ruptured atherosclerotic plaques under flow conditions [4]. Studies of P2Y$_{12}$ KO mice and of wild-type animals treated with P2Y$_{12}$ antagonists or inhibitors, using different models of experimental arterial and venous thrombosis, have clearly demonstrated the important role of this receptor in thrombogenesis *in vivo*. Experiments with P2Y$_{12}$ KO mice demonstrated a role for platelet P2Y$_{12}$ in the vessel wall response to arterial injury and thrombosis, highlighting the relationship between early thrombotic response and later neointima formation after arterial injury. In addition, drugs that inhibit the platelet P2Y$_{12}$ receptor are antithrombotic agents of proven efficacy in patients with coronary artery, peripheral artery, or cerebrovascular diseases [10].

Congenital abnormalities of the P2Y$_{12}$ receptor

First described in 1992 [11], congenital, severe P2Y$_{12}$ deficiency is an autosomal recessive disorder, characterized by lifelong history of excessive bleeding, prolonged bleeding time, reversible aggregation in response to weak agonists, and impaired aggregation in response to low concentrations of collagen or thrombin. The most typical feature is that ADP, even at very high concentrations ($>10\,\mu M$), does not induce full and irreversible platelet aggregation. Other abnormalities of platelet function include the following: (i) no inhibition by ADP of stimulated platelet AC, but normal inhibition by epinephrine; (ii) normal shape change and borderline-normal mobilization of cytoplasmic Ca^{2+} induced by ADP; and (iii) presence of approximately 30% of the normal number of ADP binding sites [4]. Severe deficiency of P2Y$_{12}$ is usually associated with mutations of the encoding gene that result in frameshifts and premature truncation of the protein [4].

Congenital dysfunctions of P2Y$_{12}$, associated with point mutations in regions of the molecule that are important for ligand recognition of signal transduction, have also been described [4].

Patients with defects of P2Y$_{12}$ experience mucocutaneous bleeding and excessive postsurgical or posttraumatic blood loss. The severity of their bleeding diathesis is variable. The degree of prolongation of their bleeding times is also variable, reflecting the severity of their clinical bleeding scores [4]. A young patient with heterozygous P2Y$_{12}$ deficiency did not manifest spontaneous pathological bleeding; due to his young age, he had not yet experienced situations that could challenge the hemostatic system; his bleeding time, despite the mild defect of P2Y$_{12}$, was prolonged (13 min) [4].

Four polymorphisms of the P2Y$_{12}$ gene were identified, which were in total linkage disequilibrium, determining haplotypes H1 and H2, with respective allelic frequencies of 0.86 and 0.14. H2 haplotype is a gain-of-function haplotype, associated with increased ADP-induced platelet aggregation. The P2Y$_{12}$ H2 haplotype does not affect the platelet response to clopidogrel [12].

Conclusions

Several lines of evidence indicate that the interaction of ADP with P2Y$_{12}$ plays a key role in the formation of the hemostatic plug and the pathogenesis of arterial thrombi: (i) ADP is present in high concentrations in platelet dense granules and released when platelets are stimulated by other agents such as thrombin or collagen, thus modulating platelet aggregation; (ii) drugs that inhibit ADP–P2Y$_{12}$-induced platelet aggregation are very effective antithrombotic drugs; and (iii) patients with defects of P2Y$_{12}$ or lacking ADP in platelet granules have a bleeding diathesis.

References

1 Jacobson, K.A., Deflorian, F., Mishra, S., and Costanzi, S. (2011) Pharmacochemistry of the platelet purinergic receptors. *Purinergic Signal*, **7**, 305–324.

2 Wang, L., Ostberg, O., Wihlborg, A.K. *et al.* (2003) Quantification of ADP and ATP receptor expression in human platelets. *Journal of Thrombosis and Haemostasis*, **1**, 330–336.

3 Cattaneo, M. and Gachet, C. (1999) ADP Receptors and clinical bleeding disorders. *Arteriosclerosis, Thrombosis, and Vascular Biology*, **19**, 2281–2285.

4 Cattaneo, M. (2011) The platelet P2Y$_{12}$ receptor for adenosine diphosphate: congenital and drug-induced defects. *Blood*, **117**, 2102–2112.

5 Jin, J. and Kunapuli, S.P. (1998) Coactivation of two different G protein-coupled receptors is essential for ADP-induced platelet aggregation. *Proceedings of the National Academy of Sciences of the United States of America*, **95**, 8070–8074.

6 Cattaneo, M. (2011) Molecular defects of the platelet P2 receptors. *Purinergic Signal*, **7**, 333–339.

7 Hollopeter, G., Jantzen, H.M., Vincent, D. *et al.* (2001) Identification of the platelet ADP receptor targeted by antithrombotic drugs. *Nature*, **409**, 202–207.

8 Cattaneo, M. and Lecchi, A. (2007) Inhibition of the platelet P2Y$_{12}$ receptor for adenosine diphosphate potentiates the antiplatelet effect of prostacyclin. *Journal of Thrombosis and Haemostasis*, **5**, 577–582.

9 Mahaffey, K.W., Wojdyla, D.M., Carroll, K. *et al.* (2011) Ticagrelor compared with clopidogrel by geographic region in the Platelet Inhibition and Patient Outcomes (PLATO) trial. *Circulation*, **124**, 544–554.

10 Cattaneo, M. (2010) New P2Y(12) inhibitors. *Circulation*, **121**, 171–179.

11 Cattaneo, M., Lecchi, A., Randi, A.M., Gregor, J.L., and Mannucci, P.M. (1992) Identification of a new congenital defect of platelet function characterized by severe impairment of platelet responses to adenosine diphosphate. *Blood*, **80**, 2787–2796.

12 von Beckerath, N., von Beckerath, O., Koch, W., Eichinger, M., Schömig, A., and Kastrati, A. (2005) $P2Y_{12}$ gene H2 haplotype is not associated with increased adenosine diphosphate-induced platelet aggregation after initiation of clopidogrel therapy with a high loading dose. *Blood Coagulation and Fibrinolysis*, **16**, 199–204.

4 Platelet Receptors and Drug Targets: GP IIb/IIIa

Eliano Pio Navarese[1,2] and Jacek Kubica[1,2]

[1]Ludwik Rydygier Collegium Medicum, Nicolaus Copernicus University, Bydgoszcz, Poland
[2]Systematic Investigation and Research on Interventions and Outcomes (SIRIO)-MEDICINE
Research Network

Introduction

The platelet glycoprotein (GP) IIb/IIIa receptor has been identified as a target for control of the platelet response to vascular injury [1]. During the last decade, intensive efforts have been made to evaluate the role of the GPIIb/IIIa complex in platelet-mediated thrombus formation.

Biology of the receptor

GPIIb/IIIa is a calcium-dependent complex consisting of two components: α-subunit (GPIIb) and β-subunit (GPIIIa), noncovalently associated together. GPIIIa is a simple chain, while GPIIb is formed by two polypeptide chains connected by one or more disulfide bounds [2, 3]; both the α- and β-subunits are noncovalently bound to each other, and calcium is required to maintain the heterodimeric structure. The complex, also known as αIIbβ3 integrin, belongs to a group of cell-surface receptors initiating multiple cell–cell and cell-surface adhesions. Over 70% of the GPIIb/IIIa is placed on the plasma membrane of platelets, while the rest is stored between membranes of the surface and cytoplasmic α-granules, from which it is released after stimulation of the platelet [4].

Glycoprotein IIb/IIIa receptor in platelet physiology

Activated platelets play a pivotal role in thrombotic processes. There are three phases in the response of platelets to tissue injury. Phase 1 is adhesion, commonly triggered by plaque rupture, which stimulates platelets to adhere to the subendothelial matrix; during acute coronary

Antiplatelet Therapy in Cardiovascular Disease, First Edition. Edited by Ron Waksman, Paul A. Gurbel, and Michael A. Gaglia, Jr.
© 2014 John Wiley & Sons, Ltd. Published 2014 by John Wiley & Sons, Ltd.

syndrome (ACS) or percutaneous coronary intervention (PCI), intimal injury can be generated causing damage to endothelium and leading to exposure of collagen and subendothelial molecules. Platelets adhere to exposed collagen, von Willebrand factor (vWF), and fibrinogen by specific cell receptors. Adherent platelets can then be activated by thrombin, collagen, thromboxane, serotonin, epinephrine, and adenosine diphosphate (ADP) – phase 2. Activated platelets degranulate and secrete various substances, including chemotaxins, clotting factors, vasoconstrictors, platelet activators (such as thromboxane A_2 (TXA_2), serotonin, ADP, and epinephrine), and mediators of inflammation and vascular repair. Platelet activation also includes changes in the platelet surface that promote coagulation and aggregation – phase 3. Regardless of the mode of platelet activation, GPIIb/IIIa serves as the receptor on platelets that binds plasma-borne adhesive proteins, such as fibrinogen and vWF, thus permitting platelet aggregation. GPIIb/IIIa receptor antagonists act by inhibiting this final common pathway of platelet aggregation.

Platelet aggregation phase

Platelet activation causes modifications in the shape of platelets and conformational changes in the GPIIb/IIIa receptor, transforming it from a ligand-unreceptive to a ligand-receptive state. The GPIIb/IIIa receptors on most platelet surfaces are presented as deactivated forms that require activation by thrombin, collagen, or TXA_2; platelet aggregation begins when an aggregating agent interacts with its receptor(s) on the platelet surface. Ligand-receptive GPIIb/IIIa receptors bind fibrinogen molecules, which establish bridges between adjacent platelets and facilitate platelet aggregation (Figure 4.1). Although binding of fibrinogen to GPIIb/IIIa receptors is the principal mechanism for platelet aggregation, other adhesive GPs including vWF, fibronectin, and vitronectin also bind to these receptors. Fibrinogen and vWF are able to form bridges between stimulated platelets and therefore are responsible for generation of platelet aggregates; specifically, platelet aggregation involves cross-linking of activated GPIIb/IIIa receptors on two adjacent platelets by a single molecule of plasma fibrinogen [5]. Several efforts have been made to explain the molecular basis for binding of the soluble adhesive proteins of vWF and fibrinogen to platelets; the GPIIb/IIIa receptor has two peptide sequences, through which the agonists bind to it. One is the Arg–Gly–Asp (RGD); the other sequence is Lys–Gln–Ala–Gly–Asp–Val (KQAGDV). The RGD sequence is present in fibrinogen, vWF, and vitronectin. Unlike RGD, KQAGDV sequence is found only in fibrinogen and is probably the predominant site for the binding of fibrinogen to GPIIb/IIIa receptors.

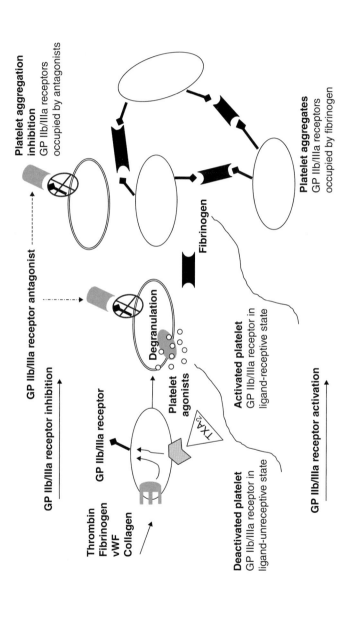

Figure 4.1 Role of GPIIb/IIIa receptor in platelet physiology and inhibition of platelet activation–aggregation by GPIIb/IIIa antagonists. GP, glycoprotein; vWF, von Willebrand factor.

"Inside-out" and "outside-in" GPIIb/IIIa signaling phenomenon

GPIIb/IIIa receptor expression and function are dynamic and responsive to the state of internal activation of platelets. "Inside-out" GPIIb/IIIa signaling has been described to trigger platelet activation and increase receptor expression and binding affinity [6].

First platelet–platelet contacts that initiate aggregation occur after fibrinogen and vWF binding to the GPIIb/IIIa receptor. These contacts are initially reversible, but at further stages, they lead to "outside-in" GPIIb/IIIa signaling that eventually stabilizes the platelet aggregates [7]. Indeed, it has been shown that the binding of the GPIIb/IIIa receptor initiates an outside-to-inside signal that prompts platelets to release the contents of their cytoplasmic granules which include adhesive molecules, growth factors, and procoagulant substances as well as to synthesize and release TXA_2. This process leads to further recruitment and activation of adjacent platelets. Platelet-activated second-messenger signals also cause a structural change to the platelet, transforming it from a discoid shape to an irregular form with multiple projections. As platelets continue to aggregate, further changes to the cytoskeleton occur. These, in turn, are involved in reinforcement and contraction of the clot. Activated platelets in thrombus can generate thrombin that promotes further platelet activation and adhesion. Inhibition of this pathway enables prevention of stable platelet aggregate formation [8].

Glycoprotein IIb/IIIa receptor and thrombus formation

One of the central tenets of thrombus formation has been the concept of primary, platelet-mediated, hemostasis in the formation of a hemostatic plug, followed by secondary hemostasis, that is, the generation of a fibrin meshwork to stabilize the platelet thrombus. Crucial to the conversion of fibrinogen to fibrin is the activation of coagulation cascade. Thrombin is a proteolytic enzyme with several important activities such as the proteolytic cleavage of fibrinogen to form soluble molecules of fibrin and activation of factor XIII which forms covalent bonds between the soluble fibrin molecules converting them into an insoluble meshwork – the clot. Additionally, thrombin is one of the most potent platelet activators. The primary thrombin receptor on the platelet is the protease-activated receptor 1 (PAR-1). Thrombin directly activates the platelet through G protein-coupled receptors, leading to platelet aggregation and granule release [9].

Unactivated platelets are unable to form thrombus, since they have almost no prothrombin expression on their surface [10]. Apart from fibrinogen binding, GPIIb/IIIa receptors on nonstimulated platelets are also involved in binding of prothrombin, an interaction that increases the rate of prothrombin conversion to the activated thrombin. Therefore, the antiplatelet and anticoagulant properties of GPIIb/IIIa receptor antagonists derive from reducing the generation of thrombin, with subsequent prolongation of clot formation.

Glycoprotein IIb/IIIa receptor antagonists

Since the GPIIb/IIIa receptor is the final common pathway by which platelet aggregation occurs, direct inhibition of this receptor is likely to prove superior to selective blockers of preceding pathways such as aspirin or clopidogrel. Platelet activation increases both receptor expression and binding affinity. Pharmacotherapy combining the receptor antagonists with other antiplatelet agents (e.g., aspirin, clopidogrel) became the mainstay of treatment in patients with ACS. The GPIIb/IIIa receptor is a part of "final common pathway" that leads to platelet aggregation; therefore, GPIIb/IIIa receptor antagonists strongly inhibit platelet aggregation. This class of drugs has been widely studied in patients with ACS undergoing PCI.

Three GPIIb/IIIa receptor antagonists have been approved for use in the treatment of ACS:

- Abciximab, a Fab fragment of humanized 7E3, is a GPIIb/IIIa monoclonal antibody. Over 80% of platelet GPIIb/IIIa receptors are blocked within 2 h of the administration of a 0.25 mg/kg abciximab bolus. Saturation is maintained during a 10 mg/min infusion (usually continued over 12–24 h), with gradual recovery of platelet function after the infusion is stopped. Short plasma half-life determined by the rapid binding to GPIIb/IIIa receptors is a characteristic feature of abciximab. This fact results in strong inhibition of platelet aggregation, while adhesion and secretion are preserved. The efficacy of abciximab may be influenced by numerous factors, such as thrombocytosis, basal platelet activation, or agonist stimulation. For example, thrombin, which is involved in the thrombus generation, upregulates the number of available GPIIb/IIIa receptors. Abciximab can be safely used in patients with kidney dysfunction, as it is not excreted by the kidney [11].
- Tirofiban is a synthetic small-molecule GPIIb/IIIa antagonist. Its dosage is 0.4 μg/kg/min for 30 min, followed by 0.10 μg/kg/min for 18 h. Tirofiban is mainly cleared from plasma by renal excretion. Approximately 65% of the dose is recovered in urine and 25% in feces mainly as unchanged drug (its metabolism is limited).
- Eptifibatide, a synthetic heptapeptide modeled on the active side of barbourin, is a disintegrin found in the venom of the southeastern pigmy rattlesnake. The dosage of this drug is 180 μg/kg body weight for 10 min, followed by 2 μg/kg/min for 18 h; 98% of eptifibatide is renally eliminated [12].

These agents bind to GPIIb/IIIa (on both stimulated and nonstimulated platelets) and thus downregulate the GPIIb/IIIa receptor activation

Table 4.1 Pharmacokinetic and pharmacodynamic properties of GPIIb/IIIa antagonists.

	Abciximab	Tirofiban	Eptifibatide
Dose in ACS	0.25 mg/kg	0.4 µg/kg/min for 30 min	180 µg/kg for 10 min
Infusion	10 mg/min for 12–24 h	0.10 µg/kg/min for 18 h	2 µg /kg/min for 18 h
Route of administration	IV or IC	IV	IV
Affinity to GP IIb/IIIa	High	Low	Low
End of anti-platelet effect	72 h	3–4 h	4 h
Half-life			
Plasma	20–30 min		
Platelet	4 h	1.5–2 h	2–3 h
Elimination	Reticuloendothelial system	60–70% renal	98% renal
		20–30 % biliar	Partialy metabolized
Dose-adjustments	Hepatic failure, elderly patients	Renal insufficiency	Renal insufficiency

ACS, acute coronary syndrome; h, hours; IC, intracoronary; IV, intravenous.

during platelet stimulation, eventually blocking platelet aggregation. Their pharmacodynamic and pharmacokinetic properties are described in Table 4.1.

Intravenous versus oral preparations: clinical aspects

Intravenous (IV) preparations of GPIIb/IIIa antagonists are used in acute setting where the rapid onset of effect is a crucial point of the therapy. These agents usually have more predictable pharmacokinetic and pharmacodynamic profiles, as they are not dependent on gastrointestinal absorption which may be impaired in acute illness. The effects of IV agents usually can be immediately resolved with infusion discontinuation. This might be valuable at the end of therapy or when a complication (bleeding) occurs. The benefits of these drugs have been demonstrated to be related to patient risk profile during PCI for ST-elevation myocardial infarction: the higher the patient's risk, the higher the benefits from IV therapy [13].

IV antiplatelet drugs have also some disadvantages. Their use is confined to the acute care setting, as it requires venous access; special storage, handling, and preparation of the product; and the necessary delivery equipment, such as IV pumps.

Antiplatelet therapies delivered orally overcome most of these limitations and can be used in a wide variety of healthcare settings.

The validity of oral drug delivery is limited in patients with concomitant gastrointestinal symptoms (nausea, vomiting).

IV GPIIb/IIIa inhibitors have a proven role in the management of patients with ischemic heart disease. Recently, intracoronary (IC) administration of GPIIb/IIIa antagonists, mainly abciximab, has been tested. Plasma concentration of available abciximab rapidly decreases after administration due to its rapid binding to GPIIb/IIIa receptors. As soon as 10 min after bolus delivery of this compound, more than 80% of GP receptors are occupied resulting in a decrease of platelet aggregation by 80%. Because of the short plasma half-life of abciximab, its IV administration does not allow one to obtain suitable concentrations at the culprit lesion and in the coronary distal bed of the culprit vessel. In contrast to IV injection, IC route of administration allows one to obtain much higher concentrations within the coronary thrombus at the culprit lesion. Not only does high local concentration of abciximab decrease platelet activity, it also results in the dissolution of existing platelet-rich thrombi at the ruptured plaque and dispersion of newly formed platelet aggregates, thus reducing distal microembolization [14, 15]. Marciniak *et al.* [14] have shown that abciximab at lower concentrations (1.5–3.0 mg/mL) prevents further aggregate formation; however, achieving concentrations of 10 mg/mL results in extensive dispersion of platelet aggregates. IC administration of abciximab has been compared to the standard IV route in several recent RCTs with contrasting results, mainly due to the low number of patients enrolled. On the other hand, IC route proved to be at least noninferior to the IV administration with potential survival advantages [16] that, on the other hand, need to be confirmed in future appropriately powered RCTs.

Acknowledgment

We thank Michalina Kolodziejczak and Natalia Kotlarek from the SIRIO-MEDICINE Research Network for their help in the preparation of the manuscript.

References

1 Gresele, P., Page, C.P., Fuster, V., and Vermylen, J. (2002) *Platelets in Thrombotic and Non-thrombotic Disorders: Pathophysiology, Pharmacology and Therapeutics*, pp. 3–24. Cambridge University Press, Cambridge.

2 Philips, D.R., Charo, I.F., Parise, L.V., and Fitzgerald, L.A. (1988) The platelet membrane glycoprotein IIb-IIIa complex. *Blood*, **71**, 831–843.

3 Fitzgerald, L.A. and Phillips, D.R. (1985) Calcium regulation of the platelet membrane glycoprotein IIb-IIIa complex. *The Journal of Biological Chemistry*, **260**, 11366–11374.

4 Stenberg, P.E., Shuman, M.A., Levine, S.P., and Bainton, D.F. (1984) Redistribution of alpha-granules and their contents in thrombin-stimulated platelets. *The Journal of Cell Biology*, **98**, 748–760.

5 Bevers, E.M., Comfurius, P., van Rijn, J.L., Hemke, H.C., and Zwaal, R.F. (1982) Generation of prothrombin-converting activity and the exposure of

phosphatidylserine at the outer surface of platelets. *European Journal of Biochemistry*, **122**, 429–436.

6 Parise, L.V. (1999) Integrin alpha IIb beta 3 signaling in platelet adhesion and aggregation. *Cell Biology*, **11**, 597–601.

7 Shattil, S.J. (1999) Signaling through platelet integrin alpha IIb beta 3: inside-out, outside-in, and sideways. *Thrombosis and Haemostasis*, **82**, 318–325.

8 Du, X.P., Plow, E.F., Frelinger, A.L., 3rd, O'Toole, T.E., Loftus, J.C., and Ginsberg, M.H. (1991) Ligands "activate" integrin alpha IIb beta 3 (platelet GPIIb-IIIa). *Cell*, **65**, 409–416.

9 Sambrano, G.R., Weiss, E.J., Zheng, Y.W., Huang, W., and Coughlin, S.R. (2001) Role of thrombin signalling in platelets in haemostasis and thrombosis. *Nature*, **413**, 74–78.

10 Swords, N., Tracy, P., and Mann, K. (1993) Intact platelet membranes, not platelet-released microvesicles, support the procoagulant activity of adherent platelets. *Arteriosclerosis and Thrombosis*, **13**, 1613–1622.

11 Kubica, A., Kozinski, M., Navarese, E.P., Grzesk, G., Goch, A. and Kubica, J., (2011) Intracoronary versus intravenous abciximab administration in STEMI patients: overview of current status and open questions. *Current Medical Research and Opinion*, **27**, 2133–2144.

12 Moser, M., Bertram, U., Karlheinz, P., Bode, C., and Rue, J. (2003) Abciximab, eptifibatide, and tirofiban exhibit dose-dependent potencies to dissolve platelet aggregates. *Journal of Cardiovascular Pharmacology*, **41 (4)**, 586–592.

13 De Luca, G., Navarese, E. ,and Marino, P. (2009) Risk profile and benefits from Gp IIb-IIIa inhibitors among patients with ST-segment elevation myocardial infarction treated with primary angioplasty: a meta-regression analysis of randomized trials. *European Heart Journal*, **30**, 2705–2713.

14 Marciniak, S.J., Jr, Mascelli, M.A., Furman, M.I. *et al.* (2002) An additional mechanism of action of abciximab: dispersal of newly formed platelet aggregates. *Thrombosis and Haemostasis*, **87**, 1020–1025.

15 Collet, J.P., Mishal, Z., Soria, J. *et al.* (2001) Disaggregation of in vitro platelet-rich clots by abciximab increases fibrinogen exposure and promotes fibrinolysis. *Arteriosclerosis, Thrombosis, and Vascular Biology*, **21**, 142–148.

16 Navarese, E.P., Kozinski, M., Obonska, K. *et al.* (2012) Clinical efficacy and safety of intracoronary vs. intravenous abciximab administration in STEMI patients undergoing primary percutaneous coronary intervention: a meta-analysis of randomized trials. *Platelets*, **23**, 274–281.

5 Platelet Receptors and Drug Targets: PAR1, Collagen, vWF, Thromboxane, and Other Novel Targets

Ping Zhang, Lidija Covic, and Athan Kuliopulos

Tufts University School of Medicine, Boston, MA, USA

Introduction

Atherothrombotic disease and acute arterial thrombosis are the leading causes of acute coronary syndromes (ACS) and cardiovascular death [1]. Platelets comprise the major component of the arterial thrombi, and effective antiplatelet therapy is critical to prevent ischemic complications of acute arterial thrombosis. Current treatment of patients undergoing percutaneous coronary interventions (PCI) and secondary prevention of ischemic events is a combination of dual antiplatelet therapy consisting of acetylsalicylic acid (ASA, aspirin) to block thromboxane synthesis and a $P2Y_{12}$ adenosine diphosphate (ADP) receptor inhibitor such as clopidogrel [2]. Dual antiplatelet therapy attenuates short- and long-term ischemic event occurrence during ACS and PCI; however, the persistence of cardiovascular events and the increased risk of bleeding remain major concerns [3, 4, 5, 6, 7, 8]. The most potent $P2Y_{12}$ receptor blockers are associated with only a 20% relative risk reduction with 10% of patients still suffering from recurrent ischemic events within 1 year of treatment [4, 5]. This indicates that there may be a ceiling effect in a strategy limited to aspirin and $P2Y_{12}$ receptor inhibition for the prevention of thrombosis in ACS and PCI patients. Intravenous GPIIb–IIIa inhibitors (abciximab, eptifibatide, tirofiban), which block the final common pathway of platelet activation and aggregation, exhibit potent antiplatelet activity but also significantly increase the risk of bleeding proportional to their potency [9]. Therefore, the new platelet inhibitors described in the succeeding text may provide alternative therapeutic efficacy versus hemorrhagic profiles to provide added benefit to patients suffering from life-threatening ischemic arterial disease.

Antiplatelet Therapy in Cardiovascular Disease, First Edition. Edited by Ron Waksman, Paul A. Gurbel, and Michael A. Gaglia, Jr.
© 2014 John Wiley & Sons, Ltd. Published 2014 by John Wiley & Sons, Ltd.

Protease-activated receptor 1 (PAR1)

The serine protease thrombin is the most potent platelet activator and plays a critical role in thrombosis and in the maintenance of hemostasis following vascular injury [10]. As direct thrombin inhibitors block thrombin-mediated cleavage of fibrinogen, targeting the downstream platelet thrombin receptors instead should theoretically result in a safer bleeding profile. Of the four PAR family members, only PAR1 and PAR4 are expressed on human platelets (Figure 5.1) and can form heterodimers on the platelet surface, which together account for the entire thrombin signal in platelets [11]. Thrombin activates the PARs by cleaving a specific peptide bond in the receptor extracellular domain: R41–S42 for PAR1 and R47–G48 for PAR4 [12]. The signal from the high-affinity PAR1 thrombin receptor is fast and transient [13], whereas the lower-affinity PAR4 [12] evokes a prolonged signal that contributes to irreversible platelet aggregation [11, 13, 14]. PAR1 is the major receptor for thrombin in human platelets and has become an intensively studied antiplatelet target in clinical trials. Conversely, PAR4 is considered to be a secondary thrombin receptor due to its lower affinity for thrombin, and there has been considerably less development of PAR4 inhibitors [11, 13, 15]. More recent studies have identified other proteases such as matrix metalloprotease-1 (MMP1), MMP13, plasmin, and activated protein C (APC) as direct activators of PAR1 [16]. Collagen activation of MMP1–PAR1 signaling may be an important new mechanism of platelet activation during the early steps of platelet thrombogenesis at the site of vessel injury [17]. PAR1 is also important in the vascular remodeling processes in unstable atherosclerotic plaques and in restenosis that may occur after PCI [10, 16, 18]. Chronic blockade of PAR1 in patients with ACS and atherothrombotic disease may therefore provide suppressive effects on both platelets and in culprit lesions undergoing pathological remodeling and inflammation.

A number of PAR1 antagonists have been developed including SCH 530348 [19], E5555 [20], FR-17113 [21], F16618 [22, 23], F16357 [24], PZ-128 [25], RWJ-56110 and RWJ-58259 [26, 27, 28], and BMS-200261 [29]. Vorapaxar (SCH 530348) and atopaxar (E5555) have been extensively evaluated in phase III and phase II clinical trials, respectively.

Vorapaxar (SCH 530348), an orally active, synthetic analog of himbacine with high affinity ($K_i = 3-8\,nM$) [30] to PAR1, has an exceptionally long elimination half-life of 6.6–13 days [31] and a functionally irreversible binding mode [32]. The pharmacodynamic half-life typically exceeds the entire lifespan of a circulating platelet with 50% recovery of platelet function by 4–8 weeks after a single 20 or 40 mg loading dose of vorapaxar [33]. The onset of inhibition of vorapaxar on PAR1 activity occurs by 2 h after receiving the loading dose. The lowest 10 mg dose gave 43% inhibition of TRAP

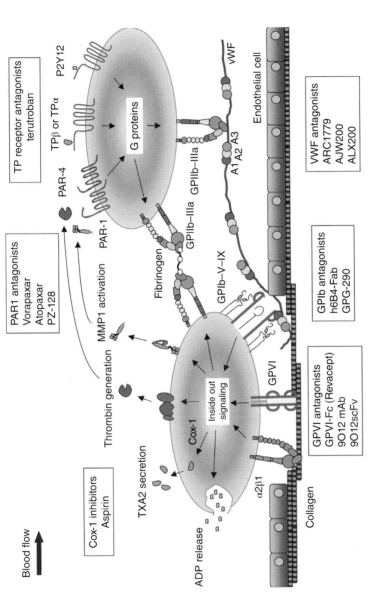

Figure 5.1 Mechanisms involved in platelet activation and emerging antiplatelet drugs. Following disruption of an atherosclerotic lesion, platelets initially adhere to exposed collagen and von Willebrand factor (vWF) from the vessel wall via GPIb–V–IX on the surface under high shear force conditions. Collagen mediates firm adhesion of platelets in a two-step mechanism in which "outside-in" signaling from the collagen receptor, GPVI, and the $\alpha2\beta1$ integrin results in the formation of a platelet monolayer. This collagen-mediated adhesion and activation of platelets leads to the release of adenosine diphosphate (ADP) and thromboxane A2 (TXA2) production via COX-1, matrix metalloprotease-1 (MMP1) activation, and thrombin generation on the surface of activated platelets. These autocrine mediators recruit additional platelets through the major fibrinogen receptor GPIIb–IIIa and activate nearby platelets to cause platelet aggregation via G protein-coupled receptors (GPCRs), PAR1, PAR4, TP, and P2Y$_{12}$.

(PAR1 peptide agonist)-induced platelet aggregation at 2 h, whereas a 40 mg dose resulted in 96% inhibition within 2 h [31]. The safety and tolerability of vorapaxar were evaluated in a phase II randomized trial, Thrombin Receptor Antagonist Percutaneous Coronary Intervention (TRA-PCI), comparing three vorapaxar oral loading doses 10, 20, and 40 mg versus placebo plus standard of care in 1030 patients undergoing nonurgent PCI [34]. The PCI cohort also received unfractionated heparin, low-molecular-weight heparin, or bivalirudin and a loading dose of clopidogrel (300–600 mg) and aspirin (162–325 mg oral or IV 150–500 mg). Patients who underwent PCI were further randomized to one of the three oral daily maintenance doses of vorapaxar (0.5, 1.0, 2.5 mg, or placebo). After 60 days of maintenance of vorapaxar, greater than 80% platelet inhibition to TRAP was seen at all three doses. Patients were evaluated at 60 days for safety (primary end point TIMI major/minor bleeding) and efficacy (MACE – nonfatal MI, nonfatal stroke, hospitalization for recurrent ischemia, or urgent coronary revascularization). The incidence of TIMI major and minor bleeding was similar in all three vorapaxar cohorts as compared to patients receiving placebo, with a dose-dependent trend toward more bleeding at the higher doses. Although not significant, vorapaxar appeared to reduce the occurrence of periprocedural myocardial infarctions (MIs) when added to dual antiplatelet therapy in patients who received PCI [34].

The safety and efficacy of vorapaxar were also evaluated in Japanese patients ($n = 117$) with a history of non-ST-segment elevation (NSTE) ACS who were receiving standard-of-care therapy (aspirin, ticlopidine, and heparin) [35]. Patients were randomized to receive a loading dose (20 or 40 mg) or placebo and daily oral maintenance doses (1 or 2.5 mg) or placebo for 60 days post-PCI. The primary end point was bleeding (TIMI criteria), and the exploratory end point included all-cause death and MACE (nonfatal MI, nonfatal stroke, hospitalization for recurrent ischemia, or urgent coronary revascularization). Periprocedural MI was defined as an elevated CK-MB or troponin-I (above three times the upper limit of normal with >50% increase above baseline) that was measured at baseline, 8, 16, and 24 h after PCI. Vorapaxar did not result in excess bleeding in the Japanese patients with NSTE ACS and significantly ($p = 0.013$) reduced the incidence of periprocedural MI by 2.5-fold in subjects undergoing PCI. The majority of MIs that did occur were asymptomatic elevations of CK-MB and troponin-I that were documented during the periprocedural period shortly after PCI.

The safety of vorapaxar was evaluated in Japanese patients ($n = 90$) with a history of ischemic cerebral infarction [36]. All patients received 1.0 or 2.5 mg vorapaxar or placebo once daily for 60 days plus aspirin (75–150 mg/day). The primary end point was overall incidence of adverse events (AE excluding MACE). The AE rate was not significantly different with the dual vorapaxar/aspirin regimen at either dose. The secondary end point of bleeding (TIMI categorized) was similar between placebo and vorapaxar [36].

The PAR1 antagonist atopaxar (E5555) is a second orally active small molecule that inhibits PAR1 activation on platelets. Atopaxar has a much shorter half-life (22–26 h) [37] than vorapaxar. E5555 nearly completely inhibited platelet activation at 20 ng/mL and caused 10–15% inhibition of ADP- and collagen-dependent platelet activation [20]. E5555 also inhibited the expression of the platelet inflammatory markers P-selectin and CD40 ligand.

Atopaxar was investigated in several phase II clinical trials including Lesson from Antagonizing the Cellular Effect of Thrombin Acute Coronary Syndromes (LANCELOT) ACS trial ($n = 603$) [37] and two smaller trials with a Japanese ACS (UA and NSTEMI) patient population (J-LANCELOT) ($n = 241$) [38] and in patients with coronary artery disease (CAD) (LANCELOT-CAD) ($n = 263$) on top of standard antiplatelet therapy [39]. ACS patients were pretreated with a 400 mg loading dose of E5555 or placebo followed by 50, 100, or 200 mg daily atopaxar for 12 weeks. Subjects with CAD were treated for 24 weeks without a loading dose with daily 50, 100, and 200 mg atopaxar or placebo on top of aspirin. The LANCELOT-ACS subjects reached maximal platelet inhibition 6 h after the loading dose of atopaxar. The primary end point was the occurrence of bleeding (CURE and TIMI), and the secondary end point was MACE including cardiovascular death, MI, and recurrent ischemia. The LANCELOT-ACS trial results demonstrated that atopaxar significantly reduced Holter-detected ischemia without a clear increase in bleeding compared with placebo. Atopaxar resulted in more minor bleeding in the 200 mg daily dose group and numerically, but not statistically significant, fewer ischemic events in patients with CAD [39]. Atopaxar was generally well tolerated; however, a transient rise in liver enzymes was observed in 3–6% of subjects ($p < 0.0001$), and prolongation of the QTc interval was observed in some individuals at the higher dose levels [37, 39]. Phase III studies will be required before the efficacy and safety of atopaxar can be fully determined.

The efficacy and long-term safety of vorapaxar over 1–2.5-year treatment periods were evaluated in two large phase III randomized trials. The effects of vorapaxar in preventing MI and stroke in patients ($n = 26,449$) with atherothrombotic disease (either post-MI, a history of stroke, or peripheral arterial disease) were assessed in the Thrombin Receptor Antagonist TRA 2°P-TIMI 50 study [40]. In addition, a second trial assessed the ability of vorapaxar to prevent MI and stroke in patients ($n = 12,944$) with chronic ACS (TRACER) [41]. Due to elevated bleeding rates, TRA 2°P-TIMI 50 was terminated early in patients that had experienced a stroke before or during the trial (17% of the enrolled patients) [40], and TRACER was terminated in all patients due to significantly increases in the risk of moderate and severe bleeding, including intracranial hemorrhage [42]. When added to standard of care in patients with non-ST elevation ACS and high use of aspirin and P2Y$_{12}$ inhibition, vorapaxar did not significantly reduce the composite of cardiovascular death, MI, stroke, hospitalization for ischemia, or urgent revascularization. However, vorapaxar did reduce the secondary end point of cardiovascular death, MI, or stroke with a significantly increased incidence of bleeding, including major bleeding and intracranial hemorrhage [42].

For patients with stable atherothrombotic disease (<75 years old and >60 kg), however, inhibition of PAR1 with a loading dose of 40 mg followed by daily 2.5 mg treatment with vorapaxar decreased the risk of cardiovascular death or ischemic events by 13% ($p < 0.001$) when added to standard dual antiplatelet treatment [40]. The subgroup of patients with prior MI also demonstrated a reduction in cardiovascular death and ischemic events [43]. However, the long half-life of 6–13 days for vorapaxar and only 50% recovery of platelet function at 4 weeks after treatment discontinuation [44] may pose a bleeding risk, especially for patients that may need to undergo subsequent coronary artery bypass (CABG) surgery. Patients with prior MI appear to be most likely to have a net clinical benefit from vorapaxar therapy, and Merck is requesting regulatory approval in patients with prior MI and no history of stroke in the USA and Europe.

The ability to rapidly and reversibly inhibit PAR1 signaling by a parenteral strategy would be an ideal in the high-risk patient undergoing PCI. Establishing rapid receptor blockade with a parenterally administered PAR1 blocker should translate into a superior reduction in adverse post-PCI thrombotic event occurrence. Similarly, the use of a more reversible agent than vorapaxar may also facilitate patient care by attenuating bleeding risk in the setting of unanticipated surgery. A fast-acting, shorter half-life pepducin-based drug, PZ-128, is currently being evaluated in human phase I studies. Pepducins are lipidated peptides that target the cytoplasmic surface of their cognate receptor [45, 46]. The PAR1 pepducin, PZ-128 (P1pal-7), is administered by an intravenous infusion during the PCI procedure. PZ-128 consists of a seven-amino-acid peptide derived from the third intracellular loop of PAR1 that is conjugated to palmitate lipid [10, 15, 45]. The solution structure of PZ-128 was determined by NMR, and the peptide was found to form a well-defined α-helix extending from the palmitate lipid. PZ-128 was found to form a highly similar structure as the corresponding region of PAR1 (residues 307–313) in the off-state with an RMSD of 1.4 Å [25]. PZ-128 showed excellent dose- and concentration-dependent inhibition of PAR1 platelet aggregation and arterial thrombosis in baboons. At the 3 mg/kg dose in baboons, PAR1-dependent aggregation was inhibited by 85% at the 1 h and 2 h time points, but was not appreciably inhibited (10%) at the 24 h time point. At the 6 mg/kg dose in baboon, PAR1-dependent aggregation was inhibited by 100% at the 1 h and 2 h time points, 90% at 6 h, but was completely recovered by the 24 h time point. Inhibition of PAR1 by PZ-128 was reversible, as evidenced by loss of inhibition with higher concentrations of SFLLRN agonist at both the 3 mg/kg and 6 mg/kg doses. PZ-128 gave no significant inhibition (0–10%) of either ADP or PAR4 platelet responses at any time point including at 1, 2, or 24 h [25]. Dose-dependent protection against arterial thrombosis with an EC_{50} of 0.075 mg/kg PZ-128 was determined in guinea pig, and synergistic protective effects were observed with oral clopidogrel. The pharmacokinetic and antiplatelet pharmacodynamic properties of PZ-128 indicate that this lipopeptide reaches maximal activity during (<15 min) and immediately after intravenous infusion and is completely eliminated from plasma by the next day. PZ-128 had no effect on bleeding or coagulation parameters in primates or in blood from PCI patients [25]. The rapid onset of platelet inhibition and reversible properties of PZ-128 are well suited to the acute interventional setting of PCI and may provide an alternative to long-acting small-molecule inhibitors of PAR1 during PCI.

Collagen

Platelet–collagen interactions are critical for the initiation of platelet adhesion and early platelet activation on subendothelial matrices at the medium and high shear rates found in arteries. Activation of platelets by collagen occurs through an initial interaction with the integrin α2β1 and activation of glycoprotein GPVI (Figure 5.1). Coupled to the γ chain of the Fc receptor (FcRγ), GPVI triggers a signal cascade via tyrosine phosphorylation events ending in protein kinase C (PKC) activation and mobilization of intracellular calcium stores. α2β1 plays a significant role in the adhesion of platelets to collagen fibers [47]. Fibrillar collagen also converts surface-bound MMP1 zymogen to active MMP1 on platelet surface, which can activate PAR1-dependent shape change and early platelet thrombogenesis [17]. Collagen is also a potent agonist that induces platelet procoagulant activity and thrombin generation [48, 49].

GPVI–collagen interactions can be disrupted by GPVI mimics and antibodies. The soluble immunoadhesion molecule GPVI–Fc (revacept) is composed of two extracellular domains of GPVI fused to the constant domain (Fc) of human IgG1. A recent phase I study demonstrated that revacept efficiently inhibited *ex vivo* collagen-induced platelet aggregation with no adverse impact on primary hemostasis in 30 healthy human volunteers [50]. Inhibitory antibodies that do not alter GPVI surface expression have also been identified. 9O12 is a high-affinity (1 nM) mAb for human GPVI. Numerous preclinical studies have been conducted with 9O12 that indicate that targeting GPVI provides good antithrombotic efficacy with no observed bleeding side effects [51, 52]. In addition to inhibition of platelet adhesion and aggregation, 9O12 also reduced collagen–GPVI platelet procoagulant activity by preventing exposure of phosphatidylserine [51, 53]. Platelet-bound 9O12 was detected from 30 min to 24 h after injection without inducing depletion of GPVI [52]. Due to the immunogenicity of murine antibody fragments, a humanized 9O12scFv that retained GPVI binding affinity is also being developed [54].

vWF

von Willebrand factor (vWF) contributes to initial platelet adhesion by acting as a bridging element between exposed collagen and the platelet GPIb receptor (Figure 5.1). vWF is a multimeric glycoprotein and interacts with collagen/GPIb via A3 and A1 domains [55]. The binding site in A1 domain is normally cryptic, preventing spontaneous binding to GPIb. High shear stress ($\geq 1000\,s^{-1}$) induces a conformational change of vWF exposing the A1 domain, and efficient vWF–GPIb interactions occur under high shear in stenotic segments of arteries [56]. Deficiency of multimeric vWF in plasma is responsible for the most common bleeding disease, namely, von Willebrand disease (vWD). The lack of GPIb on the platelet surface leads to a severe bleeding disorder termed Bernard–Soulier syndrome (BSS). Conversely, the presence of ultralarge vWF multimers causes life-threatening thrombotic thrombocytopenic purpura (TTP) due to deficiency (or antibodies against) of the vWF-cleaving protease ADAMTS13 [55, 57]. vWF levels typically rise during MI [58], and vWF may be involved in later steps of platelet thrombogenesis via binding to GPIIb–IIIa [59].

There are several large molecules that target vWF including antibodies (AJW200 and 82D6A3), nanobodies (ALX-0081 and ALX-0681), and aptamers (ARC1779 and ARC15105) [60]. These agents target A1 domain–GPIb interactions with the exception of 82D6A3 that targets the A3 domain–collagen complex. Two antibodies (h6B4-Fab and SZ2) and one chimeric protein (GPG-290) containing the N-terminal 290 amino acids of GPIba linked to human IgG1 Fc were designed to target GPIb. Preclinical and phase I results have been reported for three of these compounds: ARC1779, AJW200, and ALX-0081.

ARC1779 is a synthetic aptamer conjugated to a polyethylene glycol moiety at the 5′ terminus with a core 40-mer modified-DNA/RNA oligonucleotide. ARC1779 interferes with vWF–A1 domain interactions, and the aptamer can be neutralized by complementary antidotes if adverse effects occur. A dose-dependent effect on occlusion time in the PFA-100 device was observed in a phase I study, and 0.3 mg/kg ARC1779 was able to completely inhibit platelet function for up to 4 h with recovery by 8–12 h [61]. Several phase II studies were subsequently conducted to investigate the clinical efficacy of ARC1779 as an antithrombotic agent. In patients undergoing carotid endarterectomy, intravenous treatment with ARC1779 reduced cerebral embolization [62]. Treatment of TTP patients with ARC1779 significantly inhibited vWF activity and vWF-dependent platelet activation and increased platelet counts [63, 64, 65, 66, 67]. ARC1779 also prevented thrombocytopenia in patients with type 2B vWD [66, 68] with no excess bleeding noted in these trials. However, preclinical studies documented an increase in template bleeding time in cynomolgus macaques in a dose-dependent manner [69].

AJW200 is an IgG4 humanized monoclonal antibody to human vWF. Preclinical data showed that AJW200 specifically inhibited high shear stress-induced platelet aggregation in a concentration-dependent manner in blood from volunteers [70]. Sustained inhibition of platelet aggregation was observed over 24 h after a single bolus injection of 0.3 mg/kg AJW200 in cynomolgus monkeys with moderate prolongation of the bleeding time [70]. AJW200 has a much longer half-life (~24 h) than ARC1779. Pharmacodynamic efficacy judged by the prolongation of occlusion times by PFA-100 lasted for 3–6 h at low dose and up to 12 h for high dose. No clinically significant AE were reported nor evidence of immunogenicity [71].

ALX-0081 is a bivalent nanobody that specifically targets the GPIb binding site of vWF. vWF-bound ALX-0081 stays in circulation with an apparent half-life of 17–30 h in cynomolgus monkeys [72]. ALX-0081 was able to abolish platelet adhesion to collagen under flow conditions and completely inhibited *ex vivo* ristocetin-induced platelet aggregation in blood from patients undergoing PCI [73]. ALX-0081 abolished cyclic flow reductions in a baboon Folts model [74]. A phase II trial comparing the efficacy and safety of ALX-0081 to abciximab is currently ongoing in high-risk PCI patients [74].

Thromboxane and other receptors

Arachidonic acid, generated from membrane phospholipids by phospholipase A_2, is metabolized to an unstable endoperoxide intermediate prostaglandin H2 (PGH2) by COX-1 and COX-2, which can be further metabolized to prostaglandins by PG synthase or TX by thromboxane synthase. ASA is a member of the nonsteroidal anti-inflammatory drug (NSAID) family that reduces thromboxane A2 (TXA2) synthesis by irreversible inhibition of COX-1. A large body of data demonstrates that ASA monotherapy provides modest protection against occurrence of ischemic events especially in high-risk patients [75], but some patients do not respond to ASA with a prevalence of "ASA resistance" of 5–40% [76].

Thromboxane synthase inhibitors (TXSI) and thromboxane receptor antagonists (TXRA) have the potential to provide more efficacy than ASA due to their different mechanisms of action. After binding the TXA2 receptors (either TPα or TPβ variants), TXA2 causes increases in intracellular Ca^{2+} levels. TP receptors are activated not only by TXA2 but also by prostaglandins (PGD2, PGE2, PGF2α, PGH2), PG endoperoxides (i.e., 20-HETE), and isoprostanes, all representing ASA-insensitive mechanisms of TP receptor activation. Thus, targeting the TP receptor, a common downstream pathway for TXA2 as well as for endoperoxides and isoprostanes, may be a useful antithrombotic strategy in clinical settings such as diabetes mellitus, characterized by persistently enhanced thromboxane-dependent platelet activation through isoprostane formation and low-grade inflammation.

Terutroban, a selective TP antagonist, is an orally active drug in clinical development for use in secondary prevention of thrombotic events in cardiovascular disease. Terutroban was at least as effective as ASA in inhibition of platelet aggregation induced by arachidonic acid and collagen in patients with peripheral arterial disease [77] and was superior to ASA in inhibition of platelet aggregation and thrombus formation in an *ex vivo* model of thrombosis in blood from patients at risk for ischemic stroke [78]. Terutroban has been tested for the secondary prevention of acute thrombotic complications in the phase III clinical trial PERFORM that compared terutroban 30 mg/day with ASA 100 mg/day in patients who had a cerebral ischemic event [79]. Despite great expectations, the PERFORM trial failed to demonstrate superiority of terutroban over ASA in secondary prevention of cerebrovascular and cardiovascular events in approximately 20,000 patients with stroke, showing similar rates in the primary end point without safety advantages over ASA. In a trial of patients with primary pulmonary hypertension, terutroban was associated with severe leg pain [80]. Ridogrel, a combined TXSI and TXA2/PG endoperoxide receptor antagonist, was compared with ASA in patients with MI receiving streptokinase in the RAPT trial. Ridogrel did not improve angiographic patency and the primary end point (TIMI flow grades 2 and 3) of the trial [81]. Specific clinical settings in which selective TP blockade might confer an advantage over low-dose ASA await further investigation. Other drugs under development and evaluation include new phosphodiesterase inhibitors and compounds that target various intracellular platelet signaling pathways.

References

1 Roger, V.L., Go, A.S., Lloyd-Jones, D.M. *et al.* (2012) Heart disease and stroke statistics: 2012 update: A report from the American heart association. *Circulation*, **125 (1)**, e2–e220.

2 Gurbel, P.A. and Tantry, U.S. (2010) Combination antithrombotic therapies. *Circulation*, **121 (4)**, 569–583.

3 Yusuf, S., Zhao, F., Mehta, S.R., Chrolavicius, S., Tognoni, G., and Fox, K.K. (2001) Effects of clopidogrel in addition to aspirin in patients with acute coronary syndromes without ST-segment elevation. *New England Journal of Medicine*, **345 (7)**, 494–502.

4 Wiviott, S.D., Braunwald, E., McCabe, C.H. *et al.* (2007) Prasugrel versus clopidogrel in patients with acute coronary syndromes. *New England Journal of Medicine*, **357 (20)**, 2001–2015.

5 Wallentin, L., Becker, R.C., Budaj, A. *et al.* (2009) Ticagrelor versus clopidogrel in patients with acute coronary syndromes. *New England Journal of Medicine*, **361 (11)**, 1045–1057.

6 Harrington, R.A., Stone, G.W., McNulty, S. *et al.* (2009) Platelet inhibition with cangrelor in patients undergoing PCI. *New England Journal of Medicine*, **361 (24)**, 2318–2329.

7 Moshfegh, K., Redondo, M., Julmy, F. *et al.* (2000) Antiplatelet effects of clopidogrel compared with aspirin after myocardial infarction: enhanced inhibitory effects of combination therapy. *Journal of the American College of Cardiology*, **36 (3)**, 699–705.

8 Gori, A.M., Marcucci, R., Migliorini, A. *et al.* (2008) Incidence and clinical impact of dual nonresponsiveness to aspirin and clopidogrel in patients with drug-eluting stents. *Journal of the American College of Cardiology*, **52 (9)**, 734–739.

9 Scarborough, R.M., Kleiman, N.S., and Phillips, D.R. (1999) Platelet glycoprotein IIb/IIIa antagonists. What are the relevant issues concerning their pharmacology and clinical use? *Circulation*, **100 (4)**, 437–444.

10 Leger, A.J., Covic, L., and Kuliopulos, A. (2006) Protease-activated receptors in cardiovascular diseases. *Circulation*, **114 (10)**, 1070–1077.

11 Leger, A.J., Jacques, S.L., Badar, J. *et al.* (2006) Blocking the protease-activated receptor 1–4 heterodimer in platelet-mediated thrombosis. *Circulation*, **113 (9)**, 1244–1254.

12 Jacques, S.L. and Kuliopulos, A. (2003) Protease-activated receptor-4 uses dual prolines and an anionic retention motif for thrombin recognition and cleavage. Biochem J., **376 (Pt. 3)**, 733–740.

13 Covic, L., Gresser, A.L. and Kuliopulos, A. (2000) Biphasic kinetics of activation and signaling for PAR1 and PAR4 thrombin receptors in platelets. *Biochemistry*, **39 (18)**, 5458–5467.

14 Covic, L., Singh, C., Smith, H., and Kuliopulos, A. (2002) Role of the PAR4 thrombin receptor in stabilizing platelet-platelet aggregates as revealed by a patient with Hermansky-Pudlak syndrome. *Thrombosis and Haemostasis*, **87 (4)**, 722–727.

15 Covic, L., Misra, M., Badar, J., Singh, C., and Kuliopulos, A. (2002) Pepducin-based intervention of thrombin-receptor signaling and systemic platelet activation. *Nature Medicine*, **8 (10)**, 1161–1165.

16 Austin, K.M., Covic, L., and Kuliopulos, A. (2013) Matrix metalloproteases and PAR1 activation. *Blood*, **121 (3)**, 431–439.

17 Trivedi, V., Boire, A., Tchernychev, B. *et al.* (2009) Platelet matrix metalloprotease-1 mediates thrombogenesis by activating PAR1 at a cryptic ligand site. *Cell*, **137 (2)**, 332–343.

18 Sevigny, L.M., Austin, K.M., Zhang, P. *et al.* (2011) Protease-activated receptor-2 modulates protease-activated receptor-1-driven neointimal hyperplasia. *Arteriosclerosis, Thrombosis, and Vascular Biology*, **31 (12)**, e100–e106.

19 Oestreich, J. (2009) SCH-530348, a thrombin receptor (PAR-1) antagonist for the prevention and treatment of atherothrombosis. *Current Opinion in Investigational Drugs*, **10 (9)**, 988–996.

20 Serebruany, V.L., Kogushi, M., Dastros-Pitei, D., Flather, M., and Bhatt, D.L. (2009) The in-vitro effects of E5555, a protease-activated receptor (PAR)-1 antagonist, on platelet biomarkers in healthy volunteers and patients with coronary artery disease. *Thrombosis and Haemostasis*, **102 (1)**, 111–119.

21 Kato, Y., Kita, Y., Hirasawa-Taniyama, Y. *et al.* (2003) Inhibition of arterial thrombosis by a protease-activated receptor 1 antagonist, FR171113, in the guinea pig. *European Journal of Pharmacology*, **473 (2–3)**, 163–169.

22 Chieng-Yane, P., Bocquet, A., Letienne, R. *et al.* (2011) Protease-activated receptor-1 antagonist F 16618 reduces arterial restenosis by down-regulation of tumor necrosis factor alpha and matrix metalloproteinase 7 expression, migration, and proliferation of vascular smooth muscle cells. *Journal of Pharmacology and Experimental Therapeutics*, **336 (3)**, 643–651.

23 Perez, M., Lamothe, M., Maraval, C. *et al.* (2009) Discovery of novel protease activated receptors 1 antagonists with potent antithrombotic activity in vivo. *Journal of Medicinal Chemistry*, **52 (19)**, 5826–5836.

24 Planty, B., Pujol, C., Lamothe, M. *et al.* (2010) Exploration of a new series of PAR1 antagonists. *Bioorganic and Medicinal Chemistry Letters*, **20 (5)**, 1735–1739.

25 Zhang, P., Gruber, A., Kasuda, S. *et al.* (2012) Suppression of arterial thrombosis without affecting hemostatic parameters with a cell-penetrating PAR1 pepducin. *Circulation*, **126 (1)**, 83–91.

26 Derian, C.K., Damiano, B.P., Addo, M.F. *et al.* (2003) Blockade of the thrombin receptor protease-activated receptor-1 with a small-molecule antagonist prevents thrombus formation and vascular occlusion in nonhuman primates. *Journal of Pharmacology and Experimental Therapeutics*, **304 (2)**, 855–861.

27 Damiano, B.P., Derian, C.K., Maryanoff, B.E., Zhang, H.C., and Gordon, P.A. (2003) RWJ-58259: a selective antagonist of protease activated receptor-1. *Cardiovascular Drug Reviews*, **21 (4)**, 313–326.

28 Andrade-Gordon, P., Maryanoff, B.E., Derian, C.K. *et al.* (1999) Design, synthesis, and biological characterization of a peptide-mimetic antagonist for a tethered-ligand receptor. *Proceedings of the National Academy of Sciences of the United States of America*, **96 (22)**, 12257–12262.

29 Bernatowicz, M.S., Klimas, C.E., Hartl, K.S., Peluso, M., Allegretto, N.J., and Seiler, S.M. (1996) Development of potent thrombin receptor antagonist peptides. *Journal of Medicinal Chemistry*, **39 (25)**, 4879–4887.

30 Chackalamannil, S., Wang, Y., Greenlee, W.J. *et al.* (2008) Discovery of a novel, orally active himbacine-based thrombin receptor antagonist (SCH 530348) with potent antiplatelet activity. *Journal of Medicinal Chemistry*, **51 (11)**, 3061–3064.

31 TRA*CER EaSC. (2009) The thrombin receptor antagonist for clinical event reduction in acute coronary syndrome (TRA*CER) trial: study design and rationale. *American Heart Journal*, **158(3)**, 327–334, e4.

32 Zhang, C., Srinivasan, Y., Arlow, D.H. *et al.* (2012) High-resolution crystal structure of human protease-activated receptor 1. *Nature*, **492 (7429)**, 387–392.

33 Kosoglou, T., Reyderman, L., Tiessen, R.G. *et al.* (2012) Pharmacodynamics and pharmacokinetics of the novel PAR-1 antagonist vorapaxar (formerly SCH 530348) in healthy subjects. *European Journal of Clinical Pharmacology*, **68**, 249–258.

34 Becker, R.C., Moliterno, D.J., Jennings, L.K. *et al.* (2009) Safety and tolerability of SCH 530348 in patients undergoing non-urgent percutaneous coronary intervention: a randomised, double-blind, placebo-controlled phase II study. *Lancet*, **373 (9667)**, 919–928.

35 Goto, S., Yamaguchi, T., Ikeda, Y., Kato, K., Yamaguchi, H. and Jensen, P. (2010) Safety and exploratory efficacy of the novel thrombin receptor (PAR-1) antagonist SCH530348 for non-ST-segment elevation acute coronary syndrome. *Journal of Atherosclerosis and Thrombosis*, **17 (2)**, 156–164.

36 Shinohara, Y., Goto, S., Doi, M., and Jensen, P. (2012) Safety of the novel protease-activated receptor-1 antagonist vorapaxar in Japanese patients with a history of ischemic stroke. *Journal of Stroke and Cerebrovascular Diseases*, **21 (4)**, 318–324.

37 O'Donoghue, M.L., Bhatt, D.L., Wiviott, S.D. *et al.* (2011) Safety and tolerability of atopaxar in the treatment of patients with acute coronary syndromes: the lessons from antagonizing the cellular effects

of Thrombin-Acute Coronary Syndromes Trial. *Circulation*, **123 (17)**, 1843–1853.

38 Goto, S., Ogawa, H., Takeuchi, M., Flather, M.D., and Bhatt, D.L. (2010) Double-blind, placebo-controlled Phase II studies of the protease-activated receptor 1 antagonist E5555 (atopaxar) in Japanese patients with acute coronary syndrome or high-risk coronary artery disease. *European Heart Journal*, **31 (21)**, 2601–2613.

39 Wiviott, S.D., Flather, M.D., O'Donoghue, M.L. *et al.* (2011) Randomized trial of atopaxar in the treatment of patients with coronary artery disease: the lessons from antagonizing the cellular effect of Thrombin-Coronary Artery Disease Trial. *Circulation*, **123 (17)**, 1854–1863.

40 Morrow, D.A., Braunwald, E., Bonaca, M.P. *et al.* (2012) Vorapaxar in the secondary prevention of atherothrombotic events. *New England Journal of Medicine*, **366 (15)**, 1404–1413.

41 TRA*CER Executive and Steering Committees. (2009) The thrombin receptor antagonist for clinical event reduction in acute coronary syndrome (TRA*CER) trial: study design and rationale. *American Heart Journal*, **158 (3)**, 327–334, e4.

42 Tricoci, P., Huang, Z., Held, C. *et al.* (2012) Thrombin-receptor antagonist vorapaxar in acute coronary syndromes. *New England Journal of Medicine*, **366 (1)**, 20–33.

43 Scirica, B.M., Bonaca, M.P., Braunwald, E. *et al.* (2012) Vorapaxar for secondary prevention of thrombotic events for patients with previous myocardial infarction: a prespecified subgroup analysis of the TRA 2 degrees P-TIMI 50 trial. *Lancet*, **380 (9850)**, 1317–1324.

44 Angiolillo, D.J., Capodanno, D., and Goto, S. (2010) Platelet thrombin receptor antagonism and atherothrombosis. *European Heart Journal*, **31 (1)**, 17–28.

45 Covic, L., Gresser, A.L., Talavera, J., Swift, S. and Kuliopulos, A. (2002) Activation and inhibition of G protein-coupled receptors by cell-penetrating membrane-tethered peptides. *Proceedings of the National Academy of Sciences of the United States of America*, **99 (2)**, 643–648.

46 Covic, L., Tchernychev, B., Jacques, S., and Kuliopulos, A. (2007) Pharmacology and in vivo efficacy of pepducins in hemostasis and arterial thrombosis. In: U. Langel (ed), Handbook of Cell-Penetrating Peptides. 2nd, New York: Taylor and Francis, pp. 245–257.

47 Gruner, S., Prostredna, M., Aktas, B. *et al.* (2004) Anti-glycoprotein VI treatment severely compromises hemostasis in mice with reduced alpha2beta1 levels or concomitant aspirin therapy. *Circulation*, **110 (18)**, 2946–2951.

48 Bevers, E.M., Comfurius, P., van Rijn, J.L., Hemker, H.C., and Zwaal, R.F. (1982) Generation of prothrombin-converting activity and the exposure of phosphatidylserine at the outer surface of platelets. *European Journal of Biochemistry*, **122 (2)**, 429–436.

49 Kimmelstiel, C., Zhang, P., Kapur, N.K. *et al.* (2011) Bivalirudin is a dual inhibitor of thrombin and collagen-dependent platelet activation in patients undergoing percutaneous coronary intervention. *Circulation. Cardiovascular Interventions*, **4 (2)**, 171–179.

50 Ungerer, M., Rosport, K., Bultmann, A. *et al.* (2011) Novel antiplatelet drug revacept (Dimeric Glycoprotein VI-Fc) specifically and efficiently inhibited collagen-induced platelet aggregation without affecting general hemostasis in humans. *Circulation*, **123 (17)**, 1891–1899.

51 Lecut, C., Feeney, L.A., Kingsbury, G. *et al.* (2003) Human platelet glycoprotein VI function is antagonized by monoclonal antibody-derived Fab fragments. *Journal of Thrombosis and Haemostasis*, **1 (12)**, 2653–2662.

52 Ohlmann, P., Hechler, B., Ravanat, C. *et al.* (2008) Ex vivo inhibition of thrombus formation by an anti-glycoprotein VI Fab fragment in non-human primates without modification of glycoprotein VI expression. *Journal of Thrombosis and Haemostasis*, **6 (6)**, 1003–1011.

53 Lecut, C., Feijge, M.A., Cosemans, J.M., Jandrot-Perrus, M. and Heemskerk, J.W. (2005) Fibrillar type I collagens enhance platelet-dependent thrombin generation via glycoprotein VI with direct support of alpha2beta1 but not alphaIIbbeta3 integrin. *Thrombosis and Haemostasis*, **94 (1)**, 107–114.

54 Muzard, J., Bouabdelli, M., Zahid, M. *et al.* (2009) Design and humanization of a murine scFv that blocks human platelet glycoprotein VI in vitro. *FEBS Journal*, **276 (15)**, 4207–4222.

55 Sadler JE. (2002) BIOMEDICINE: Contact – how platelets touch von Willebrand factor. *Science*, **297(5584)**, 1128–1129.

56 Lenting, P.J., Pegon, J.N., Groot, E., and de Groot, P.G. (2010) Regulation of von Willebrand factor-platelet interactions. *Thrombosis and Haemostasis*, **104 (3)**, 449–455.

57 Zhang, P., Pan, W., Rux, A.H., Sachais, B.S., and Zheng, X.L. (2007) The cooperative activity between the carboxyl-terminal TSP1 repeats and the CUB domains of ADAMTS13 is crucial for recognition of von Willebrand factor under flow. *Blood*, **110 (6)**, 1887–1894.

58 Spiel, A.O., Gilbert, J.C., and Jilma, B. (2008) Willebrand factor in cardiovascular disease: focus on acute coronary syndromes. Circulation, **117 (11)**, 1449–1459.

59 Gawaz, M., Langer, H. and May, A.E. (2005) Platelets in inflammation and atherogenesis. *Journal of Clinical Investigation*, **115 (12)**, 3378–3384.

60 Firbas, C., Siller-Matula, J.M., and Jilma, B. (2010) Targeting von Willebrand factor and platelet glycoprotein Ib receptor. *Expert Review of Cardiovascular Therapy*, **8 (12)**, 1689–1701.

61 Gilbert, J.C., DeFeo-Fraulini, T., Hutabarat, R.M. *et al.* (2007) First-in-human evaluation of anti von Willebrand factor therapeutic aptamer ARC1779 in healthy volunteers. *Circulation*, **116 (23)**, 2678–2686.

62 Markus, H.S., McCollum, C., Imray, C., Goulder, M.A., Gilbert, J., and King, A. (2011) The von Willebrand inhibitor ARC1779 reduces cerebral embolization after carotid endarterectomy: a randomized trial. *Stroke*, **42 (8)**, 2149–2153.

63 Knobl, P., Jilma, B., Gilbert, J.C., Hutabarat, R.M., Wagner, P.G., and Jilma-Stohlawetz, P. (2009) Anti-von Willebrand factor aptamer ARC1779 for refractory thrombotic thrombocytopenic purpura. *Transfusion*, **49 (10)**, 2181–2185.

64 Mayr, F.B., Knobl, P., Jilma, B. *et al.* (2010) The aptamer ARC1779 blocks von Willebrand factor-dependent platelet function in patients with thrombotic thrombocytopenic purpura ex vivo. *Transfusion*, **50 (5)**, 1079–1087.

65 Jilma-Stohlawetz, P., Gorczyca, M.E., Jilma, B., Siller-Matula, J., Gilbert, J.C., and Knobl, P. (2011) Inhibition of von Willebrand factor by ARC1779 in patients with acute thrombotic thrombocytopenic purpura. *Thrombosis and Haemostasis*, **105 (3)**, 545–552.

66 Jilma-Stohlawetz, P., Knobl, P., Gilbert, J.C., and Jilma, B. (2012) The anti-von Willebrand factor aptamer ARC1779 increases von Willebrand factor levels

and platelet counts in patients with type 2B von Willebrand disease. *Thrombosis and Haemostasis*, **108 (2)**, 284–290.

67 Cataland, S.R., Peyvandi, F., Mannucci, P.M. *et al.* (2012) Initial experience from a double-blind, placebo-controlled, clinical outcome study of ARC1779 in patients with thrombotic thrombocytopenic purpura. *American Journal of Hematology*, **87 (4)**, 430–432.

68 Jilma, B., Paulinska, P., Jilma-Stohlawetz, P., Gilbert, J.C., Hutabarat, R., and Knobl, P. (2010) A randomised pilot trial of the anti-von Willebrand factor aptamer ARC1779 in patients with type 2b von Willebrand disease. *Thrombosis and Haemostasis*, **104 (3)**, 563–570.

69 Diener, J.L., Daniel Lagasse, H.A., Duerschmied, D. *et al.* (2009) Inhibition of von Willebrand factor-mediated platelet activation and thrombosis by the anti-von Willebrand factor A1-domain aptamer ARC1779. *Journal of Thrombosis and Haemostasis*, **7 (7)**, 1155–1162.

70 Kageyama, S., Yamamoto, H., Nakazawa, H. *et al.* (2002) Pharmacokinetics and pharmacodynamics of AJW200, a humanized monoclonal antibody to von Willebrand factor, in monkeys. *Arteriosclerosis, Thrombosis, and Vascular Biology*, **22 (1)**, 187–192.

71 Siller-Matula, J.M., Krumphuber, J., and Jilma, B. (2010) Pharmacokinetic, pharmacodynamic and clinical profile of novel antiplatelet drugs targeting vascular diseases. *British Journal of Pharmacology*, **159 (3)**, 502–517.

72 Lenting, P.J., Westein, E., Terraube, V. *et al.* (2004) An experimental model to study the in vivo survival of von Willebrand factor. Basic aspects and application to the R1205H mutation. *Journal of Biological Chemistry*, **279 (13)**, 12102–12109.

73 van Loon, J.E., de Jaegere, P.P., Ulrichts, H. *et al.* (2011) The in vitro effect of the new antithrombotic drug candidate ALX-0081 on blood samples of patients undergoing percutaneous coronary intervention. *Thrombosis and Haemostasis*, **106 (1)**, 165–171.

74 Ulrichts, H., Silence, K., Schoolmeester, A. *et al.* (2011) Antithrombotic drug candidate ALX-0081 shows superior preclinical efficacy and safety compared with currently marketed antiplatelet drugs. *Blood*, **118 (3)**, 757–765.

75 Eikelboom, J.W., Hirsh, J., Spencer, F.A., Baglin, T.P., and Weitz, J.I. (2012) Antiplatelet drugs: antithrombotic therapy and prevention of thrombosis, 9th ed: American college of chest physicians evidence-based clinical practice guidelines. *Chest*, **141** (2 Suppl), e89S–e119S.

76 Gum, P.A., Thamilarasan, M., Watanabe, J., Blackstone, E.H., and Lauer, M.S. (2001) Aspirin use and all-cause mortality among patients being evaluated for known or suspected coronary artery disease: a propensity analysis. *JAMA*, **286 (10)**, 1187–1194.

77 Fiessinger, J.N., Bounameaux, H., Cairols, M.A. *et al.* (2010) Thromboxane antagonism with terutroban in peripheral arterial disease: the TAIPAD study. *Journal of Thrombosis and Haemostasis*, **8 (11)**, 2369–2376.

78 Bal Dit Sollier, C., Crassard, I., Simoneau, G., Bergmann, J.F., Bousser, M.G., and Drouet, L. (2009) Effect of the thromboxane prostaglandin receptor antagonist terutroban on arterial thrombogenesis after repeated administration in patients treated for the prevention of ischemic stroke. *Cerebrovasc Dis*, **28 (5)**, 505–513.

79 Bousser, M.G., Amarenco, P., Chamorro, A. *et al.* (2011) Terutroban versus aspirin in patients with cerebral ischaemic events (PERFORM): a randomised, double-blind, parallel-group trial. *Lancet*, **377 (9782)**, 2013–2022.

80 Langleben, D., Christman, B.W., Barst, R.J. *et al.* (2002) Effects of the thromboxane synthetase inhibitor and receptor antagonist terbogrel in patients with primary pulmonary hypertension. *American Heart Journal*, **143 (5)**, E4.

81 RAPT Investigations (1994) Randomized trial of ridogrel, a combined thromboxane A2 synthase inhibitor and thromboxane A2/prostaglandin endoperoxide receptor antagonist, versus aspirin as adjunct to thrombolysis in patients with acute myocardial infarction. The Ridogrel Versus Aspirin Patency Trial (RAPT). *Circulation*, **89 (2)**, 588–595.

6 Role of Inflammation and Hypercoagulability in Thrombosis

Paul A. Gurbel[1,2,3], Nachiket Apte[1,2], and Udaya S. Tantry[1]
[1]Sinai Hospital of Baltimore, Baltimore, MD, USA
[2]Johns Hopkins University School of Medicine, Baltimore, MD, USA
[3]Duke University School of Medicine, Durham, NC, USA

The development of atherothrombosis is strongly influenced by the complex interplay between platelet function, inflammation, and hypercoagulability. The progression of a stable plaque to a vulnerable state leading to occlusive thrombus generation in selected patients is a discontinuous and unpredictable process. Transition from an asymptomatic disease state to the sudden occurrence of myocardial infarction may be preceded by inflammation and the development of blood vulnerability characterized by measurements of heightened platelet function and hypercoagulability. The characterization of mechanisms responsible for the transition from an asymptomatic disease state to an unstable disease state and identification of "thrombogenic" phenotype is an important goal in the treatment and prevention of acute thrombotic complications. Therefore, linking vulnerable blood ("thrombogenic" phenotype) to the vulnerable patient who is at risk for thrombotic complications is important in the optimal diagnosis and treatment of patients with coronary artery disease (CAD) [1].

Systemic and local inflammation has been strongly implicated in the initiation, progression, and vulnerability of an atherosclerotic plaque. Various prospective studies have established that C-reactive protein (CRP) is an important systemic inflammation marker predictive of future myocardial infarction and stroke. Elevated CRP has been associated with CAD risk in a generally healthy population with an odds ratio of 1.45, and data from 25 prospective cohort studies in subjects with and without documented heart disease have demonstrated that high-sensitivity CRP (hs-CRP) concentrations are independently associated with the future risk of cardiovascular events [2, 3]. Experimental, clinical, and epidemiological evidences support the hypothesis that CRP is a "marker" as well as an active participant in the development of atherothrombotic complications [4, 5, 6]. *In vitro* studies suggest a direct

Antiplatelet Therapy in Cardiovascular Disease, First Edition. Edited by Ron Waksman, Paul A. Gurbel, and Michael A. Gaglia, Jr.
© 2014 John Wiley & Sons, Ltd. Published 2014 by John Wiley & Sons, Ltd.

influence of CRP on endothelial and platelet function. It has been reported that CRP stimulates procoagulant activity by stimulating tissue factor (TF) release or by reducing fibrinolysis [6]. In autopsy studies, CRP immune reactivity was demonstrated in atherosclerotic but not normal arteries, and also, the presence of high levels of CRP was demonstrated in fibrous tissue and atheroma of atherectomy specimens from patients with unstable angina and myocardial infarction compared to patients with stable angina [7]. CRP is an important regulator of endothelial cell activation and dysfunction. CRP can upregulate the surface expression of proinflammatory adhesion molecules such as intracellular cell adhesion molecule (ICAM)-1, vascular cell adhesion molecule (VCAM)-1, and E-selectin in addition to TF on endothelial cells, vascular smooth muscle cells, and monocytes. Thus, CRP can induce the adhesion of platelets and monocytes to endothelial cells to promote atherothrombotic processes. In addition, CRP is known to induce MCP-1 and TF from monocytes. Finally, the inhibition of nitric oxide, prostaglandin I_2 (PGI_2), and plasminogen activator inhibitor type 1 (PAI-1) release may also contribute to the prothrombotic actions of CRP. These effects of CRP have been attributed to the binding of monomeric CRP that results from the conformational rearrangement of native CRP to FcγRIII (CD16) receptor and complement protein (C1q) [7]. A strong association between CRP and hypercoagulability (high thrombin-induced platelet–fibrin clot strength measured by thrombelastography) at different stages of CAD has been demonstrated supporting the significant role of CRP in plaque instability and subsequent thrombotic complications [1].

In addition to elevated CRP, elevated CD40 ligand (CD40L), selected interleukins (ILs), myeloperoxidase, tumor necrosis factors (TNFs), adhesion molecules (soluble intercellular adhesion molecule [sICAM-1], and soluble VCAM-1 have also been associated with ischemic event occurrences. The CD40L expressed on activated platelets has been shown to activate endothelial cells and promote the release of IL-6, IL-8, and TF. IL-6 is an important procoagulant cytokine, whereas IL-8 is a pivotal molecule influencing leukocyte recruitment. IL-6 has been shown not only to increase platelet reactivity but is also associated with elevated plasma concentrations of fibrinogen and CRP. In patients undergoing stenting, high thrombin-induced platelet–fibrin clot strength (highest quartile) was associated with greater levels of ADP-induced platelet aggregation, CRP, epidermal growth factor (EGF), vascular endothelial growth factor (VEGF), and IL-8 and also associated with significantly greater 2-year ischemic event occurrence than patients with low thrombin-induced platelet–fibrin clot strength. These data suggest that a link is present between inflammation and heightened thrombogenicity measured preprocedurally in the patient at high risk for recurrent ischemic events after stenting [8].

In a study of symptomatic CAD patients undergoing PCI, a correlation was observed between plasma levels of inflammation markers (IL-6, RANTES, and CRP) and ADP- and arachidonic acid-induced aggregation measured by multiplate analyzer. In a retrospective analysis of patients with CAD undergoing PCI, high baseline CRP and high on-treatment platelet reactivity were independent predictors for combined major events and stent thrombosis after multivariate adjustment [9]. Furthermore, a significant association between IL-10, IF-gamma, IL-4, and AA- and ADP-induced platelet aggregation in ACS patients undergoing PCI on dual antiplatelet therapy was demonstrated after adjustment for age, sex, cardiovascular risk factors, ejection fraction, body mass index, von Willebrand factor (vWF), and CRP [10].

More rapid progression of CAD has been associated with elevated levels of matrix metalloproteinase (MMP)-9, whereas other studies have demonstrated that MMP-2 and MMP-9 are involved in various acute complications of cardiovascular disease. Plaque destabilization as well as vascular remodeling by collagen metabolism in the fibrous cap was associated with MMP-2, MMP-3, and MMP-9. Moreover, it was demonstrated that patients undergoing elective PCI for stable angina pectoris exhibit a specific biomarker fingerprint with elevated levels of MMP's that significantly differ from patients with long-term quiescent disease, including those with a history of remote revascularization. In addition to increased MMP levels, increased TIMP-1 and α2-macroglobulin levels were also found in symptomatic patients compared to asymptomatic patients, suggesting the presence of an active counterbalancing mechanism in patients undergoing stenting [11].

Hypercoagulability characterized by elevated levels of fibrinogen, D-dimer, vWF, and tissue plasminogen activator inhibitor has also been linked to CAD progression. A distinct stepwise increment in hypercoagulability as measured by thrombin-induced platelet–fibrin clot strength and the strongest correlation between thrombin-induced platelet–fibrin clot strength and other prothrombotic markers, inflammation markers, and CRP at all levels of CAD acuity has been demonstrated (Figure 6.1). Since tissue plasminogen activator is an important physiological regulator of arterial thrombosis, increases in PAI-1 expression may contribute to cardiovascular ischemic complications by attenuating fibrinolysis. PAI-1 is released from endothelial cells in response to inflammation and activated platelets are also a rich source of PAI-1. In addition to PAI-1, significantly elevated levels of growth factors, EGF and VEGF, were observed in patients with high-MA suggesting a common underlying pathobiology associated with a high risk for the occurrence of ischemic events after PCI. The latter demonstration of significant correlations between inflammation, platelet function, and hypercoagulability markers strengthens the hypothesis that cross talk between these processes plays an important role in the development of progressive and unstable CAD [1]. In a recent study of patients with established CAD undergoing coronary stenting, elevated post-PCI CRP levels were associated with heightened maximal plasma fibrin clot strength as compared with those with low CRP, which is independent of association between fibrinogen and CRP levels [12]. In another study of stable patients ($n = 1223$) on chronic antiplatelet

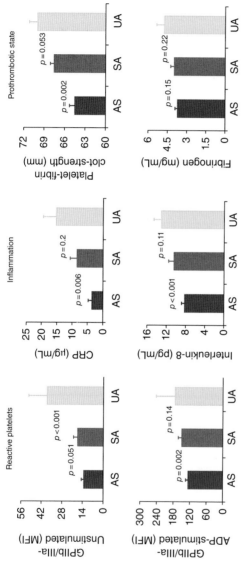
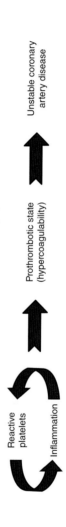

A distinct pathophysiological state of heightened platelet reactivity to ADP, platelet activation, inflammation, and hypercoagulability may mark the transition from stable cardiovascular disease to an unstable and symptomatic condition.

Figure 6.1 Relation between platelet function, coagulation, inflammation, and disease state. Results from the Thrombosis Risk Progression (TRIP) Study. AS, asymptomatic CAD patients; MFI, mean fluorescence intensity; SA, stable angina; UA, unstable angina. (*Platelets*, 2010, **21**, 360–367. © Informa.)

treatment with aspirin and clopidogrel undergoing stenting, elevated levels of CRP, WBC count, and fibrinogen were significantly associated with high platelet reactivity [13].

These observations may lay the foundation for future larger investigations to identify patients at risk based on a specific biomarker profile including high platelet reactivity, hypercoagulability, coagulation factors, and inflammation markers and also suggest that early and potentially serial implementation of a similar biomarker analysis may identify the at-risk patient and facilitate early intervention with a personalized therapeutic strategy.

References

1 Tantry, U.S., Bliden, K.P., Suarez, T.A., Kreutz, R.P., Dichiara, J. & Gurbel, P.A. (2010) Hypercoagulability, platelet function, inflammation and coronary artery disease acuity: results of the Thrombotic RIsk Progression (TRIP) study. *Platelets*, **21**, 360–367.

2 Ridker, P.M. (2007) C-reactive protein and the prediction of cardiovascular events among those at intermediate risk: moving an inflammatory hypothesis toward consensus. *Journal of the American College of Cardiology*, **49**, 2129–2138.

3 Ridker, P.M. (2008) High-sensitivity C-reactive protein as a predictor of all-cause mortality: implications for research and patient care. *Clinical Chemistry*, **54**, 234–237.

4 Kreutz, R.P., Bliden, K.P., Tantry, U.S. & Gurbel, P.A. (2005) Viral respiratory tract infections increase platelet reactivity and activation: an explanation for the higher rates of myocardial infarction and stroke during viral illness. *Journal of Thrombosis and Haemostasis*, **3**, 2108–2109.

5 Kreutz, R.P., Tantry, U.S., Bliden, K.P. & Gurbel, P.A. (2007) Inflammatory changes during the "common cold" are associated with platelet activation and increased reactivity of platelets to agonists. *Blood Coagulation and Fibrinolysis*, **18**, 713–718.

6 Gurbel P.A., DiChiara J., Antonino M. & Tantry U.S. CRP and its role in coronary heart disease: new research developments. In: Satoshi Nagasawa (ed.) *C-Reactive Protein*. Nova Science Publications Inc., Hauppauge, pp. 39–41, 2009.

7 Norja, S., Nuutila, L., Karhunen, P.J. & Goebeler, S. (2007) C-reactive protein in vulnerable coronary plaques. *Journal of Clinical Pathology*, **60**, 545–548.

8 Gurbel, P.A., Bliden, K.P., Kreutz, R.P., Dichiara, J., Antonino, M.J. & Tantry, U.S. (2009) The link between heightened thrombogenicity and inflammation: pre-procedure characterization of the patient at high risk for recurrent events after stenting. *Platelets*, **20**, 97–104.

9 Müller, K., Aichele, S., Herkommer, M. *et al.* (2010) Impact of inflammatory markers on platelet inhibition and cardiovascular outcome including stent thrombosis in patients with symptomatic coronary artery disease. *Atherosclerosis*, **213**, 256–262.

10 Gori, A.M., Cesari, F., Marcucci, R. *et al.* (2009) The balance between pro- and anti-inflammatory cytokines is associated with platelet aggregability in acute coronary syndrome patients. *Atherosclerosis*, **202**, 255–262.

11 Gurbel, P.A., Kreutz, R.P., Bliden, K.P., DiChiara, J. & Tantry, U.S. (2008) Biomarker analysis by fluorokine multianalyte profiling distinguishes patients

requiring intervention from patients with long-term quiescent coronary artery disease: a potential approach to identify atherosclerotic disease progression. *American Heart Journal*, **155**, 56–61.

12 Kreutz, R.P., Owens, J., Breall, J.A. *et al.* (2013) C-reactive protein and fibrin clot strength measured by thrombelastography after coronary stenting. *Blood Coagulation and Fibrinolysis*, **24**, 321–326.

13 Bernlochner, I., Steinhubl, S., Braun, S. *et al.* (2010) Association between inflammatory biomarkers and platelet aggregation in patients under chronic clopidogrel treatment. *Thrombosis and Haemostasis*, **104**, 1193–1200.

Section II

Platelet Function Tests

7 Light Transmission Aggregometry

Paul A. Gurbel[1,2], Martin Gesheff[1], Kevin P. Bliden[1], and Udaya S. Tantry[1]

[1] Sinai Hospital of Baltimore, Baltimore, MD, USA
[2] Johns Hopkins University School of Medicine, Baltimore, MD, USA

Laboratory evaluation of platelet function by a simple and reliable *in vitro* method is crucial to understand the critical role of platelets during hemostasis and thrombotic complications of cardiovascular disease. This process is very challenging, since platelets can be easily activated during blood drawing and samples must be processed in a timely manner to avoid spontaneous platelet activation. An *in vitro* quantitative determination of platelet aggregation by the light transmittance aggregometry (LTA) and the important role of adenosine diphosphate (ADP) during platelet aggregation were first described by Born in 1962 [1]. Despite some important limitations, LTA (turbidimetric assay, optical aggregometry, or conventional aggregometry) with platelet-rich plasma (PRP) is still considered as the "gold standard assay" for platelet function measurement.

In the landmark study by Born, it was reported that PRP was stirred at a rate of 1000 rotations per minute using a small polyethylene-covered iron rod, and the extent of decrease in optical density following platelet aggregation was proportional to the concentration of the ADP added. It was further demonstrated that the addition of adenosine monophosphate at similar concentrations reversed the platelet aggregation induced by ADP [1]. This study laid the foundation for the development of *in vitro* methods of platelet function testing (PFT), which were widely used during the assessment of bleeding disorders. It was further used in experiments to identify important targets to inhibit platelet function and to develop antiplatelet agents directed against these targets. Currently, these antiplatelet agents such as aspirin, $P2Y_{12}$ receptor inhibitors, and glycoprotein (GP)IIb/IIIa inhibitors constitute a major pharmacological therapy in the treatment of high-risk coronary artery disease patients.

Antiplatelet Therapy in Cardiovascular Disease, First Edition. Edited by Ron Waksman, Paul A. Gurbel, and Michael A. Gaglia, Jr.

Technique

Sample collection

Before collecting blood samples for platelet aggregation to assess antiplatelet drug response, it is crucial to document all comedications. An effort should be made to minimize interference from agents that are known to influence platelet function. Moreover, information on exercise, smoking status, and dietary habits (caffeine, chocolate, fruits such as grapes and grape fruit) should also be taken into account. Due to diurnal variation, it is preferred to collect fasting blood samples at a standard time during the morning hours.

Sodium citrate (3.2% or 3.8%) at a ratio of 1 (anticoagulant):9 (blood) by volume is widely used. If the blood sample cannot be processed for more than 1–2 h, buffered anticogulant can be used to maintain the pH at 7.2–7.4. The principle behind using sodium citrate is to bring the extracellular ionized calcium concentration from 0.94–1.33 mM, which is present in normal blood sample, to 40–50 µM. At this concentration, there will be very low level of platelet activation, and the low ionized calcium concentration is sufficient for the binding of fibrinogen to GPIIb/IIIa receptor and subsequent platelet aggregation. It was also suggested that at this low citrate concentration, there is an increased aggregation response to some commonly used weak agonists, such as ADP and epinephrine, and also, the antiplatelet response to GPIIb/IIIa receptor inhibitor may be over exaggerated. Other ideal anticoagulants that do not influence Ca^{2+} concentrations are hirudin and D-phenylalanine–proline–arginine–chloromethyl ketone (PPACK). PPACK is usually recommended to assess platelet response to GPIIb/IIIa receptor inhibitors. However, these anticoagulants are not regularly used due to high cost.

Ideally, the blood sample for platelet aggregation should be collected in a 19-gauge needle through venipuncture using minimum pulling pressure to fill vacuum-evacuated or screw-capped plastic collection tubes to avoid platelet activation. The blood tube should be mixed immediately and gently by inversion.

Anticoagulated blood samples are centrifuged at low-speed centrifugation (~170 g) for 15 min to recover PRP. The centrifugation force should be standardized to ensure that the PRP is devoid of any erythrocytes and leukocytes while recovering maximum number of platelets in PRP. The remaining blood sample is again subjected to a high-speed centrifugation at approximately 700 g for 15 min to recover platelet-poor plasma (PPP, clear plasma). Recent observations indicate that adjusting the platelet count in PRP is not necessary before aggregation and ultimately may induce laboratory artifacts [2, 3]. The PRP should be incubated at 37°C for at least 2 min before adding an agonist. The light transmittance through the PPP cuvette should be set to 100% and through the PRP cuvette with constant stirring should be set to 0%. A specific agonist is then added to induce platelet aggregation.

Arachidonic acid is used to measure platelet response to aspirin, and ADP is used to measure response to ADP ($P2Y_{12}$) receptor antagonists and GPIIb/IIIa inhibitors. Protease-activated receptor-1 (PAR-1) agonist can be used to assess response to PAR-1 antagonists such as atopaxar and vorapaxar and also GPIIb/IIIa inhibitors. Following platelet aggregation, PRP becomes more transparent with an increase in the light transmittance. Change in light transmittance is recorded in real time for about 8 min and is plotted against time to generate a platelet aggregation curve. In the presence of contaminated PPP, more than 100% aggregation will be observed.

At low concentrations of ADP, there will be two waves of aggregation in the presence of citrate anticoagulant and the second wave is due to ADP-induced TxB_2 release and endogenous ADP release from platelets. However, in the presence of other anticoagulants that maintain physiological divalent cation concentrations such as heparin and hirudin, TxB_2 formation is minimal and only primary aggregation is prominent. In the absence of an antiplatelet agent or any substance that is known to influence platelet function, steady state maximal aggregation prevails following primary aggregation due to continuous ADP secretion. In the presence of an antiplatelet agent particularly $P2Y_{12}$ receptor blocker, there will be disaggregation or deaggregation that is more pronounced after 5–6 min (Figure 7.1). Therefore, some studies use aggregation levels recorded at 6 min (final aggregation or residual aggregation) to indicate antiplatelet response instead of maximal aggregation. However, other

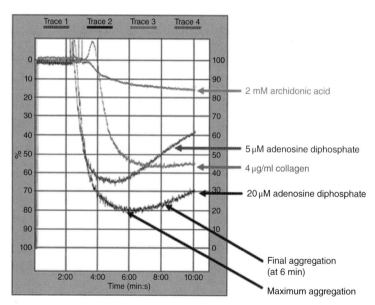

Figure 7.1 A typical aggregation curve in a patient receiving chronic 75 mg/day clopidogrel therapy.

studies have suggested that the antiplatelet response is similarly indicated with maximal aggregation and final aggregation measurements [4, 5]. It has also been suggested that initial rate of ADP-induced platelet aggregation is dependent on the downstream response from $P2Y_1$ receptor, whereas the final extent of aggregation is dependent on $P2Y_{12}$ receptor response [6]. With collagen, there is an initial reduction in light transmittance due to shape change, followed by rapid increases in light transmittance due to platelet aggregation associated with TxB_2 generation and ADP release from platelets. Therefore, platelet aggregation with low level collagen concentration (2–4 µg/mL) is used to evaluate antiplatelet drug response.

In addition to the assessment of antiplatelet drug response, LTA is also used to study bleeding disorders and congenital or acquired disorders of platelet receptors. LTA is time consuming, labor intensive, associated with more chances of introducing laboratory artifacts and poor reproducibility. Since the method is dependent on light transmittance, the effects of lipemia, hemolysis, or contamination with other blood cells that are known to modulate platelet function are major limitations. Artificial platelet activation during blood drawing and sample processing is also a major drawback.

Many of the earlier studies that attempted to link *ex vivo* measurement of platelet reactivity to clinical ischemic event occurrence using LTA were criticized for the potential introduction of artifacts by the laboratory methods and were regarded as "unconvincing" for two reasons: "the tests are crude substitutes for the … interactions … in vivo," and they "failed to satisfy … the minimal criteria to establish a causal relation … between the results of the .. test and …. a thromboembolic event." The latter position, accepted by many, impeded advances in translational studies conducted in the early 1990s that attempted to identify high platelet reactivity as a risk factor for thrombotic event occurrence [7]. However, the development of user-friendly point-of-care methods to assess ADP-induced platelet aggregation overcame some of these concerns, and recent studies have established a strong relation between the results of the PFT using POC and clinical event occurrence [8, 9].

References

1 Born, G.V. (1962) Aggregation of blood platelets by adenosine diphosphate and its reversal. *Nature*, **194**, 927–929.
2 Linnemann, B., Schwonberg, J., Mani, H., Prochnow, S., and Lindhoff-Last, E. (2008) Standardization of light transmittance aggregometry for monitoring antiplatelet therapy: an adjustment for platelet count is not necessary. *Journal of Thrombosis and Haemostasis*, **6**, 677–683.
3 Cattaneo, M., Lecchi, A., Zighetti, M.L., and Lussana, F. (2007) Platelet aggregation studies: autologous platelet-poor plasma inhibits platelet aggregation when added to platelet-rich plasma to normalize platelet count. *Haematologica*, **92**, 694–697.
4 Labarthe, B., Theroux, P., Angioi, M., and Ghitescu, M. (2005) Matching the evaluation of the clinical efficacy of clopidogrel to platelet function tests

relevant to the biological properties of the drug. *Journal of the American College of Cardiology*, **46**, 638–645.

5 Gurbel, P.A., Bliden, K.P., Etherington, A., and Tantry, U.S. (2007) Assessment of clopidogrel responsiveness: measurements of maximum platelet aggregation, final platelet aggregation and their correlation with vasodilator-stimulated phosphoprotein in resistant patients. *Thrombosis Research*, **121**, 107–115.

6 Murugappa, S. and Kunapuli, S.P. (2006) The role of ADP receptors in platelet function. *Frontiers in Bioscience*, **11**, 1977–1986.

7 Hirsh, J. (1987) Hyperactive platelets and complications of coronary artery disease. *The New England Journal of Medicine*, **316**, 1543–1544.

8 Gurbel, P.A., Becker, R.C., Mann, K.G., Steinhubl, S.R., and Michelson, A.D. (2007) Platelet function monitoring in patients with coronary artery disease. *Journal of the American College of Cardiology*, **50**, 1822–1834.

9 Tantry U.S., Bonello L., Aradi D., *et al.* (2013) Consensus and update on the definition of on-treatment platelet reactivity to ADP associated with ischemia and bleeding. *Journal of the American College of Cardiology*, **62(24)**, 2261–2273.

8 Vasodilator-Stimulated Phosphoprotein (VASP) Assay

Marc Laine, Franck Paganelli, and Laurent Bonello

Hôpital Nord, Chemin des Bourrely, Marseille, France

Introduction

Optimal platelet reactivity (PR) inhibition is critical to prevent thrombotic events (cardiovascular deaths, myocardial infarction, stent thrombosis, or stroke) in stented patients, especially in the aftermath of acute coronary syndromes (ACS). Therefore, several antiplatelet agents have been developed in order to preclude such complications.

Aspirin was the first antiplatelet agent used in patients presenting with coronary artery disease. Although effective in low-risk patients, it offered only a very limited protection in high-risk patients (ACS patients), leading to the development of new antiplatelet agents targeting another platelet activation pathway. Ticlopidine and then clopidogrel are thienopyridines targeting the platelets P2Y12 receptor to adenosine diphosphate (ADP). They were shown to reduce (in combination with aspirin) major adverse cardiac events (MACE) in ACS and patients undergoing percutaneous coronary interventions (PCI) [1, 2].

Therefore, dual antiplatelet therapy with aspirin in addition to a P2Y12 inhibitor (e.g., clopidogrel, prasugrel, or ticagrelor) was recommended in stented patients by international guidelines [3, 4, 5].

However, dual antiplatelet therapy failed to eradicate MACE following PCI. In the early days of clopidogrel, stent thrombosis at 1 month occurred in about 2% of stented patients raising concern of clinical resistance to clopidogrel [6].

Järemo *et al.* were the first to demonstrate the interindividual variability in response to clopidogrel, thanks to a flow cytometer assessing the rate of platelets bound to fibrinogen reflecting PR [7]. Nevertheless, this method lacks specificity and does not allow to analyze specifically the response to P2Y12 inhibitors such as clopidogrel. More specific tests are required.

Antiplatelet Therapy in Cardiovascular Disease, First Edition. Edited by Ron Waksman, Paul A. Gurbel, and Michael A. Gaglia, Jr.

© 2014 John Wiley & Sons, Ltd. Published 2014 by John Wiley & Sons, Ltd.

The VASP index assay

Vasodilator-stimulated phosphoprotein (VASP) is an intraplatelet actin-binding protein [8, 9] is involved in the transduction of signal between the P2Y12 ADP receptor antagonists, which participate in the amplification process of platelet aggregation. When activated, the P2Y12 ADP receptor induces a dephosphorylation of the VASP index through the inactivation of a cyclic adenosine monophosphate-dependent protein kinase or guanosine monophosphate-dependent protein kinase [10]. This dephosphorylated VASP induces the activation of glycoprotein GPIIb/IIIa, which is involved in platelet aggregation [11]. Prostaglandin E1 (PGE1)-activated adenylyl cyclase and P2Y12 inhibitors cause VASP phosphorylation [12].

The VASP index assay is a flow cytometer assessment of the ratio of phosphorylated and dephosphorylated VASP. This test is performed on a citrated blood sample. The blood is incubated with either PGE1 or with PGE1 associated with ADP for about 10 min. After being fixed with formaldehyde, platelets are permeabilized by a detergent. Afterward, platelets are marked with a fluorescent monoclonal antibody against phosphorylated VASP [8]. The median fluorescence intensity (MFI) is assessed by a flow cytometer. Thus, the VASP index is expressed in platelet reactivity index (PRI) and is determined with this calculation:

$$VASP-index = \left(\frac{MFI(PGE\,1) - MFI(PGE1 + ADP)}{MFI(PGE\,1)} \right) \times 100$$

The main limitations of this test are the need for a trained operator, the use of a flow cytometer (which can be an economic limitation), and the need for a compatible rate of red cells.

A VASP index ELISA assay has been recently validated and may overcome these limitations [13, 14].

VASP index and clinical events

Barragan *et al.* were the first to demonstrate the relation between thrombotic events (stent thrombosis) and high on-treatment platelet reactivity (HTPR) [15]. They compared the VASP index of 16 prospectively included patients with 30 stented patients free from stent thrombosis. Stent thrombosis patients had a higher VASP index than control ($63.28 \pm 9.56\%$ vs. $39.80 \pm 10.9\%$, $p < 0.0001$). Several studies followed and clearly confirmed the relation between MACE in stented patients and HTPR after the clopidogrel loading dose [16, 17, 18, 19, 20, 21].

Further, using a ROC curve analysis on the data from several studies, a consensus determined the cutoff value of VASP PRI greater than 50% to define patients presenting with high on-clopidogrel PR. A VASP index above this threshold is a risk marker of thrombotic events (i.e., stent thrombosis, myocardial infarction, or cardiovascular deaths) in stented patients. This threshold yields to this test an excellent negative predictive value although the positive predictive value is low [19, 22].

Using different tests to assess PR, recent studies suggested a link between low on-treatment PR (« hyperresponders ») and bleeding events in patients treated with dual antiplatelet therapy. These observations lead to the concept of therapeutic window for PR inhibition in patients receiving a P2Y12 ADP receptor antagonist and treated with PCI or CABG [23, 24, 25].

Alteration of antiplatelet therapy based on the VASP index

Due to the lack of appropriate large-scale randomized clinical trials, antiplatelet therapy adjustment based on PR is – to this date – not recommended by international guidelines in routine practice.

Nonetheless, several small-size studies had interesting results. Repeated loading doses of 600 mg of clopidogrel (up to four) in stented patients with a VASP index greater than 50% PRI (after a first loading dose of clopidogrel) can overcome HTPR and further significantly reduce the rate of thrombotic events without excess of hemorrhage [20, 21, 26]. This strategy remains effective in patients carrying a loss-of-function allele CYP 2C19*2, which is known to be responsible for an attenuated bioactivation of clopidogrel [27]. A recent meta-analysis by Aradi *et al.* suggested that intensified therapy based on PR assessment could improve the clinical outcome of patients receiving clopidogrel. This remains controversial since large randomized trials failed to confirm this hypothesis. However, these trials had major limitations including the inclusion of low-risk patients and ineffective therapeutic strategy to overcome HTPR.

VASP index and new oral antiplatelet agents

Most trials comparing new antiplatelet agents to clopidogrel have used the VASP index as a biological end point.

The pharmacodynamics substudy of the TRITON-TIMI 38 trial revealed that 24% of ACS patients treated with prasugrel (a third-generation thienopyridine) have HTPR (i.e., VASP index > 50%) at 1 month (vs. 43% with clopidogrel, $p = 0.033$) [28]. Interestingly, the cutoff value of 50% defining HTPR seems to remain valid for prasugrel (as determined by a ROC curve analysis). Above this threshold, patients have higher risk of thrombotic events [29]. Besides, as previously described for clopidogrel, a low VASP index in patients treated with prasugrel was associated in this study with an increased bleeding risk [30, 31].

VASP index was also used to determine the proportion of patients included in the PLATO trial that presented high on ticagrelor PR (0–8%) [32].

Conclusions

The VASP index is an excellent test, which has many assets and very few limitations. It is the most specific test assessing PR of patients under P2Y12 inhibitors (either clopidogrel, prasugrel, or ticagrelor). Unlike point-of-care assays, it is not affected by anti-glycoprotein IIb/IIIa or anticoagulants. Thanks to an abundant literature, this test is now clearly acknowledged as a risk marker of thrombotic events in stented patients. Its threshold (PRI > 50%) is associated with an excellent negative predictive value and is also validated with different antiplatelet agents.

The cutoff value defining low on-treatment PR remains to be determined, and the benefit of adjusted antiplatelet therapy according to the VASP index has to be demonstrated in specifically designed trials.

References

1 Mehta, S., Yusuf, S., Peters, R. *et al.* (2001) Effects of pretreatment with clopidogrel and aspirin followed by long-term therapy in patients undergoing percutaneous coronary intervention: the PCI-CURE study. *The Lancet*, **358 (9281)**, 527–533.

2 Yusuf, S., Zhao, F., Mehta, S.R. *et al.* (2001) Effects of clopidogrel in addition to aspirin in patients with acute coronary syndromes without ST-segment elevation. *New England Journal of Medicine*, **345 (7)**, 494–502.

3 Authors/Task Force Members, Steg, S.K., James, S.K. *et al.* (2012) ESC Guidelines for the management of acute myocardial infarction in patients presenting with ST-segment elevation: The Task Force on the management of ST-segment elevation acute myocardial infarction of the European Society of Cardiology (ESC). *European Heart Journal*, **33 (20)**, 2569–2619.

4 Hamm, C.W., Bassand, J.-P., Agewall, S. *et al.* (2011) ESC Guidelines for the management of acute coronary syndromes in patients presenting without persistent ST-segment elevation: The Task Force for the management of acute coronary syndromes (ACS) in patients presenting without persistent ST-segment elevation of the European Society of Cardiology (ESC). *European Heart Journal*, **23**, 2999–3054.

5 Wijns, W., Kolh, P., Danchin, N. *et al.* (2010) Guidelines on myocardial revascularization. *European Heart Journal*, **31 (20)**, 2501–2555.

6 Taniuchi, M., Kurz, H.I., and Lasala, J.M. (2001) Randomized comparison of ticlopidine and clopidogrel after intracoronary stent implantation in a broad patient population. *Circulation*, **104** (5), 539–543.

7 Järemo, P., Lindahl, T.L., Fransson, S.G., and Richter, A. (2002) Individual variations of platelet inhibition after loading doses of clopidogrel. *Journal of Internal Medicine*, **252** (3), 233–238.

8 Aleil, B., Ravanat, C., Cazenave, J.P., Rochoux, G., Heitz, A., and Gachet, C. (2005) Flow cytometric analysis of intraplatelet VASP phosphorylation for the detection of clopidogrel resistance in patients with ischemic cardiovascular diseases. *Journal of Thrombosis and Haemostasis*, **3** (1), 85–92.

9 Wentworth, J.K.T., Pula, G., and Poole, A.W. (2006) Vasodilator-stimulated phosphoprotein (VASP) is phosphorylated on Ser157 by protein kinase C-dependent and -independent mechanisms in thrombin-stimulated human platelets. *Biochemical Journal*, **393** (Pt. 2), 555–564.

10 Waldmann, R., Nieberding, M., and Walter, U. (1987) Vasodilator-stimulated protein phosphorylation in platelets is mediated by cAMP- and cGMP-dependent protein kinases. *European Journal of Biochemistry*, **167** (3), 441–448.

11 Horstrup, K., Jablonka, B., Hönig-Liedl, P., Just, M., Kochsiek, K., and Walter, U. (1994) Phosphorylation of focal adhesion vasodilator-stimulated phosphoprotein at Ser157 in intact human platelets correlates with fibrinogen receptor inhibition. *European Journal of Biochemistry*, **225** (1), 21–27.

12 Geiger, J., Brich, J., Hönig-Liedl, P. *et al.* (1999) Specific impairment of human platelet P2Y(AC) ADP receptor-mediated signaling by the antiplatelet drug clopidogrel. *Arteriosclerosis, Thrombosis, and Vascular Biology*, **19** (8), 2007–2011.

13 Barragan, P., Paganelli, F., Camoin-Jau, L. *et al.* (2010) Validation of a novel ELISA-based VASP whole blood assay to measure P2Y12-ADP receptor activity. *Journal of Thrombosis and Haemostasis*, **104** (2), 410–411.

14 Jakubowski, J.A., Payne, C.D., Li, Y.G. *et al.* (2008) The use of the VerifyNow P2Y12 point-of-care device to monitor platelet function across a range of P2Y12 inhibition levels following prasugrel and clopidogrel administration. *Journal of Thrombosis and Haemostasis*, **99** (2), 409–415.

15 Barragan, P., Bouvier, J.-L., Roquebert, P.-O. *et al.* (2003) Resistance to thienopyridines: clinical detection of coronary stent thrombosis by monitoring of vasodilator-stimulated phosphoprotein phosphorylation. *Catheterization and Cardiovascular Interventions*, **59** (3), 295–302.

16 Aradi, D., Komócsi, A., Vorobcsuk, A. *et al.* (2010) Prognostic significance of high on-clopidogrel platelet reactivity after percutaneous coronary intervention: systematic review and meta-analysis. *American Heart Journal*, **160** (3), 543–551.

17 Blindt, R., Stellbrink, K., de Taeye, A. *et al.* (2007) The significance of vasodilator-stimulated phosphoprotein for risk stratification of stent thrombosis. *Journal of Thrombosis and Haemostasis*, **98** (6), 1329–1334.

18 Frere, C., Cuisset, T., Quilici, J. *et al.* (2007) ADP-induced platelet aggregation and platelet reactivity index VASP are good predictive markers for clinical outcomes in non-ST elevation acute coronary syndrome. *Journal of Thrombosis and Haemostasis*, **98** (4), 838–843.

19 Bonello, L., Paganelli, F., Arpin-Bornet, M. *et al.* (2007) Vasodilator-stimulated phosphoprotein phosphorylation analysis prior to percutaneous

coronary intervention for exclusion of postprocedural major adverse cardiovascular events. *Journal of Thrombosis and Haemostasis*, **5 (8)**, 1630–1636.

20 Bonello, L., Camoin-Jau, L., Arques, S. *et al.* (2008) Adjusted clopidogrel loading doses according to vasodilator-stimulated phosphoprotein phosphorylation index decrease rate of major adverse cardiovascular events in patients with clopidogrel resistance: a multicenter randomized prospective study. *Journal of the American College of Cardiology*, **51 (14)**, 1404–1411.

21 Bonello, L., Camoin-Jau, L., Armero, S. *et al.* (2009) Tailored clopidogrel loading dose according to platelet reactivity monitoring to prevent acute and subacute stent thrombosis. *American Journal of Cardiology*, **103 (1)**, 5–10.

22 Bonello, L., Tantry, U.S., Marcucci, R. *et al.* (2010) Consensus and future directions on the definition of high on-treatment platelet reactivity to adenosine diphosphate. *Journal of the American College of Cardiology*, **56 (12)**, 919–933.

23 Mangiacapra, F., Patti, G., Barbato, E. *et al.* (2012) A therapeutic window for platelet reactivity for patients undergoing elective percutaneous coronary intervention: results of the ARMYDA-PROVE (Antiplatelet therapy for Reduction of MYocardial Damage during Angioplasty-Platelet Reactivity for Outcome Validation Effort) study. *JACC: Cardiovascular Interventions*, **5 (3)**, 281–289.

24 Sibbing, D., Schulz, S., Braun, S. *et al.* (2010) Antiplatelet effects of clopidogrel and bleeding in patients undergoing coronary stent placement. *Journal of Thrombosis and Haemostasis*, **8 (2)**, 250–256.

25 Sibbing, D., Steinhubl, S.R., Schulz, S., Schömig, A. and Kastrati, A. (2010) Platelet aggregation and its association with stent thrombosis and bleeding in clopidogrel-treated patients. *Journal of the American College of Cardiology*, **56 (4)**, 317–318.

26 Bonello-Palot, N., Armero, S., Paganelli, F. *et al.* (2009) Relation of body mass index to high on-treatment platelet reactivity and of failed clopidogrel dose adjustment according to platelet reactivity monitoring in patients undergoing percutaneous coronary intervention. *American Journal of Cardiology*, **104 (11)**, 1511–1515.

27 Bonello, L., Armero, S., Ait Mokhtar, O. *et al.* (2010) Clopidogrel loading dose adjustment according to platelet reactivity monitoring in patients carrying the 2C19*2 loss of function polymorphism. *Journal of the American College of Cardiology*, **56 (20)**, 1630–1636.

28 Michelson, A.D., Frelinger, A.L., 3rd, Braunwald, E. *et al.* (2009) Pharmacodynamic assessment of platelet inhibition by prasugrel vs. clopidogrel in the TRITON-TIMI 38 trial. *European Heart Journal*, **30 (14)**, 1753–1763.

29 Bonello, L., Pansieri, M., Mancini, J. *et al.* (2011) High on-treatment platelet reactivity after prasugrel loading dose and cardiovascular events after percutaneous coronary intervention in acute coronary syndromes. *Journal of the American College of Cardiology*, **58 (5)**, 467–473.

30 Bonello, L., Mancini, J., Pansieri, M. *et al.* (2012) Relationship between post-treatment platelet reactivity and ischemic and bleeding events at 1-year follow-up in patients receiving prasugrel. *Journal of Thrombosis and Haemostasis*, **10 (10)**, 1999–2005.

31 Cuisset, T., Gaborit, B., Dubois, N. *et al.* (2013) Platelet reactivity in diabetic patients undergoing coronary stenting for acute coronary syndrome treated with clopidogrel loading dose followed by prasugrel maintenance therapy. *International Journal of Cardiology*, **168 (1)**, 523–528.

32 Bliden, K.P., Tantry, U.S., Storey, R.F. *et al.* (2011) The effect of ticagrelor versus clopidogrel on high on-treatment platelet reactivity: Combined analysis of the ONSET/OFFSET and RESPOND studies. *American Heart Journal*, **162 (1)**, 160–165.

9 VerifyNow P2Y12 and Plateletworks Assays

Matthew J. Price[1,2], Nicoline J. Breet[3], and Jurriën M. ten Berg[3]
[1] Scripps Clinic, La Jolla, CA, USA
[2] Scripps Translational Science Institute, La Jolla, CA, USA
[3] St Antonius Hospital, Nieuwegein, The Netherlands

Introduction

Several methods are available to assess the pharmacodynamic effect of antiplatelet agents, yet the incorporation of these assays into clinical use has been challenging due to several practical considerations, such as sample preparation, technical skill, and infrastructure requirements. Platelet function tests that require little formal training and can be integrated into patient care at the point-of-service or point-of-care may therefore be advantageous. Two such tests are VerifyNow P2Y12 (Accumetrics, San Diego, CA, USA) and Plateletworks (Helena Laboratories, Beaumont, TX, USA). Unique to the other platelet function tests, VerifyNow P2Y12 has been incorporated into several observational and randomized clinical trials involving in total many thousands of patients, thereby providing robust data regarding the relationship between VerifyNow P2Y12 results and clinical outcomes. Herein, we review the methodology of these two platelet function tests, the data supporting their validity in measuring the antiplatelet effect of pharmacological agents, their strengths and weaknesses, and pertinent clinical outcome data.

VerifyNow P2Y12

Methodology

The VerifyNow System is a point-of-care turbidimetric-based optical detection system that measures platelet-induced aggregation [1]. The system consists of an analyzer instrument and a disposable assay device. The instrument controls all assay sequencing, temperature, and reagent–sample mixing and performs self-diagnostics. The assay device contains a lyophilized preparation of human fibrinogen-coated beads, platelet activators, buffer, and preservative (Figure 9.1). The patient sample is

---

Antiplatelet Therapy in Cardiovascular Disease, First Edition. Edited by Ron Waksman, Paul A. Gurbel, and Michael A. Gaglia, Jr.
© 2014 John Wiley & Sons, Ltd. Published 2014 by John Wiley & Sons, Ltd.

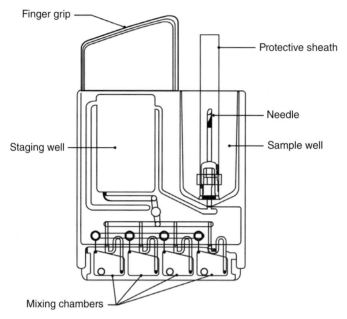

Figure 9.1 VerifyNow test device. The patient sample is whole blood, which is automatically dispensed from the citrated blood collection tube. The assay device contains a lyophilized preparation of human fibrinogen-coated beads and platelet activators in its mixing chambers, which in the case of the P2Y12 test, are ADP and PGE1. The rate and extent of agglutination of the fibrinogen-coated beads is measured through changes in light transmission, and a value is reported in P2Y12 reaction units (PRU).

whole blood, which is automatically dispensed from the citrated blood collection tube into the assay device by the instrument.

The intended use of the VerifyNow P2Y12 test is the measurement of the level of platelet P2Y$_{12}$ receptor blockade in the laboratory or point-of-care setting. The test cartridge contains 20 μmol adenosine diphosphate (ADP) and 22 nmol prostaglandin E1 (PGE1). PGE1 suppresses the ADP-induced P2Y$_1$-mediated increase in intracellular cyclic adenosine monophosphate (cAMP) and calcium levels, thereby reducing the activation contribution from P2Y$_1$ receptors and increasing the assay sensitivity to P2Y$_{12}$ receptor-mediated platelet activity. When platelets activated by ADP are exposed to the fibrinogen-coated microparticles, agglutination occurs in proportion to the number of available platelet receptors. The analyzer system measures the agglutination as an increase in light transmittance; the test result is a function of the rate and extent of agglutination and is expressed in P2Y12 reaction units (PRU). A higher PRU reflects greater ADP-induced platelet reactivity.

The earlier versions of the VerifyNow P2Y12 test reported a second result based on the rate and extent of agglutination in a separate "BASE" channel containing the agonist iso-thrombin receptor-activating peptide (iso-TRAP), also known as protease-activated receptor-1 (PAR-1)-activating peptide. The goal of this agonist is to maximally activate platelets despite blockade of the $P2Y_{12}$ receptor by $P2Y_{12}$ antagonists or the antiplatelet effect of aspirin. The device provides an estimated inhibition ("%") without a preclopidogrel sample by calculating the result of the formula $[1 - ([ADP\text{-}PGE_1 \text{ channel}]/BASE)] \times 100$. While the overall correlation was excellent between this result and the relative change in the ADP-PGE1 channel before and after exposure to a $P2Y_{12}$ antagonist (i.e., $[1 - (PRU_{pretreatment}/PRU_{posttreatment})] \times 100$) with a correlation coefficient of 0.98 [2], the accuracy was less at lower levels of treatment effect. Discordance has been reported between the results of the PAR-1 peptide channel and the results of the ADP-PGE1 channel in patients not exposed to clopidogrel [3]. In addition, studies of PAR-1-mediated platelet signaling have demonstrated that PAR-1-mediated platelet aggregation is partly dependent on $P2Y_{12}$ function and therefore is not completely insensitive to the effect of $P2Y_{12}$ receptor antagonists [4]. A revised formulation of the BASE channel uses both PAR-1- and protease-activated receptor (PAR-4)-activating peptides, and this has been shown to more accurately provide a "% inhibition" in patients treated with more effective $P2Y_{12}$ antagonists [4] and is used in devices outside of the USA.

Accurate readings with the VerifyNow System depend upon the collection of the appropriate volume of sample through a 21-gauge needle or greater. Moreover, the time between sample collection and assay performance should be at least 10 min but not more than 4 h. Since the mechanism is based upon the agglutination of fibrinogen-coated beads by activated platelets, the test is not interpretable in the presence of glycoprotein IIb/IIIa inhibitors. Patients with a platelet count less than 100,000 or hematocrit less than 30% were not included in the studies that led to Food and Drug Administration (FDA) 510(K) clearance. The mean coefficient of variation of test precision has been reported to be less than 8% in volunteers [5] and 3.2% in patients with coronary artery disease [6].

Data supporting validity of measurement

In an initial study of 147 aspirin-treated subjects with multiple vascular risk factors, the distribution of PRU values for the VerifyNow P2Y12 test displayed a separation from baseline to postclopidogrel values with some overlap due to high interindividual variations in response [7]. Figure 9.2 illustrates the ranges of PRU values that have been observed in several large, observational studies of clopidogrel-treated patients undergoing PCI. The results of the VerifyNow P2Y12 test are well correlated with ADP-induced platelet aggregation by light transmittance aggregometry (LTA) and vasophosphoprotein phosphorylation (VASP) analysis in clopidogrel- and prasugrel-treated patients [2, 5, 6, 8, 9] (Figure 9.3 and Figure 9.4). Similarly, VerifyNow P2Y12 results are consistent with those of LTA and VASP analysis in subjects treated with ticagrelor [10]. PRU levels have also been strongly correlated with clopidogrel and prasugrel active metabolite levels [8] (Figure 9.5). The dynamic range is narrower than that of LTA or VASP, and therefore, the assay may not be able to discriminate between very strong or between very weak levels of $P2Y_{12}$

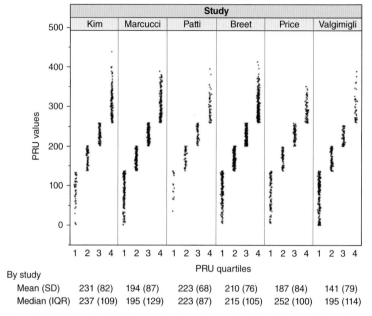

Figure 9.2 Distribution of VerifyNow P2Y12 PRU in several studies of clopidogrel-treated patients undergoing PCI. In the total pooled cohort of 3058 patients, the mean reactivity was 197±85 PRU, and the median reactivity was 200 PRU (interquartile range, 200 PRU). (Source: Adapted from Brar SS et al., 2011 [18]. Reproduced with permission of Elsevier.)

receptor inhibition [2]. Moreover, at very high levels of P2Y12 antagonism, platelet function measured by VerifyNow P2Y12 is maximally inhibited and does not reflect further changes that can be observed with VASP or LTA methods [8]. The clinical significance of this is likely minimal since the proposed thresholds for both ischemic and bleeding risk are not within the extremes of $P2Y_{12}$ effect [11, 12, 13, 14, 15, 16].

Clinical outcome data

The relationship between on-treatment reactivity according to VerifyNow P2Y12 and clinical outcomes has been explored in a large number of observational studies and in pharmacodynamics analyses of several randomized, clinical trials [11, 15, 16, 17, 18, 19, 20, 21, 22, 23]. The bulk of the data supports the supposition that among patients undergoing PCI treated with clopidogrel or prasugrel, higher values of PRU are associated with ischemic events. Although the use of receiver operating characteristic (ROC) curves can be problematic in determining the strength of a prognostic test [24], ROC curve analysis of several observational studies has shown that the VerifyNow P2Y12 can discriminate between clopidogrel patients who will and will not have a subsequent cardiovascular events after PCI, and observational studies using ROC curve analysis have consistently identified "optimal" cut points for predicting ischemic risk between

(A)

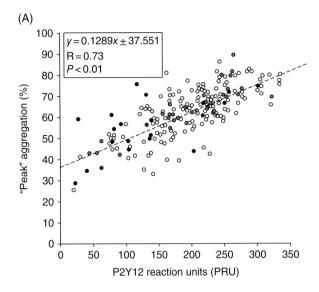

(B)

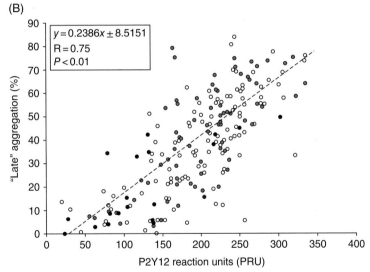

Figure 9.3 Correlation between the results of the VerifyNow P2Y12 test and light transmission aggregometry (LTA) among patients undergoing elective PCI. (A) Peak aggregation and (B) late aggregation using 20 μmol ADP. The high y intercept with peak aggregation is likely due to the addition of prostaglandin E1 (PGE1) in the VerifyNow P2Y12 test, which suppresses the additional contribution of ADP-induced activation of the P2Y1 pathway, resulting in a relatively higher magnitude of platelet reactivity with LTA. White dots, patients receiving clopidogrel 75 mg daily; gray dots, patients receiving clopidogrel 300 mg loading dose; black dots, patients receiving 600 mg loading dose. (Source: Adapted from van Werkum, JW et al., 2006 [9]. Reproduced with permission of John Wiley & Sons Ltd.)

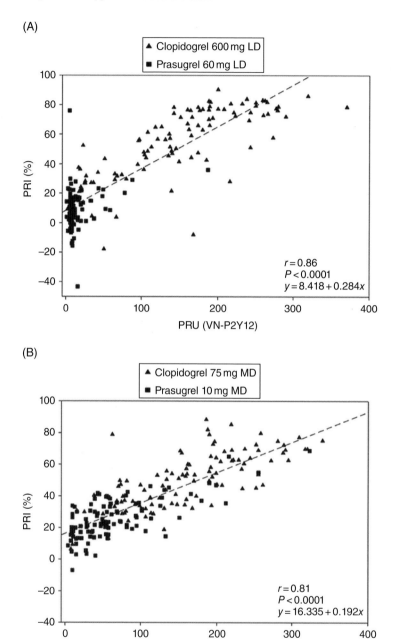

Figure 9.4 Correlation between the results of VerifyNow P2Y12 and vasophosphoprotein phosphorylation analysis (VASP) in aspirin-treated patients with coronary artery disease randomly assigned to clopidogrel or prasugrel, after (A) loading dose and (B) maintenance dosing (MD). LD, loading dose; MD, maintenance dose; PRI, platelet reactivity index; PRU, P2Y12 reaction units. (Source: Adapted from Varenhorst C et al., 2009 [8]. Reproduced with permission of Elsevier.)

(A)

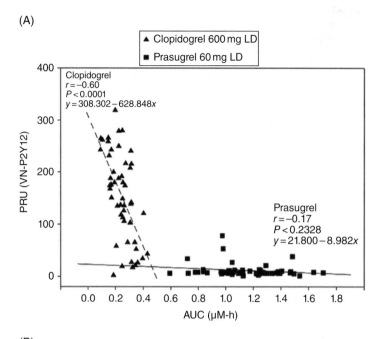

(B)

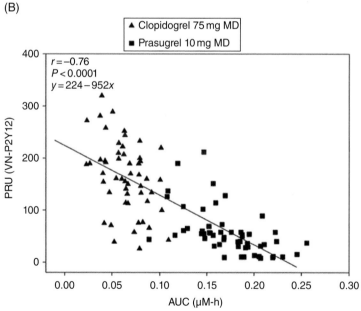

Figure 9.5 Correlation between VerifyNow P2Y12 test results and concentrations of clopidogrel or prasugrel active metabolites after (A) loading dose and (B) maintenance dosing. AUC, area under the curve; LD, loading dose; MD, maintenance dose; PRU, P2Y12 reaction units; VN, VerifyNow. (Source: Adapted from Varenhorst C et al., 2009 [8]. Reproduced with permission of Elsevier.)

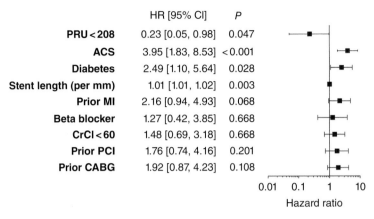

	HR [95% CI]	P
PRU < 208	0.23 [0.05, 0.98]	0.047
ACS	3.95 [1.83, 8.53]	< 0.001
Diabetes	2.49 [1.10, 5.64]	0.028
Stent length (per mm)	1.01 [1.01, 1.02]	0.003
Prior MI	2.16 [0.94, 4.93]	0.068
Beta blocker	1.27 [0.42, 3.85]	0.668
CrCl < 60	1.48 [0.69, 3.18]	0.668
Prior PCI	1.76 [0.74, 4.16]	0.201
Prior CABG	1.92 [0.87, 4.23]	0.108

Figure 9.6 Relationship between PRU and outcomes in a time-dependent analysis of the GRAVITAS trial. After adjustment for other predictors of cardiovascular events, patients who achieved a PRU less than 208 had a significantly lower risk of cardiovascular events at 60-day follow-up. ACS, acute coronary syndrome; CABG, coronary artery bypass grafting; CrCl, creatinine clearance; MI, myocardial infarction; PCI, percutaneous coronary intervention; PRU, P2Y12 reaction units.

approximately 200 and 240 PRU [11, 15, 17, 18, 21]. A *post hoc*, time-dependent analysis of the Gauging Responsiveness with A VerifyNow Assay – Impact on Thrombosis And Safety (GRAVITAS) trial found that achievement of a PRU less than 208 was significantly associated with a lower risk of cardiovascular death, myocardial infarction (MI), or stent thrombosis, even after adjustment for other predictors [25] (Figure 9.6). On-treatment reactivity above this threshold was also significantly and independently associated with stent thrombosis at 30-day and 1-year follow-up in an observational study of more than 8,000 patients treated with PCI [26]. On-treatment reactivity according to VerifyNow P2Y12 significantly improved net reclassification for major adverse cardiovascular events in a pooled patient-level meta-analysis, supporting the prognostic utility of this test in the setting of PCI [18]. The relationship between PRU and outcomes appears to depend on clinical presentation: in the platelet sub-substudy of the TRILOGY ACS trial, which randomly assigned patients recovering from ACS who did not undergo revascularization to either prasugrel or clopidogrel, there did not appear to be an association between PRU and outcomes after adjustment for a large number of other predictors [27, 28].

The results of the VerifyNow P2Y12 test have also been associated with the risk of bleeding [13, 16], although the current dataset is not quite as robust as that for ischemic events. In the recently presented ADAPT-DES registry, PRU was independently and significantly associated with bleeding events at 1-year follow-up after PCI.

Randomized clinical trials

Four randomized clinical trials have examined whether using the VerifyNow P2Y12 test can improve patient outcomes. In the double-blinded, multicenter, randomized Tailoring Treatment with Tirofiban in

Patients Showing Resistance to Aspirin and/or Resistance to Clopidogrel (3T/2R) trial, patients undergoing elective PCI who were poor responders to aspirin or clopidogrel according to the VerifyNow test were randomly assigned to receive either tirofiban or placebo on top of standard aspirin and clopidogrel therapy [29]. Patients receiving tirofiban had significantly lower rates of periprocedural MI. At late follow-up, poor response to clopidogrel was an independent predictor of worse 1-year outcome [15]. The GRAVITAS trial was a multicenter, double-blinded, active-control trial that randomly assigned 2214 patients with on-treatment reactivity ≥235 PRU after PCI to either high-dose clopidogrel (additional 600 mg loading dose followed by 150 mg daily maintenance dose [MD]) or standard-dose clopidogrel (75 mg MD) [30]. Most of the enrolled patients had stable angina or ischemia. At 6 months, the rate of death from cardiovascular causes, MI, or stent thrombosis did not differ between groups (2.3% vs. 2.3%; hazard ratio [HR], 1.01; 95% confidence interval [CI], 0.58–1.76; $p = 0.97$) The high-dose regimen provided a 22% absolute reduction in the rate of high on-treatment reactivity [30], suggesting that an insufficient antiplatelet effect of the study intervention may in part have contributed to the lack of clinical efficacy observed in the overall trial. The Testing Platelet Reactivity In Patients Undergoing Elective Stent Placement on Clopidogrel to Guide Alternative Therapy with Prasugrel (TRIGGER-PCI) trial randomly assigned clopidogrel-treated patients with stable CAD and PRU greater than 208 according to open-label platelet function testing after nonurgent PCI to either prasugrel 10 mg MD or clopidogrel 75 mg MD. The planned enrollment was 2150 patients, but the study was terminated prematurely after a nonprespecified interim analysis found a lower-than-expected event rate after 274 patients completed 6-month follow-up [31], supporting the observation from GRAVITAS that the absolute rates of cardiovascular events appear low in patients undergoing elective PCI for relatively simple coronary anatomy irrespective of platelet reactivity according to the VerifyNow P2Y12 test. The Assessment by a Double Randomization of a Conventional Antiplatelet Strategy versus a Monitoring-guided Strategy for Drug-Eluting Stent Implantation and of Treatment Interruption versus Continuation 1 Year after Stenting (ARCTIC) was a randomized, multicenter, open-label trial that examined whether the incorporation of platelet function testing (PFT) into antiplatelet therapy decision-making would be superior to conventional management without PFT in reducing ischemic events in patients undergoing PCI [32]. Approximately three quarters of the enrolled patients had stable angina or ischemia. Patients in the PFT arm were assessed for both clopidogrel and aspirin responsiveness prior to PCI and again 2–4 weeks postprocedure. The choice of antiplatelet therapy in either the PFT or conventional management arm was according to operator discretion, although general recommendations were provided for adjustment in the PFT group. Most patients with high reactivity were treated after PCI with clopidogrel 150 mg MD. At 1-year follow-up, the rate of the primary end point, a composite of death, MI, stroke or transient ischemic attack, urgent coronary revascularization, and stent thrombosis, did not differ between treatment groups (34.6% vs. 31.1%; HR, 1.13; 95% CI, 0.98–1.29) and was driven by troponin-defined periprocedural MI. The rates of stent thrombosis were low and similar between groups (0.7% vs. 1.0%; HR, 1.34; 95% CI, 0.56–3.18).

While the randomized clinical trials that have incorporated the VerifyNow P2Y12 test do not support the routine use of testing in elective PCI patients, the clinical efficacy and economic value of the VerifyNow P2Y12 test to guide therapy in patients with ACS undergoing PCI remains undefined, as this population was underrepresented in GRAVITAS and ARCTIC and not addressed in TRIGGER-PCI.

Plateletworks

Methodology

The Plateletworks® assay (Helena Laboratories, Beaumont, Texas) uses standard cell-counting hematology principles to determine the level of aggregation in response to a platelet agonist. It is based on single platelet disappearance expressed as the platelet count ratio before and after exposure to such an agonist, thereby allowing the calculation of the percentage of platelet inhibition [33, 34]. Whole blood samples are collected in tubes containing K_3-ethylenediaminetetraacetic acid (EDTA) and tubes containing D-Phe–Pro–Arg–chloromethylketone (PPACK) with either ADP, arachidonic acid (AA), or collagen. The tube containing ADP (20 μmol) is used to assess the effect of platelet $P2Y_{12}$ receptor antagonists. A routine platelet count using a cell counter is performed on each sample; the platelet count of the K_3-EDTA tube is used as a reference. In the presence of agonist, uninhibited platelets will activate and aggregate. As aggregated platelets exceed the threshold limits for platelet size (<30 fL), they are no longer counted as individual platelets. The percentage of inhibition of platelet aggregation is the ratio between the platelet count in the agonist sample and the platelet count in the reference sample, that is, [count (agonist)/count (EDTA)] × 100 (%), while (1 – count [agonist]/count [EDTA]) × 100 describes the percentage aggregation (Figure 9.7). For example, a greater antiplatelet effect will result in less agonist-induced platelet clumping and a smaller difference in platelet counts between the reference and agonist samples, resulting in less calculated platelet aggregation and greater platelet inhibition.

Strengths and weaknesses

The Plateletworks assay requires minimal sample preparation and uses a small volume of whole blood (1 mL), and the results are available within minutes. However, rapid performance of this assay within 10 min of drawing the blood sample is required since platelet aggregates formed upon ADP stimulation disaggregate after this time point, resulting in an unreliable test result in which the extent of platelet inhibition will be overestimated [34] (Figure 9.8). A possible solution to this issue may be to place a cell counter in the catheterization laboratory for rapid

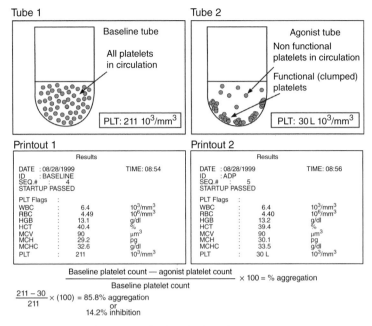

Figure 9.7 Methodological principle of the Plateletworks assay.

measurements between 5 and 10 min after blood collection. It has also been shown that the degree of platelet inhibition measured by the Plateletworks® assay is less compared with LTA. This has led to the hypothesis that LTA provides information regarding platelet macroaggregate formation only, while the platelet count ratio measures the platelet macro- and microaggregate formation [35]. However, the relevance of microaggregation as a predictor for clinical outcome has not been established.

Validity of the test in measuring antiplatelet effect and its association with clinical outcomes

Aspirin

In 50 consecutive patients undergoing elective cardiac surgery, Lennon and colleagues demonstrated that the Plateletworks® assay was not diagnostic for the detection of the effect of aspirin on platelet function when collagen is used as the agonist [36]. On ROC analysis, the area under the curve (AUC) for the identification of recent aspirin ingestion using Plateletworks® was 0.58 (95% CI, 0.42–0.75) compared with 0.77 (95% CI, 0.61–0.95) for turbidimetric platelet aggregometry; there was no significant association between platelet reactivity and perioperative blood loss. Thus, these findings suggest that the Plateletworks assay appears to be of limited use in the evaluation of aspirin response.

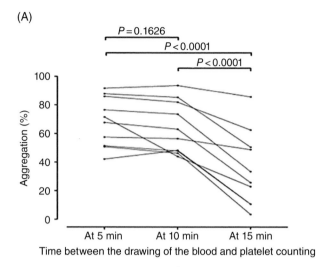

Figure 9.8 Magnitude of calculated platelet (micro)aggregation according to the Plateletworks assay at different time points after the drawing of blood in the ADP tube. (A) Patients receiving dual antiplatelet therapy with aspirin and clopidogrel and (B) healthy volunteers not on antiplatelet therapy. Delay in running the test after sample collection resulted in the underestimation of platelet aggregation and overestimation of the degree of platelet inhibition, likely due to disaggregation of the formed aggregates. (Source: Adapted from Van Werkum JJ et al., 2010 [34]. Reproduced with permission of Elsevier.)

Clopidogrel

Several studies have demonstrated that the Plateletworks® correlates with LTA [37, 38] and can be used to monitor the antiplatelet effect of clopidogrel therapy [37, 39, 40]. However, in a small prospective study of 50 clopidogrel-treated patients undergoing cardiac catheterization, high on-treatment platelet reactivity as measured with the Plateletworks® ADP

assay did not correlate with the atherothrombotic events [39].
In contradistinction to these findings, the Do Platelet Function Assays
Predict Clinical Outcomes in Clopidogrel-Pretreated Patients Undergoing
Elective PCI (POPular) study, which is the largest study to date to evaluate
this assay, demonstrated a significant relation between the results of the
Plateletworks® ADP assay and clinical outcomes in 606 patients
undergoing PCI [41]. The ROC analysis based on the primary end point
(a composite of death, MI, stent thrombosis, and stroke) at 1-year
follow-up determined an optimal cutoff value of 80.5% aggregation
(i.e., highest sum of sensitivity and specificity for cardiovascular events).
At 1-year follow-up, the primary end point occurred more frequently in
patients above this cutoff (12.6% vs. 6.1%, odds ratio 2.22 [95% CI,
1.25–3.93], $p = 0.005$). The addition of the Plateletworks® result to a model
consisting of standard cardiovascular- and procedure-related risk factors
provided the largest increase in predictive value (i.e., largest incremental
increase in AUC) of all the platelet function assays evaluated in POPular,
including LTA and VerifyNow P2Y12 [41].

Glycoprotein IIb/IIIa receptor inhibitors

Two studies have demonstrated consistent findings between the
Plateletworks® assay and LTA for measuring the magnitude of platelet
inhibition achieved by glycoprotein IIb/IIIa receptor (GP IIb/IIIa)
antagonists using ADP or collagen as the agonist [42, 43]. In the Ongoing
Tirofiban in Myocardial Evaluation (On-TIME) trial, the level of platelet
microaggregation inhibition according to the Plateletworks® assay was
measured in 463 patients presenting with ST-elevation MI undergoing
primary PCI who had been randomly assigned to either prehospital
tirofiban or initiation in the cardiac catheterization laboratory [44]. No
relationship was observed between the magnitude of inhibition and
atherothrombotic events, nor was there an association between quartile of
platelet microaggregation inhibition and distal embolization, TIMI-3 flow
and blush grade 3 after PCI, mean corrected TIMI frame count, ejection
fraction, enzymatic infarct size, and percentage ST-segment resolution.
Thus, although the correlation between other platelet function assays and
the Plateletworks® is good, the clinical utility of the device to monitor the
efficacy of GP IIb/IIIa inhibitors remains to be established.

Conclusion

Point-of-care or point-of-service PFT holds significant promise for
clinical care given the ease of integrating such testing into routine clinical
practice. The VerifyNow P2Y12 test consists of a rapid, all-in-one tabletop
system that requires little training or additional infrastructure; the
Plateletworks assay uses standard cell-counting methodology with
specialized sample collection tubes. While small studies have shown
consistency between the results of Plateletworks and platelet
aggregometry, the relationship between the clopidogrel-induced platelet

inhibition according to Plateletworks and clinical outcomes remains to be established. A large body of data from both observational and randomized studies has established that the results of the VerifyNow P2Y12 test is a significant risk factor for cardiovascular outcomes after PCI in clopidogrel-treated patients. However, the results of randomized trials that have incorporated VerifyNow P2Y12 do not support the routine use of this test to intensify antiplatelet therapy in elective PCI patients. The clinical and economic utility of the VerifyNow P2Y12 test to tailor therapy in patients with ACS undergoing revascularization has not been definitively addressed.

References

1 Price, M.J. (2009) Bedside evaluation of thienopyridine antiplatelet therapy. *Circulation*, **119 (19)**, 2625–2632.

2 Jakubowski, J.A., Payne, C.D., Li, Y.G. *et al.* (2008) The use of the VerifyNow P2Y12 point-of-care device to monitor platelet function across a range of P2Y12 inhibition levels following prasugrel and clopidogrel administration. *Thrombosis and Haemostasis*, **99 (2)**, 409–415.

3 Lordkipanidze, M., Pharand, C., Nguyen, T.A., Schampaert, E., and Diodati, J.G. (2008) Assessment of VerifyNow P2Y12 assay accuracy in evaluating clopidogrel-induced platelet inhibition. *Therapeutic Drug Monitoring*, **30 (3)**, 372–378.

4 Jakubowski, J.A., Zhou, C., Egan, B. *et al.* (2011) Modification of the VerifyNow(R) P2Y12 test BASE channel to accommodate high levels of P2Y(12) antagonism. *Platelets*, **22 (8)**, 619–625.

5 Malinin, A., Pokov, A., Swaim, L., Kotob, M., and Serebruany, V. (2006) Validation of a VerifyNow-P2Y12 cartridge for monitoring platelet inhibition with clopidogrel. *Methods and Findings in Experimental and Clinical Pharmacology*, **28 (5)**, 315–322.

6 Paniccia, R., Antonucci, E., Gori, A.M. *et al.* (2007) Different methodologies for evaluating the effect of clopidogrel on platelet function in high-risk coronary artery disease patients. *Journal of Thrombosis and Haemostasis*, **5**, 1839–1847.

7 Malinin, A., Pokov, A., Spergling, M. *et al.* (2007) Monitoring platelet inhibition after clopidogrel with the VerifyNow-P2Y12(R) rapid analyzer: the VERIfy Thrombosis risk ASsessment (VERITAS) study. *Thrombosis Research*, **119 (3)**, 277–284.

8 Varenhorst, C., James, S., Erlinge, D. *et al.* (2009) Assessment of P2Y12 inhibition with the point-of-care device VerifyNow P2Y12 in patients treated with prasugrel or clopidogrel coadministered with aspirin. *American Heart Journal*, **157**, 562.e1–562.e9.

9 van Werkum, J.W., van der Stelt, C.A., Seesing, T.H., Hackeng, C.M., and ten Berg, J.M. (2006) A head-to-head comparison between the VerifyNow P2Y12 assay and light transmittance aggregometry for monitoring the individual platelet response to clopidogrel in patients undergoing elective percutaneous coronary intervention. *Journal of Thrombosis and Haemostasis*, **4 (11)**, 2516–2518.

10 Gurbel, P.A., Bliden, K.P., Butler, K. *et al.* (2009) Randomized double-blind assessment of the ONSET and OFFSET of the antiplatelet effects of ticagrelor versus clopidogrel in patients with stable coronary artery disease: the ONSET/OFFSET study. *Circulation*, **120 (25)**, 2577–2585.

11 Bonello, L., Tantry, U.S., Marcucci, R. *et al.* (2010) Consensus and future directions on the definition of high on-treatment platelet reactivity to adenosine diphosphate. *Journal of the American College of Cardiology*, **56** (**12**), 919–933.

12 Sibbing, D., Steinhubl, S.R., Schulz, S., Schomig, A., and Kastrati, A. (2010) Platelet aggregation and its association with stent thrombosis and bleeding in clopidogrel-treated patients: initial evidence of a therapeutic window. *Journal of the American College of Cardiology*, **56** (**4**), 317–318.

13 Patti, G., Pasceri, V., Vizzi, V., Ricottini, E., and Di Sciascio, G. (2011) Usefulness of platelet response to clopidogrel by point-of-care testing to predict bleeding outcomes in patients undergoing percutaneous coronary intervention (from the Antiplatelet Therapy for Reduction of Myocardial Damage During Angioplasty-Bleeding Study). *The American Journal of Cardiology*, **107** (**7**), 995–1000.

14 Ferreiro, J.L., Sibbing, D., and Angiolillo, D.J. (2010) Platelet function testing and risk of bleeding complications. *Thrombosis and Haemostasis*, **103** (**6**), 1128–1135.

15 Campo, G., Fileti, L., de Cesare, N. *et al.* (2010) Long-term clinical outcome based on aspirin and clopidogrel responsiveness status after elective percutaneous coronary intervention: a 3T/2R (tailoring treatment with tirofiban in patients showing resistance to aspirin and/or resistance to clopidogrel) trial substudy. *Journal of the American College of Cardiology*, **56** (**18**), 1447–1455.

16 Campo, G., Parrinello, G., Ferraresi, P. *et al.* (2011) Prospective evaluation of on-clopidogrel platelet reactivity over time in patients treated with percutaneous coronary intervention relationship with gene polymorphisms and clinical outcome. *Journal of the American College of Cardiology*, **57** (**25**), 2474–2483.

17 Marcucci, R., Gori, A.M., Paniccia, R. *et al.* (2009) Cardiovascular death and nonfatal myocardial infarction in acute coronary syndrome patients receiving coronary stenting are predicted by residual platelet reactivity to ADP detected by a point-of-care assay: a 12-month follow-up. *Circulation*, **119** (**2**), 237–242.

18 Brar, S.S., ten Berg, J., Marcucci, R. *et al.* (2011) Impact of platelet reactivity on clinical outcomes after percutaneous coronary intervention: a collaborative meta-analysis of individual participant data. *Journal of the American College of Cardiology*, **58** (**19**), 1945–1954.

19 Patti, G., Nusca, A., Mangiacapra, F., Gatto, L., D'Ambrosio, A., and Di Sciascio, G. (2008) Point-of-care measurement of clopidogrel responsiveness predicts clinical outcome in patients undergoing percutaneous coronary intervention results of the ARMYDA-PRO (Antiplatelet therapy for Reduction of MYocardial Damage during Angioplasty-Platelet Reactivity Predicts Outcome) study. *Journal of the American College of Cardiology*, **52** (**14**), 1128–1133.

20 Mangiacapra, F., Barbato, E., Patti, G. *et al.* (2010) Point-of-care assessment of platelet reactivity after clopidogrel to predict myonecrosis in patients undergoing percutaneous coronary intervention. *JACC: Cardiovascular Interventions*, **3** (**3**), 318–323.

21 Price, M.J., Endemann, S., Gollapudi, R.R. *et al.* (2008) Prognostic significance of post-clopidogrel platelet reactivity assessed by a point-of-care assay on thrombotic events after drug-eluting stent implantation. *European Heart Journal*, **29** (**8**), 992–1000.

22 Park, D.W., Lee, S.W., Yun, S.C. *et al.* (2011) A point-of-care platelet function assay and C-reactive protein for prediction of major cardiovascular events after drug-eluting stent implantation. *Journal of the American College of Cardiology*, **58 (25)**, 2630–2639.

23 Cuisset, T., Hamilos, M., Sarma, J. *et al.* (2008) Relation of low response to clopidogrel assessed with point-of-care assay to periprocedural myonecrosis in patients undergoing elective coronary stenting for stable angina pectoris. *The American Journal of Cardiology*, **101 (12)**, 1700–1703.

24 Dahlen J.R., Price M.J., Parise H., Gurbel P.A. (2012) Evaluating the clinical usefulness of platelet function testing: considerations for the proper application and interpretation of performance measures. *Thrombosis and Haemostasis*. **20, 109 (2)**, 808–816.

25 Price, M.J., Angiolillo, D.J., Teirstein, P.S. *et al.* (2011) Platelet reactivity and cardiovascular outcomes after percutaneous coronary intervention: a time-dependent analysis of the gauging responsiveness with a VerifyNow P2Y12 assay: impact on thrombosis and safety (GRAVITAS) trial. *Circulation*, **124**, 1132–1137.

26 Stone, G.W. (ed) (2011) Assessment of Dual AntiPlatelet Therapy with Drug-Eluting Stents (ADAPT-DES): a large-scale, prospective, multicenter registry examining the relationship between platelet responsiveness and stent thrombosis after DES implantation. Paper presented at Transcatheter Cardiovascular Therapeutics, November 10, 2011, San Francisco.

27 Roe, M.T., Armstrong, P.W., Fox, K.A. *et al.* (2012) Prasugrel versus clopidogrel for acute coronary syndromes without revascularization. *The New England Journal of Medicine*, **367 (14)**, 1297–1309.

28 Price, M.J. (2012) Measured drug effect and cardiovascular outcomes in patients receiving platelet P2Y12 receptor antagonists: clarifying the time and place for intensive inhibition. *JAMA*, **308 (17)**, 1806–1808.

29 Valgimigli, M., Campo, G., de Cesare, N. *et al.* (2009) Intensifying platelet inhibition with tirofiban in poor responders to aspirin, clopidogrel, or both agents undergoing elective coronary intervention: results from the double-blind, prospective, randomized Tailoring Treatment with Tirofiban in Patients Showing Resistance to Aspirin and/or Resistance to Clopidogrel study. *Circulation*, **119 (25)**, 3215–3222.

30 Price, M.J., Berger, P.B., Teirstein, P.S. *et al.* (2011) Standard- vs high-dose clopidogrel based on platelet function testing after percutaneous coronary intervention: the GRAVITAS randomized trial. *JAMA*, **305 (11)**, 1097–1105.

31 Trenk, D., Stone, G.W., Gawaz, M. *et al.* (2012) A randomized trial of prasugrel versus clopidogrel in patients with high platelet reactivity on clopidogrel after elective percutaneous coronary intervention with implantation of drug-eluting stents: results of the TRIGGER-PCI (Testing Platelet Reactivity In Patients Undergoing Elective Stent Placement on Clopidogrel to Guide Alternative Therapy With Prasugrel) study. *Journal of the American College of Cardiology*, **59 (24)**, 2159–2164.

32 Collet, J.P., Cuisset, T., Range, G. *et al.* (2012) Bedside monitoring to adjust antiplatelet therapy for coronary stenting. *The New England Journal of Medicine*, **367 (22)**, 2100–2109.

33 Carville, D.G., Schleckser, P.A., Guyer, K.E., Corsello, M., and Walsh, M.M. (1998) Whole blood platelet function assay on the ICHOR point-of-care hematology analyzer. *The Journal of Extra-Corporeal Technology*, **30 (4)**, 171–177.

34 van Werkum, J.W., Kleibeuker, M., Postma, S. *et al.* (2010) A comparison between the Plateletworks-assay and light transmittance aggregometry for monitoring the inhibitory effects of clopidogrel. *International Journal of Cardiology*, **140 (1)**, 123–126.

35 Storey, R.F., Wilcox, R.G. and Heptinstall, S. (1998) Differential effects of glycoprotein IIb/IIIa antagonists on platelet microaggregate and macroaggregate formation and effect of anticoagulant on antagonist potency. Implications for assay methodology and comparison of different antagonists. *Circulation*, **98 (16)**, 1616–1621.

36 Lennon, M.J., Gibbs, N.M., Weightman, W.M., McGuire, D., and Michalopoulos, N. (2004) A comparison of plateletworks and platelet aggregometry for the assessment of aspirin-related platelet dysfunction in cardiac surgical patients. *Journal of Cardiothoracic and Vascular Anesthesia*, **18 (2)**, 136–140.

37 Craft, R.M., Chavez, J.J., Snider, C.C., Muenchen, R.A., and Carroll, R.C. (2005) Comparison of modified Thrombelastograph and Plateletworks whole blood assays to optical platelet aggregation for monitoring reversal of clopidogrel inhibition in elective surgery patients. *The Journal of Laboratory and Clinical Medicine*, **145 (6)**, 309–315.

38 Nicholson NS, Panzer-Knodle SG, Haas NF, *et al.* (1998) Assessment of platelet function assays. *American Heart Journal.* **135**(5 Pt. 2, Suppl.): S170–S178.

39 Mobley, J.E., Bresee, S.J., Wortham, D.C., Craft, R.M., Snider, C.C., and Carroll, R.C. (2004) Frequency of nonresponse antiplatelet activity of clopidogrel during pretreatment for cardiac catheterization. *The American Journal of Cardiology*, **93 (4)**, 456–458.

40 Lau, W.C., Waskell, L.A., Watkins, P.B. *et al.* (2003) Atorvastatin reduces the ability of clopidogrel to inhibit platelet aggregation: a new drug–drug interaction. *Circulation*, **107 (1)**, 32–37.

41 Breet, N.J., van Werkum, J.W., Bouman, H.J. *et al.* (2010) Comparison of platelet function tests in predicting clinical outcome in patients undergoing coronary stent implantation. *JAMA*, **303 (8)**, 754–762.

42 White, M.M., Krishnan, R., Kueter, T.J., Jacoski, M.V., and Jennings, L.K. (2004) The use of the point of care Helena ICHOR/Plateletworks and the Accumetrics Ultegra RPFA for assessment of platelet function with GPIIB-IIIa antagonists. *Journal of Thrombosis and Thrombolysis*, **18 (3)**, 163–169.

43 Lakkis, N.M., George, S., Thomas, E., Ali, M., Guyer, K., and Carville, D. (2001) Use of ICHOR-platelet works to assess platelet function in patients treated with GP IIb/IIIa inhibitors. *Catheterization and Cardiovascular Interventions*, **53 (3)**, 346–351.

44 Smit, J.J., Ernst, N.M., Slingerland, R.J. *et al.* (2006) Platelet microaggregation inhibition in patients with acute myocardial infarction pretreated with tirofiban and relationship with angiographic and clinical outcome. *American Heart Journal*, **151 (5)**, 1102–1107.

10 Multiplate Analyzer

Martin Orban and Dirk Sibbing

Klinikum der Universität München, Ludwig-Maximilians-Universität München, Munich, Germany

Historical background

Light transmission aggregometry (LTA), first described by Born in 1962 [1], was the established gold standard of platelet function measurement for decades. This method requires translucent suspensions like platelet-rich plasma (PRP) and measures platelet function in an artificial milieu. Besides optical aggregometry, another principle to assess platelet aggregation in whole blood and using electrical impedance was first described in 1979 by Cardinal and Flower [2]. The original method, however, lacks standardization, is relatively complicated, needs skilled personnel, and is therefore labor and time consuming – features that make them impractical to be incorporated into everyday clinical routine.

Principles of the Multiplate® analyzer

To overcome the shortcomings of the latter – laboratory-based – methods, the Multiplate® analyzer (Verum Diagnostica GmbH, Roche, Germany) was developed in the last decade and was introduced in clinical practice. The Multiplate® analyzer is a benchtop multiple electrode impedance aggregometer (MEA) (Figure 10.1B), which measures changes in electrical impedance over time. The name Multiplate arises from the multiplicity of channels and sensors per channel of the device. One Multiplate® test cell incorporates two independent sensor units that serve as internal control at each test. One unit consists of two silver-coated highly conductive copper wires with a length of 3.2 mm (Figure 10.1A). After dilution (1:2 with 0.9% NaCl solution) of anticoagulated whole blood (hirudin is recommended for anticoagulation) and stirring for 3 min in the test cuvettes at 37°C, the testing reagents are added and aggregation is continuously recorded for

---

Antiplatelet Therapy in Cardiovascular Disease, First Edition. Edited by Ron Waksman, Paul A. Gurbel, and Michael A. Gaglia, Jr.
© 2014 John Wiley & Sons, Ltd. Published 2014 by John Wiley & Sons, Ltd.

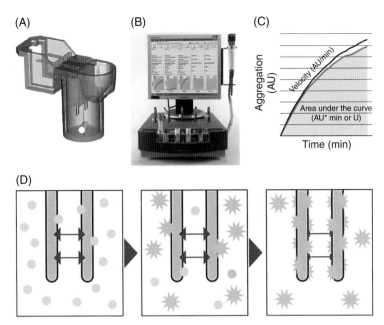

Figure 10.1 The Multiplate analyzer. The figure shows the components and principles of the electrical impedance aggregometer Multiplate® analyzer. (A) shows a Multiplate® test cell with two independent sensor units consisting of two pairs of electrodes, (B) shows the whole Multiplate® benchtop device, (C) shows the output of the device for platelet aggregation measurements that are plotted against time (in AU*min), and (D) shows an example of platelets clotting on the metal surface of the two electrodes of one sensor unit. By doing so, electrical impedance is rising between the two electrodes, and less current is flowing between the electrodes (arrows). (Source: Images kindly provided by Verum Diagnostica, Munich, Germany.)

a defined time span. During stimulation, platelets adhere to the metal surface of the electrodes, get activated, and aggregate (see Figure 10.1D and Figure 10.2). The increase of impedance due to the attachment of platelets to the electrodes is detected for each sensor unit separately during 6 min and transformed to aggregation units (AU) that are plotted against time (see Figure 10.1C). Approximately 8 AU correspond to 1 Ω. Aggregation measured with MEA is quantified as AU and area under the curve (AUC) of AU (AU*min). Electrical detection of impedance is calibrated by the manufacturer during production, and liquid controls are used to ensure quality control of impedance detection on-site.

Currently, there are five certified testing stimuli available, which are (i) ASPI test (arachidonic acid) for the effect of aspirin, (ii) ADP test (adenosine diphosphate) for P2Y12 ADP antagonists, (iii) TRAP test (thrombin receptor-activating peptide-6) for GPIIb/IIIa inhibitors, (iv) COL test (collagen) for aspirin and GPIIb/IIIa inhibitors, and (v) RISTO test (ristocetin) for the detection of severe von Willebrand disease and Bernard–Soulier syndrome.

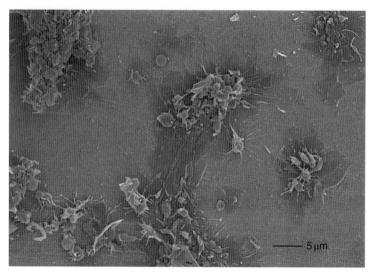

Figure 10.2 Electron microscopic imaging of a disposable Multiplate® analyzer test. Electron microscopic imaging (2000× magnified) of a disposable Multiplate® analyzer test cell showing platelets sticking on the surface of the electrode after a standard test. (Source: Image was kindly provided by Prof. Dr. Armin Reininger.)

Advantages

The Multiplate® analyzer resembles a near-patient, semiautomated device and is well standardized, easy, and reliable to use, and the results can be available within 10 min after starting the testing process [3]. By using whole blood, which displays the natural environment of all blood components, it does not miss complex cellular interactions that can influence platelet function. The principle of platelet aggregation on a metal surface is likely to resemble the physiological process after plaque rupture or percutaneous coronary intervention (PCI). The method correlates well with the gold standard LTA [4] and is able to detect the effect of the commonly and most widely used antiplatelet agents, which are (i) the cyclooxygenase-1 inhibitor aspirin; (ii) the ADP receptor antagonists clopidogrel, prasugrel, and ticagrelor; and (iii) GPIIb/IIIa inhibitors.

Disadvantages

As the Multiplate® analyzer is a semiautomated device – in contrast to real point-of-care systems like the VerifyNow® system – it still requires sample preparation and pipetting. In addition, measurements are dependent on the hematocrit level and platelet count such that extreme values of these parameters may result in an imprecise assessment of platelet function. Similar as for other methods like LTA and the VerifyNow® system, the

ADP test cannot be used to quantify P2Y12 receptor-directed platelet inhibition if GPIIb/IIIa inhibitors were administered before blood sampling.

Clinical studies in cardiovascular medicine

Different antagonists of the P2Y12 ADP receptor are in focus of contemporary research and clinical use of antiplatelet therapy monitoring because they are widely and extensively used; a status of high on-P2Y12 inhibitor treatment platelet reactivity (HPR) has been detected and is a known risk factor for ischemic events after PCI in elective patients and patients suffering from an acute coronary syndrome (ACS) [5]. The first studies that showed that higher platelet reactivity on clopidogrel treatment in patients undergoing PCI was linked to an elevated frequency of ischemic events in the past used predominantly the laboratory-based LTA [6, 7, 8]. Selected studies in which platelet reactivity was measured using the Multiplate® analyzer are presented in the following section (see Table 10.1). Toth *et al.* were among the first who performed a comparison between MEA assessed with the Multiplate® analyzer and single platelet counting (SPC) to measure platelet aggregation and inhibition by aspirin and apyrase in whole blood [9]. Platelet inhibition by apyrase and aspirin was comparable between MEA and SPC. The study also showed that the use of hirudin as an anticoagulant for MEA is preferable to the use of citrate. In 2009, we compared the ADP-induced platelet aggregation assessed with MEA and LTA in 149 patients undergoing PCI after clopidogrel loading with 600 mg. We were able to show a significant correlation (Spearman rank correlation coefficient = 0.71, $p < 0.0001$) between both methods. In a large prospectively designed study, we assessed the correlation between

Table 10.1 Selected studies in cardiology using the Multiplate® analyzer

Study	N	Setting	Focus on
Hazarbasanov et al. [16]	192	PCI with DES implantations	MACE
Penz et al. [3]		Healthy subjects	Platelet function
Sibbing et al. [4]	149	PCI with DES implantations	Platelet function
Sibbing et al. [27]	2533	PCI with DES implantations	Bleeding (in hospital)
Sibbing et al. [10]	1608	PCI with DES implantations (elective and ACS)	Definite ST (30 days)
Sibbing et al. [13]	564	PCI (ACS)	MACE (30 days)
Siller-Matula et al. [11]	416	PCI (all comers)	ST (6 months)
Siller-Matula et al. [17]	798	PCI (all comers)	ST (6 months)
Toth et al. [9]		Healthy subjects	Platelet function

ACS, acute coronary syndrome; MACE, major adverse cardiovascular event; PCI, percutaneous coronary intervention; and ST, stent thrombosis.

platelet reactivity measured with the Multiplate® analyzer after a high clopidogrel loading dose and the frequency of stent thrombosis (ST) in 1608 consecutive patients undergoing PCI. Clopidogrel low responders were defined as the upper quintile of platelet reactivity. Patients who showed a low response to clopidogrel had a significantly higher risk of suffering from an ST within 30 days after PCI compared to normal responders (2.2% vs. 0.2%; OR, 9.4; 95% CI, 3.1–28.4; $p < 0.0001$). The optimal cutoff value to predict an increased risk of the event of ST according to ROC analysis was ≥468 AU*min. The sensitivity and specificity of this cutoff value were 70% and 84%, respectively [10]. Siller-Matula and coworkers also found a correlation between HPR and ST in 416 patients undergoing PCI [11]. In their work, they could show that HPR detected by the Multiplate® analyzer can distinguish better between patients with or without ST compared to the laboratory-based VASP assay (area under the ROC curve, 0.92 for the Multiplate® analyzer, $p = 0.012$, and 0.60 for VASP, $p = 0.55$). With a sensitivity of 100% for both methods, specificity of the Multiplate® analyzer was higher (86% vs. 37%). Further selected studies that assessed platelet function using the Multiplate® analyzer in respect to adjunctive antithrombotic therapy, to newer ADP receptor antagonists, or in cardiogenic shock condition are described in this section. The Intracoronary Stenting and Antithrombotic Regimen: Rapid Early Action for Coronary Treatment-4 (ISAR-REACT-4) [12] platelet substudy [13] investigated the impact of HPR following clopidogrel loading (600 mg) in patients with NSTEMI undergoing PCI treated either with the combination of the GPIIb/IIIa inhibitor abciximab with unfractionated heparin (UFH) or bivalirudin. The 30-day incidence of a combined efficacy end point (death, myocardial infarction, urgent target vessel revascularization) was similar in HPR versus no-HPR patients in the abciximab with UFH group. For bivalirudin, the incidence of the efficacy end point was significantly higher in HPR versus no-HPR patients. By using the Multiplate® analyzer on intensive care units in cardiogenic shock patients undergoing urgent PCI due to acute myocardial infarction, cases have been reported showing a delayed onset of action of the prodrugs clopidogrel and prasugrel, which was linked to the occurrence of ST [14, 15]. Studies that assessed a personalized antiplatelet treatment using the Multiplate® analyzer are available as well. Hazarbasanov and colleagues showed that the incidence of cardiac death, myocardial infarction, ischemic stroke, or definite/probable ST during 6 months after PCI in 192 patients was significantly lower in the tailored antiplatelet therapy group (repeated loading dose of clopidogrel and maintenance dose of 150 mg/day) as compared to the standard therapy group (0% vs. 5.3%, $p = 0.03$) [16]. Just recently, in the MADONNA study, Siller-Matula *et al.* investigated the efficacy and safety of an individualized antiplatelet therapy in 789 patients undergoing PCI [17]. Patients in the individualized arm (401 patients with switching to prasugrel or increasing the dosage of clopidogrel) showed significantly less ST compared to the conventional group (0.2% vs. 1.9%, $p = 0.027$).

Studies in cardiovascular surgery

Perioperative bleeding complications can be caused by antiplatelet treatment. Several clinical studies have shown the predictivity of platelet function measurement with regard to bleeding events and the requirement of blood products using the Multiplate® analyzer (see Table 10.2). In 2008, Rahe-Meyer *et al.* compared the assessment of aspirin intake by patient self-reporting versus measurement of platelet function using the Multiplate® analyzer with regard to transfusion requirements in 100 patients undergoing coronary artery bypass surgery. Patients with reduced aggregation values before surgery (<51 U) required significantly more platelet transfusions than patients with normal aggregation values (1.1 U compared to 0.3 U, $p = 0.001$) [18]. The same group correlated platelet function before cardiac surgery in 60 patients with the transfusion of platelet concentrates (PC) in 2009. Patients within the lowest tertile of preoperative platelet aggregation values need significantly more PC [19]. Görlinger and colleagues showed in a retrospective analysis of 3865 patients undergoing cardiovascular surgery that the implementation of a coagulation management algorithm based on point-of-care platelet function testing and the first-line therapy with coagulation factors was associated with decreased requirements of blood transfusions [20]. In 2011, Reece *et al.* were able to detect an impaired periprocedural platelet function in 44 patients undergoing coronary artery bypass surgery *per se* [21]. This effect was even more pronounced in patients receiving packed red blood cells (PRBC). Just recently, Weber *et al.* investigated the efficacy of conventional coagulation versus point-of-care platelet function testing in a prospective, randomized clinical trial to improve hemostatic therapy in 100 patients undergoing cardiac surgery [22]. Patients randomized to the platelet function-guided group required less PRBC compared to the conventional group (3 vs. 5 PRBC, $p < 0.001$).

Table 10.2 Selected studies in cardiovascular surgery using the Multiplate® analyzer

Study	N	Setting	Focus on
Görlinger *et al.* [20]	3865	Cardiovascular surgery	Transfusion requirements
Rahe-Meyer *et al.* [18]	100	Coronary artery bypass grafting	Transfusion of packed erythrocytes
Rahe-Meyer *et al.* [19]	60	Routine cardiac surgery	Transfusion of platelet concentrates (PC)
Reece *et al.* [21]	44	Coronary artery bypass grafting	Platelet function
Weber *et al.* [22]	152	Cardiac surgery	Transfusion of packed erythrocytes

Transfusions comprise packed red blood cells (PRBC), fresh frozen plasma, and PC.

The Multiplate® analyzer has also proved useful for the detection of Glanzmann's disease and Bernard–Soulier syndrome [23]. Furthermore, cases have been published that functional detection of the heparin-induced thrombocytopenia (HIT) – using the Multiplate® analyzer – is possible [24, 25].

Consensus definitions and cutoff values concerning platelet reactivity

The "Working Group on High On-treatment Platelet Reactivity" provided a consensus definition of HPR to ADP for four platelet function devices in 2010, including the Multiplate® analyzer [5]. The specific cutoff value defining HPR and its association with thrombotic events was set to ≥468 AU*min for the Multiplate® analyzer [10, 26]. In addition, evidence is accumulating that an enhanced response on P2Y12 receptor inhibitor treatment or a low on-treatment platelet reactivity (LPR) is associated with a higher frequency of bleeding events [27, 28, 29, 30]. The respective cutoff value for low platelet aggregation that proofed its association with an increase of post-PCI bleeding events in a prior large observational study in 2533 clopidogrel-treated patients undergoing PCI is ≤188 AU × min for the Multiplate® analyzer [27]. Both cutoff values determine a potential therapeutic window of platelet inhibition as patients with aggregation values in the range of 189–467 AU*min showed remarkably low risk for the occurrence of both bleeding and ST [30].

Summary

The Multiplate® analyzer measures platelet aggregation in whole blood and is well standardized, easy, and reliable to use, and the results can be available fast within minutes. Specific cutoff values (≥468 AU*min for thrombotic events after PCI and ≤188 AU*min for periprocedural bleeding complications) were recently established. Therefore, the Multiplate® analyzer could be highly valuable for future studies and clinical practice to determine patients at risk for thrombotic and bleeding events. As a future perspective, platelet function monitoring may guide the attending physician which available drug to choose for the individual patient to maneuver antiplatelet therapy between thrombotic and bleeding events. The more antiplatelet agents become available for treatment of patients undergoing PCI or cardiac surgery, the higher the need for platelet function monitoring to determine the best drug for the individual patient.

Acknowledgment

Electron microscopic imaging (Figure 10.2) was kindly provided by Prof. Dr. Armin Reininger.

References

1 Born, G.V. (1962) Aggregation of blood platelets by adenosine diphosphate and its reversal. *Nature*, **194**, 927–929.

2 Cardinal, D.C. and Flower, R.J. (1980) The electronic aggregometer: a novel device for assessing platelet behavior in blood. *Journal of Pharmacological Methods*, **3**, 135–158.

3 Penz, S.M., Bernlochner, I., Toth, O., Lorenz, R., Calatzis, A., and Siess, W. (2010) Selective and rapid monitoring of dual platelet inhibition by aspirin and p2y12 antagonists by using multiple electrode aggregometry. *Thrombosis Journal*, **8**, 9.

4 Sibbing, D., Braun, S., Jawansky, S. *et al.* (2008) Assessment of adp-induced platelet aggregation with light transmission aggregometry and multiple electrode platelet aggregometry before and after clopidogrel treatment. *Thrombosis and Haemostasis*, **99**, 121–126.

5 Bonello, L., Tantry, U.S., Marcucci, R. *et al.* (2010) Consensus and future directions on the definition of high on-treatment platelet reactivity to adenosine diphosphate. *Journal of the American College of Cardiology*, **56**, 919–933.

6 Buonamici, P., Marcucci, R., Migliorini, A. *et al.* (2007) Impact of platelet reactivity after clopidogrel administration on drug-eluting stent thrombosis. *Journal of the American College of Cardiology*, **49**, 2312–2317.

7 Hochholzer, W., Trenk, D., Bestehorn, H.P. *et al.* (2006) Impact of the degree of peri-interventional platelet inhibition after loading with clopidogrel on early clinical outcome of elective coronary stent placement. *Journal of the American College of Cardiology*, **48**, 1742–1750.

8 Geisler, T., Langer, H., Wydymus, M. *et al.* (2006) Low response to clopidogrel is associated with cardiovascular outcome after coronary stent implantation. *European Heart Journal*, **27**, 2420–2425.

9 Toth, O., Calatzis, A., Penz, S., Losonczy, H., and Siess, W. (2006) Multiple electrode aggregometry: a new device to measure platelet aggregation in whole blood. *Thrombosis and Haemostasis*, **96**, 781–788.

10 Sibbing, D., Braun, S., Morath, T. *et al.* (2009) Platelet reactivity after clopidogrel treatment assessed with point-of-care analysis and early drug-eluting stent thrombosis. *Journal of the American College of Cardiology*, **53**, 849–856.

11 Siller-Matula, J.M., Christ, G., Lang, I.M., Delle-Karth, G., Huber, K., and Jilma, B. (2010) Multiple electrode aggregometry predicts stent thrombosis better than the vasodilator-stimulated phosphoprotein phosphorylation assay. *Journal of Thrombosis and Haemostasis*, **8**, 351–359.

12 Kastrati, A., Neumann, F.J., Schulz, S. *et al.* (2011) Abciximab and heparin versus bivalirudin for non-ST-elevation myocardial infarction. *The New England Journal of Medicine*, **365**, 1980–1989.

13 Sibbing, D., Bernlochner, I., Schulz, S. *et al.* (2012) Prognostic value of a high on-clopidogrel treatment platelet reactivity in bivalirudin versus abciximab treated non-ST-segment elevation myocardial infarction patients. ISAR-REACT 4 (intracoronary stenting and antithrombotic regimen: rapid early action for coronary treatment-4) platelet substudy. *Journal of the American College of Cardiology*, **60**, 369–377.

14 Orban, M., Byrne, R.A., Hausleiter, J., Laugwitz, K.L. and Sibbing, D. (2011) Massive thrombus burden with recurrence of intracoronary thrombosis early after stenting and delayed onset of prasugrel action in a patient with

ST-elevation myocardial infarction and cardiac shock. *Thrombosis and Haemostasis*, **106**, 555–558.

15 Orban, M., Riegger, J., Joner, M. *et al.* (2012) Dual thienopyridine low-response to clopidogrel and prasugrel in a patient with stemi, cardiogenic shock and early stent thrombosis is overcome by ticagrelor. *Platelets*, **23**, 395–398.

16 Hazarbasanov, D., Velchev, V., Finkov, B. *et al.* (2012) Tailoring clopidogrel dose according to multiple electrode aggregometry decreases the rate of ischemic complications after percutaneous coronary intervention. *Journal of Thrombosis and Thrombolysis*, **34**, 85–90.

17 Siller-Matula, J.M., Francesconi, M., Dechant, C. *et al.* (2013) Personalized antiplatelet treatment after percutaneous coronary intervention: the madonna study. *International Journal of Cardiology*, **167** (5), 2018–2023.

18 Rahe-Meyer, N., Winterhalter, M., Hartmann, J. *et al.* (2008) An evaluation of cyclooxygenase-1 inhibition before coronary artery surgery: aggregometry versus patient self-reporting. *Anesthesia and Analgesia*, **107**, 1791–1797.

19 Rahe-Meyer, N., Winterhalter, M., Boden, A. *et al.* (2009) Platelet concentrates transfusion in cardiac surgery and platelet function assessment by multiple electrode aggregometry. *Acta Anaesthesiologica Scandinavica*, **53**, 168–175.

20 Görlinger, K., Dirkmann, D., Hanke, A.A. *et al.* (2011) First-line therapy with coagulation factor concentrates combined with point-of-care coagulation testing is associated with decreased allogeneic blood transfusion in cardiovascular surgery: a retrospective, single-center cohort study. *Anesthesiology*, **115**, 1179–1191.

21 Reece, M.J., Klein, A.A., Salviz, E.A. *et al.* (2011) Near-patient platelet function testing in patients undergoing coronary artery surgery: a pilot study. *Anaesthesia*, **66**, 97–103.

22 Weber, C.F., Görlinger, K., Meininger, D. *et al.* (2012) Point-of-care testing: a prospective, randomized clinical trial of efficacy in coagulopathic cardiac surgery patients. *Anesthesiology*, **117**, 531–547.

23 Awidi, A., Maqablah, A., Dweik, M., Bsoul, N., and Abu-Khader, A. (2009) Comparison of platelet aggregation using light transmission and multiple electrode aggregometry in Glanzmann thrombasthenia. *Platelets*, **20**, 297–301.

24 Elalamy, I., Galea, V., Hatmi, M., and Gerotziafas, G.T. (2009) Heparin-induced multiple electrode aggregometry: a potential tool for improvement of heparin-induced thrombocytopenia diagnosis. *Journal of Thrombosis and Haemostasis*, **7**, 1932–1934.

25 Morel-Kopp, M.C., Aboud, M., Tan, C.W., Kulathilake, C., and Ward, C. (2010) Whole blood impedance aggregometry detects heparin-induced thrombocytopenia antibodies. *Thrombosis Research*, **125**, e234–e239.

26 Siller-Matula, J.M., Delle-Karth, G., Lang, I.M. *et al.* (2012) Phenotyping vs. genotyping for prediction of clopidogrel efficacy and safety: the PEGASUS-PCI study. *Journal of Thrombosis and Haemostasis*, **10**, 529–542.

27 Sibbing, D., Schulz, S., Braun, S. *et al.* (2010) Antiplatelet effects of clopidogrel and bleeding in patients undergoing coronary stent placement. *Journal of Thrombosis and Haemostasis*, **8**, 250–256.

28 Cuisset, T., Cayla, G., Frere, C. *et al.* (2009) Predictive value of post-treatment platelet reactivity for occurrence of post-discharge bleeding after non-st elevation acute coronary syndrome. Shifting from antiplatelet resistance to bleeding risk assessment? *EuroIntervention*, **5**, 325–329.

29 Serebruany, V., Rao, S.V., Silva, M.A. *et al.* (2010) Correlation of inhibition of platelet aggregation after clopidogrel with post discharge bleeding events: assessment by different bleeding classifications. *European Heart Journal*, **31**, 227–235.

30 Sibbing, D., Steinhubl, S.R., Schulz, S., Schomig, A., and Kastrati, A. (2010) Platelet aggregation and its association with stent thrombosis and bleeding in clopidogrel-treated patients: initial evidence of a therapeutic window. *Journal of the American College of Cardiology*, **56**, 317–318.

11 Shear Stress-Based Platelet Function Tests

Nicoline J. Breet and Jurriën M. ten Berg
St Antonius Hospital, Nieuwegein, The Netherlands

PFA-100

Description of the test: General concepts

The PFA-100® system (Siemens Healthcare Diagnostics Products GmbH, Germany) measures platelet function, in particular adhesion and aggregation, in whole blood under high shear conditions (5000/s) [1]. A constant vacuum of 40 mBar is maintained in the system that mimics the pressure in a capillary in the human body [2].

The time needed to form a platelet plug occluding the aperture cut into a membrane coated with an agonist is determined and reported as closure time (CT) in seconds, which is inversely related to platelet reactivity. If the formed clot is too weak, the CT cannot be measured and the results are presented as greater than 300 s [2] (Figure 11.1).

Various types of cartridges are available. The membrane of the classic cartridge is coated with either collagen and epinephrine (COL/EPI) or collagen and adenosine diphosphate (COL/ADP) as agonists. The COL/EPI test cartridge detects intrinsic platelet defects, von Willebrand disease, as well as exposure to platelet-inhibiting agents such as aspirin. The COL/ADP test cartridge is less influenced by aspirin use. Recently, a novel PFA-100® test cartridge has been introduced, the final prototype of INNOVANCE® PFA P2Y*. This novel test cartridge intents to measure the effect of P2Y12 receptor blockers on platelet function [3].

Strengths and weaknesses of the test

The PFA-100 is a simple and semiautomated assay that uses whole blood. It mimics the *in vivo* process of thrombus formation by inducing shear stress. However, several studies have demonstrated that the COL/ADP cartridge is relatively insensitive to the effect of P2Y12 receptor blocker treatment [4]. This might be attributed to the relatively high local concentration of collagen (6 µg/mL) and ADP (0.5 mmol/L) in the cartridge, under which circumstances clopidogrel might be unable to

Antiplatelet Therapy in Cardiovascular Disease, First Edition. Edited by Ron Waksman, Paul A. Gurbel, and Michael A. Gaglia, Jr.
© 2014 John Wiley & Sons, Ltd. Published 2014 by John Wiley & Sons, Ltd.

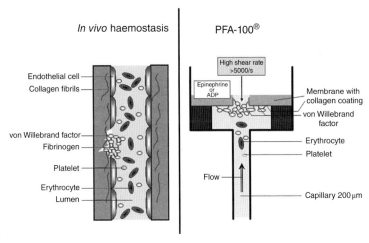

Figure 11.1 Schematic presentation of the PFA-100 system. The time needed to form a platelet plug occluding the aperture cut into a collagen/epinephrine (COL/EPI) or collagen/ADP (COL/ADP)-coated membrane is determined and reported as closure time (CT) in seconds.

inhibit the formation of the platelet plug [5, 6]. Furthermore, since the assay is highly affected by the levels of von Willebrand factor (vWF) and hematocrit [5, 6], high vWF levels might mask the inhibitory effects of clopidogrel because the shear stress will lead to instant binding of vWF to glycoprotein (GP)IIb/IIIa [5].

Validity of the test in measuring antiplatelet effect and predicting clinical outcomes
Aspirin
The relation between the PFA COL/EPI cartridge and the arachidonic acid (AA)-induced light transmittance aggregometry is good [7]. Multiple studies have described the ability of the PFA COL/EPI cartridge in monitoring the efficacy of aspirin-induced antiplatelet effect [8, 9, 10, 11, 12, 13, 14, 15]. Nevertheless, contrasting results have been reported concerning the predictive accuracy of this cartridge. Some studies demonstrated a two- to fivefold [16, 17, 18] higher risk in aspirin-treated patients with a shorter CT, using either a cutoff value of 193 or 300 s, whereas the largest study thus far demonstrated no association at all between high on-aspirin platelet reactivity (HAPR) according to the PFA COL/EPI and adverse clinical outcome [19].

A meta-analysis on the predictive value of a short CT as established by the PFA COL/EPI cartridge in aspirin-treated patients demonstrated an odds ratio of 2.1 (95% CI, 1.4–3.4) of HAPR in the eight prospective studies of varying patient populations with different clinical scenarios, using cutoff values varying between 170 and 203 ($n = 1227$). In contrast, in the meta-analysis on nonprospective studies, no association between HAPR according to the PFA COL/EPI and clinical outcome was established ($n = 1466$) [16].

Some issues merit careful consideration. Since there are no recommended cutoffs, the cutoff values in the studies included in this meta-analysis were not based on clinical outcome and thus can be questioned. In addition, the study with the highest odds ratio used the relatively subjective clinical end point angina (either as single end point or as part of a combined end point) [15]. Furthermore, the studies establishing a higher odds ratio in patients with HAPR all included higher-risk patients (presenting with an acute coronary syndrome (ACS)). In addition, the largest studies thus far that demonstrated no association between HAPR according to the PFA COL/EPI and adverse clinical outcome were not included in the current meta-analysis [19, 20]. In the first study, a prospective study of 700 aspirin-treated patients presenting for angiographic evaluation of coronary artery disease, it was demonstrated that HAPR as assessed by the PFA COL/EPI cartridge using the manufacturer's advised cutoff of 193 s did not correlate with the subsequent major adverse cardiovascular events (defined as all-cause death, cardiovascular death, and a combined end point including cardiovascular death, myocardial infarction (MI), hospitalization for revascularization, or ACS). This is in line with the observations of the POPular study ($n = 719$), in which the PFA COL/EPI was also unable to discriminate between patients with and without primary end point (a composite of all-cause death, nonfatal myocardial, stent thrombosis (ST), and ischemic stroke), both using the currently accepted cutoff value of 193 s as the cutoff established by receiver operating characteristic (ROC) curve analysis and set at 277 s. Both studies were performed in a relatively low-risk population, undergoing elective PCI with stent implantation, and excluded higher-risk patients (in particular ST-elevation MI). As the PFA-100 mimics the *in vivo* process of thrombus formation by inducing shear stress, it might be considered a better model for ACS rather than stable ischemia.

Clopidogrel

Clinical evaluation of the PFA-100 COL/ADP in monitoring P2Y12 receptor blocker therapy is limited.

Several studies have demonstrated a slight but nonsignificant prolongation of the CT with the COL/ADP cartridge after clopidogrel administration, suggesting that this cartridge might not be suitable for monitoring therapy with P2Y12 receptor blockers [4, 21, 22, 23]. This is in line with the observation of the POPular study, the only study thus far describing performance data of the cartridge in a large cohort of patients undergoing elective PCI [24]. The PFA-100 COL/ADP cartridge ($n = 812$) was unable to discriminate between patients with and without ischemic events at 1-year follow-up.

The POPular study was the first to report performance data of the prototype INNOVANCE® PFA P2Y, which in its final design became available halfway through the inclusion period. Although the sample size has insufficient statistical power ($n = 588$), the survival analysis demonstrated a lower incidence of the primary end point in patients without high on-treatment platelet reactivity. However, the addition of high on-treatment platelet reactivity as measured with INNOVANCE® PFA P2Y to a statistical model containing traditional Framingham and procedural risk factors did not improve the predictability of the risk model (as measured by an increase in the area under the curve). Thus, the novel cartridge seems promising for the evaluation of the efficacy of P2Y12 inhibition [24], but its utility as a predictor of cardiovascular events still requires further investigation.

Glycoprotein IIb/IIIa receptor inhibitors

To date, little data are available on the PFA-100® system in patients on GPIIb/IIIa receptor inhibitors (GPIIb/IIIa inhibitors) [25, 26]. Madan *et al.* demonstrated that the PFA-100 provides similar qualitative information on platelet inhibition as light transmission aggregometry [27]. Still, as almost all patients achieved a maximal CT, the useful range of the assay is limited [28]. In addition, there are no studies available addressing the relation between CT as established by the PFA COL/EPI or PFA COL/ADP and clinical outcome in patients on GPIIb/IIIa inhibitors.

Conclusion

Although this test can be used in the catheterization laboratory and the reproducibility between laboratories is good, data on its predictive value in patients on aspirin is conflicting. In addition, its use in predicting clinical outcome patients on P2Y12 receptor blockers seems promising but remains to be confirmed by other studies. Therefore, we consider the PFA not suitable for use in daily clinical practice yet.

IMPACT-R

Description of the test: General concepts

The IMPACT-R device (DiaMed, Cressier, Switzerland) is based on the cone and plate(let) analyzer technology [29] and intents to mimic the interaction of platelets with the subendothelium under flow conditions with similar shear forces [30]. Citrated whole blood samples are prestimulated with a suboptimal concentration AA (0.32 mM) or ADP (1.38 μmol/L) and gently mixed (10 RPM) for 1 min. Prestimulation with the agonist leads to the formation of microaggregates in patients not using aspirin or in whom aspirin does not effectively inhibit platelet function (using AA) or in those on clopidogrel or in whom clopidogrel is ineffective (using ADP) [31]. These microaggregated platelets temporarily lose their adhesive properties. Aliquots of the preincubated whole blood sample (130 μL) are transferred to a polystyrene well and subjected to shear (1800/s for 2 min) using a rotating cone. Under these test conditions, vWF and fibrinogen are instantly immobilized on the polystyrene surface, serving as a substrate for platelet adhesion and subsequent aggregation. The wells are washed and stained with May–Grünwald stain and analyzed with an inverted light microscope

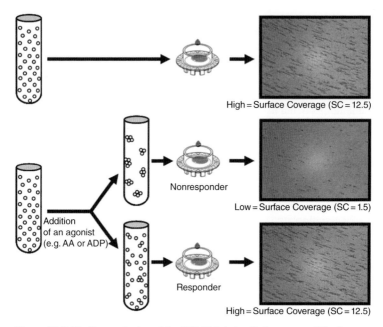

Figure 11.2 Working mechanism of the IMPACT-R device. Testing a normal blood sample with the IMPACT-R results in aggregates formation on the well surface (normal SC: upper part). However, pre-incubating the blood sample under gentle mixing (10 rpm) for 1 min with an appropriate platelet agonist (e.g.: ADP, AA) induces microaggregates formation when platelets are insufficiently inhibited by clopidogrel and/or aspirin. These activated platelets lose their adhesion properties temporary until spontaneous disaggregation occurs.

that is connected to an image analysis system. Platelet adhesion and aggregation on the surface are evaluated by examining the percentage of total area covered with platelet designated as surface coverage (SC) and the average size of surface-bound objects (i.e., platelet aggregates). The percentage SC is inversely correlated with the magnitude of AA- or ADP-induced platelet activation (Figure 11.2).

Strengths and weaknesses of the test

The IMPACT-R is based on shear stress. This is potentially advantageous because shear is of utmost importance in the pathophysiology of thrombus formation. The method needs a low sample whole blood volume. However, the accuracy of the test might be hampered because the device requires multiple sample preparation proceedings, which might lead to a relatively high coefficient of variation (CV) of the device. In our laboratory, the intra-assay CV for the IMPACT-R varied between 3.7% and 23.1%, and an external validation of the IMPACT-R demonstrated an intra-assay variability for SC ranging from 21% to 36%. The interassay variability was less than 10% [32]. Furthermore, because of this extensive sample handling, it cannot be considered as a true point-of-care assay [2].

Validity of the test in measuring antiplatelet effect and predicting clinical outcomes
Aspirin

In a study on healthy volunteers, the correlation between light transmittance aggregometry and the IMPACT-R AA was good [33]. Patients with an SC less than 2.5% were considered to exhibit HAPR. However, the relation between the IMPACT-R AA and serum thromboxane B2, which is, being the stable metabolite of TXA2, considered the most specific measurement of platelet COX-1 activity in identifying patients with HAPR, is poor [34].

In a small study of 63 patients presenting with ACS (both ST-elevation MI and non-ST-elevation MI), using light transmittance aggregometry and the IMPACT-R AA, patients with good laboratory response to aspirin before but not after PCI had a significantly lower major cardiovascular event rate during a 15-month follow-up in multivariate analysis using light transmittance aggregometry. Using the IMPACT-R AA, a trend toward a better prognosis at 6 months was shown in those with a good response to AA, but this only holds true in univariate analysis [35].

The largest study to date to investigate the association between HAPR according to the IMPACT-R AA and adverse clinical outcome was the POPular study ($n = 791$), in which the cutoff value to identify patients with HAPR was determined by ROC curve analysis and set at 7.2% SC. In this prospective study in patients undergoing elective PCI with stent implantation, the IMPACT-R was not able to segregate patients with and without HAPR or to identify patients at higher risk of atherothrombotic events, neither using our cutoff nor the one derived from the literature [20, 31].

Clopidogrel

Matetzky and coworkers evaluated the response to clopidogrel therapy among 60 patients undergoing PCI with stenting for ST-elevation MI. Platelet reactivity was assessed using the IMPACT-R, and patients were stratified into quartiles according to the magnitude of platelet reactivity. Patients in the highest quartile of platelet reactivity were considered to have high on-clopidogrel platelet reactivity. At a 6-month follow-up, eight CV events occurred. Seven of these events (88%) were observed in those patients exhibiting high on-treatment platelet reactivity. Since the sample size of this study is relatively small, it does not allow definite conclusions [36].

It is presumed that platelet function testing under "physiological" high shear conditions reflects the physiological milieu more precisely than *ex vivo* aggregation-based platelet function tests. However, in a study evaluating the IMPACT-R ADP, it was established that the IMPACT-R ADP is relatively insensitive to the effects of clopidogrel as a high percentage of healthy volunteers was classified as clopidogrel responsive while they were not on antiplatelet therapy. In addition, the correlation between the IMPACT-R ADP and both light transmittance aggregometry and the flow cytometric VASP analysis was only modest [37]. In addition, a recent study has demonstrated that the magnitude of platelet reactivity as measured by the IMPACT-R ADP is inversely correlated with the active thiol metabolite of clopidogrel ($r = -0.48$, $p = 0.03$) and is therefore not suitable to determine the *in vivo* bioavailability of the active metabolite of clopidogrel [38]. Furthermore, the POPular study recently demonstrated in a large cohort of patients that the IMPACT-R was not able to predict the combined end point of death, MI, ST, and stroke (7.5% vs. 9.8%, $p = 0.21$, using IMPACT-R [$n = 910$] and 7.9% vs. 8.6%, $p = 0.68$, using IMPACT-R ADP [$n = 905$]) nor its single components [24].

Glycoprotein IIb/IIIa receptor inhibitors

A good correlation between IMPACT-R and light transmittance aggregometry was observed in patients with an ACS [39]. Surprisingly, in patients undergoing carotid stenting with adjuvant abciximab therapy, using light transmittance aggregometry platelet function remained inhibited for only 1 day after abciximab therapy, while using the IMPACT-R showed prolonged platelet inhibition with gradual recovery from GPIIb/IIIa receptor blockade in the first week after abciximab administration. In addition, the IMPACT-R showed a better correlation with the percentage of free GPIIb/IIIa receptors. These data suggest that testing platelet function under high shear conditions reflects GPIIb/IIIa inhibition in a more precise way and that the IMPACT-R is more sensitive to detect lower levels of platelet inhibition as compared to light transmittance aggregometry [40]. However, to date, the IMPACT-R has not (yet) been validated against clinical outcomes in patients on GPIIb/IIIa receptor inhibitors.

Conclusion

The correlation between the IMPACT-R and other platelet function tests is low. In addition, there is no relation between the active metabolite of clopidogrel and the magnitude of platelet reactivity as measured by the IMPACT-R. Of even more importance, there is no relation between the magnitude of platelet reactivity according to the IMPACT-R and clinical outcome. Thus, there is no evidence for using this platelet function assay in clinical practice.

References

1 Favaloro, E.J. (2002) Clinical application of the PFA-100. *Current Opinion in Hematology*, **9**, 407–415.
2 van Werkum, J.W., Hackeng, C.M., Smit, J.J., van't Hof, A.W., Verheugt, F., and Ten Berg, J.M. (2008) Monitoring antiplatelet therapy with point-of-care platelet function assays: a review of the evidence. *Future Cardiology*, **8**, 33–55.
3 Pittens, C.A., Bouman, H.J., van Werkum, J.W., Ten Berg, J.M., and Hackeng, C.M. (2009) Comparison between hirudin and citrate in monitoring the inhibitory effects of P2Y12 receptor antagonists with different platelet function tests. *Journal of Thrombosis and Haemostasis*, **7**, 1929–1932.
4 Golanski, J., Pluta, J., Baraniak, J., and Watala, C. (2004) Limited usefulness of the PFA-100 for the monitoring of ADP receptor antagonists – in vitro experience. *Clinical Chemistry and Laboratory Medicine*, **42**, 25–29.

5 Chakroun, T., Gerotziafas, G., Robert, F. *et al.* (2004) In vitro aspirin resistance detected by PFA-100 closure time: pivotal role of plasma von Willebrand factor. *British Journal of Haematology*, **124**, 80–85.

6 Haubelt, H., Anders, C., Vogt, A., Hoerdt, P., Seyfert, U.T., and Hellstern, P. (2005) Variables influencing platelet function analyzer-100 closure times in healthy individuals. *British Journal of Haematology*, **130**, 759–767.

7 Tantry, U.S., Bliden, K.P., and Gurbel, P.A. (2005) Overestimation of platelet aspirin resistance detection by thrombelastograph platelet mapping and validation by conventional aggregometry using arachidonic acid stimulation. *Journal of the American College of Cardiology*, **46**, 1705–1709.

8 Sambola, A., Heras, M., Escolar, G. *et al.* (2004) The PFA-100 detects sub-optimal antiplatelet responses in patients on aspirin. *Platelets*, **15**, 439–446.

9 Angiolillo, D.J., Fernandez-Ortiz, A., Bernardo, E. *et al.* (2006) Influence of aspirin resistance on platelet function profiles in patients on long-term aspirin and clopidogrel after percutaneous coronary intervention. *The American Journal of Cardiology*, **97**, 38–43.

10 Macchi, L., Christiaens, L., Brabant, S. *et al.* (2002) Resistance to aspirin in vitro is associated with increased platelet sensitivity to adenosine diphosphate. *Thrombosis Research*, **107**, 45–49.

11 Andersen, K., Hurlen, M., Arnesen, H., and Seljeflot, I. (2002) Aspirin non-responsiveness as measured by PFA-100 in patients with coronary artery disease. *Thrombosis Research*, **108**, 37–42.

12 Abaci, A., Caliskan, M., Bayram, F. *et al.* (2006) A new definition of aspirin non-responsiveness by platelet function analyzer-100 and its predictors. *Platelets*, **17**, 7–13.

13 Alberts, M.J., Bergman, D.L., Molner, E., Jovanovic, B.D., Ushiwata, I., and Teruya, J. (2004) Antiplatelet effect of aspirin in patients with cerebrovascular disease. *Stroke*, **35**, 175–178.

14 Roller, R.E., Dorr, A., Ulrich, S., and Pilger, E. (2002) Effect of aspirin treatment in patients with peripheral arterial disease monitored with the platelet function analyzer PFA-100. *Blood Coagulation and Fibrinolysis*, **13**, 277–281.

15 Gianetti, J., Parri, M.S., Sbrana, S., *et al.* (2005) Platelet activation predicts recurrent ischemic events after percutaneous coronary angioplasty: a 6 months prospective study. *Thrombosis Research*, **118**, 487–493.

16 Reny, J.L., de Moerloose, P., Dauzat, M., and Fontana, P. (2008) Use of the PFA-100 closure time to predict cardiovascular events in aspirin-treated cardiovascular patients: a systematic review and meta-analysis. *Journal of Thrombosis and Haemostasis*, **6**, 444–450.

17 Fuchs, I., Frossard, M., Spiel, A., Riedmuller, E., Laggner, A.N., and Jilma, B. (2006) Platelet function in patients with acute coronary syndrome (ACS) predicts recurrent ACS. *Journal of Thrombosis and Haemostasis*, **4**, 2547–2552.

18 Christie, D.J., Kottke-Marchant, K., and Gorman, R.T. (2008) Hypersensitivity of platelets to adenosine diphosphate in patients with stable cardiovascular disease predicts major adverse events despite antiplatelet therapy. *Platelets*, **19**, 104–110.

19 Frelinger, A.L., III, Li, Y., Linden, M.D. *et al.* (2009) Association of cyclooxygenase-1-dependent and -independent platelet function assays with adverse clinical outcomes in aspirin-treated patients presenting for cardiac catheterization. *Circulation*, **120**, 2586–2596.

20 Breet, N.J., van Werkum, J.W., Bouman, H.J., Kelder, J.C., Ten Berg, J.M., and Hackeng, C.M. (2010) High on-aspirin platelet reactivity as measured with aggregation based, COX-1 inhibition sensitive platelet function tests is associated with the occurrence of atherothrombotic events. *Journal of Thrombosis and Haemostasis*, **8**, 2140–2148.

21 Hezard, N., Metz, D., Nazeyrollas, P., Droulle, C., Potron, G., and Nguyen, P. (2002) PFA-100 and flow cytometry: can they challenge aggregometry to assess antiplatelet agents, other than GPIIbIIIa blockers, in coronary angioplasty? *Thrombosis Research*, **108**, 43–47.

22 Grau, A.J., Reiners, S., Lichy, C., Buggle, F., and Ruf, A. (2003) Platelet function under aspirin, clopidogrel, and both after ischemic stroke: a case-crossover study. *Stroke*, **34**, 849–854.

23 Raman, S. and Jilma, B. (2004) Time lag in platelet function inhibition by clopidogrel in stroke patients as measured by PFA-100. *Journal of Thrombosis and Haemostasis*, **2**, 2278–2279.

24 Breet, N.J., van Werkum, J.W., Bouman, H.J. *et al.* (2010) Comparison between platelet function tests in predicting clinical outcome in patients undergoing coronary stent placement. *JAMA*, **303**, 754–762.

25 Coller, B.S., Lang, D., and Scudder, L.E. (1997) Rapid and simple platelet function assay to assess glycoprotein IIb/IIIa receptor blockade. *Circulation*, **95**, 860–867.

26 Smith, J.W., Steinhubl, S.R., Lincoff, A.M. *et al.* (1999) Rapid platelet-function assay: an automated and quantitative cartridge-based method. *Circulation*, **99**, 620–625.

27 Madan, M., Berkowitz, S.D., Christie, D.J. *et al.* (2001) Rapid assessment of glycoprotein IIb/IIIa blockade with the platelet function analyzer (PFA-100) during percutaneous coronary intervention. *American Heart Journal*, **141 (2)**, 226–233.

28 Kereiakes, D.J., Mueller, M., Howard, W. *et al.* (1999) Efficacy of abciximab induced platelet blockade using a rapid point of care assay. *Journal of Thrombosis and Thrombolysis*, **7**, 265–276.

29 Varon, D., Savion N. (2006) Impact cone and plate(let) analyzer. In: Michelson A.D., ed. *Platelets*; 2nd ed. Elsevier, San Diego, pp. 535–544.

30 Varon, D., Dardik, R., Shenkman, B. *et al.* (1997) A new method for quantitative analysis of whole blood platelet interaction with extracellular matrix under flow conditions. *Thrombosis Research*, **85**, 283–294.

31 Savion, N. and Varon, D. (2006) Impact – the cone and plate(let) analyzer: testing platelet function and anti-platelet drug response. *Pathophysiology of Haemostasis and Thrombosis*, **35**, 83–88.

32 Peerschke, E.I., Silver, R.T., Weksler, B., Grigg, S.E., Savion, N., and Varon, D. (2004) Ex vivo evaluation of erythrocytosis-enhanced platelet thrombus formation using the cone and plate(let) analyzer: effect of platelet antagonists. *British Journal of Haematology*, **127**, 195–203.

33 Spectre, G., Brill, A., Gural, A. *et al.* (2005) A new point-of-care method for monitoring anti-platelet therapy: application of the cone and plate(let) analyzer. *Platelets*, **16**, 293–299.

34 Gremmel, T., Steiner, S., Seidinger, D., Koppensteiner, R., Panzer, S., and Kopp, C.W. (2011) Comparison of methods to evaluate aspirin-mediated platelet inhibition after percutaneous intervention with stent implantation. *Platelets*, **22**, 188–195.

35 Spectre, G., Mosseri, M., Abdelrahman, N.M. *et al.* (2011) Clinical and prognostic implications of the initial response to aspirin in patients with

acute coronary syndrome. *The American Journal of Cardiology*, **108**, 1112–1118.

36 Matetzky, S., Shenkman, B., Guetta, V. *et al.* (2004) Clopidogrel resistance is associated with increased risk of recurrent atherothrombotic events in patients with acute myocardial infarction. *Circulation*, **109**, 3171–3175.

37 van Werkum, J.W., Bouman, H.J., Breet, N.J., Ten Berg, J.M., and Hackeng, C.M. (2010) The cone-and-plate(let) analyzer is not suitable to monitor clopidogrel therapy: a comparison with the flowcytometric VASP assay and optical aggregometry. *Thrombosis Research*, **126**, 44–49.

38 Bouman, H.J., Parlak, E., van Werkum, J.W. *et al.* (2010) Which platelet function test is suitable to monitor clopidogrel responsiveness? A pharmacokinetic analysis on the active metabolite of clopidogrel. *Journal of Thrombosis and Haemostasis*, **8**, 482–488.

39 Shenkman, B., Savion, N., Dardik, R., Tamarin, I., and Varon, D. (2000) Testing of platelet deposition on polystyrene surface under flow conditions by the cone and plate(let) analyzer: role of platelet activation, fibrinogen and von Willebrand factor. *Thrombosis Research*, **99**, 353–361.

40 Osende, J.I., Fuster, V., Lev, E.I. *et al.* (2001) Testing platelet activation with a shear-dependent platelet function test versus aggregation-based tests: relevance for monitoring long-term glycoprotein IIb/IIIa inhibition. *Circulation*, **103**, 1488–1491.

12 Thrombelastography and Other Novel Techniques

Udaya S. Tantry[1], Vijay A. Doraiswamy[3], Glenn Stokken[3], Marvin J. Slepian[3], and Paul A. Gurbel[1,2,4]

[1] Sinai Hospital of Baltimore, Baltimore, MD, USA
[2] Johns Hopkins University School of Medicine, Baltimore, MD, USA
[3] University of Arizona, Tucson, AZ, USA
[4] Duke University School of Medicine, Durham, NC, USA

Recent implementation of user-friendly, point-of-care (POC) and near-POC platelet function assays in translational research studies enhanced interest in the personalized antiplatelet therapy concept [1]. However, these *ex vivo* laboratory assays have limitations. In these assays, platelet function is measured in response to a specific agonist, and therefore, these assays may be adequate to assess pharmacodynamic response to an antiplatelet agent. Secondly, platelet function is measured in the presence of an anticoagulant, completely ignoring the contribution of thrombin and fibrin to thrombotic risk. The generation of thrombin and fibrin plays important roles in the formation of stable clot at the site of vascular injury in the presence of high arterial shear and subsequent ischemic event occurrence. Moreover, the positive predictive value of POC assays in identifying patients destined to have ischemic event occurrences is low, indicating that the assessment of platelet function alone may not be adequate to optimally identify high-risk patients for personalized antiplatelet therapy strategies. Therefore, in addition to the measurement of platelet response to a particular agonist, analyses of thrombin generation and viscoelastic characteristics of platelet–fibrin clot generation may enhance the prognostic value of the functional test.

Thrombelastograph refers to the graphic display produced from measurement of the viscoelastic properties of platelet–fibrin clot generated in the whole blood under conditions of low shear. Viscoelastic properties can be determined by thrombelastography using the TEG (Haemonetics Corp, Braintree, MA, USA) or ROTEM (Tern International GmbH, Munich, Germany) devices. In the TEG assay, the change in clot strength is measured by the rotation of a torsion wire, whereas in the ROTEM assay, it is determined by an optical detector. Thrombelastography has been used extensively to monitor hemostasis during major surgical interventions such as liver transplantations, cardiovascular procedures, trauma, and neurosurgery [2].

In the TEG assay, blood anticoagulated with citrate is recalcified with the addition of calcium chloride and then activated by kaolin.

The kaolin-activated blood is then placed in a cylindrical cup. Fibrin strands in the blood sample during clot formation first link the rotating cylindrical cup to a stationary pin suspended by the torsion wire. Changes in the viscoelasticity of the blood are transmitted to the pin. Pin movement is converted to an electrical signal by a transducer, and the magnitude of the electrical signal generated by the torque is plotted as a function of time [3] (Figure 12.1).

The platelet–fibrin clot assessment is dependent on (i) cellular (mainly platelets) and plasma components (procoagulant and fibrinolytic factors) and (ii) the activity and concentration of coagulation elements. The TEG trace can therefore provide continuous real-time information on the viscoelastic properties of the evolving clot from the time of initial fibrin formation through platelet aggregation, fibrin cross-linkage, and clot strengthening to clot lysis. In this assay, (i) the speed of clot generation,

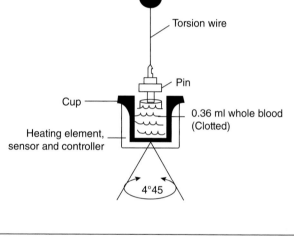

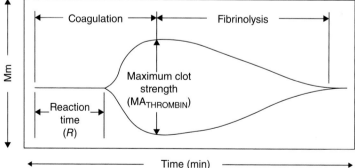

Figure 12.1 Schematic of thrombelastograph system: a torsion wire suspending a pin that is immersed in blood. As the clot forms while the cup is rotated 45°, the pin will rotate depending on the strength of the platelet–fibrin bonds. Signal is discharged continuously that reflects the onset of clotting (reaction time [R]) and the clot strength (MA). (Source: Adapted from Gurbel PA et al., 2005 [3]. Reproduced with permission of Elsevier.)

(ii) its strength, and (iii) its stability are calculated by a computer-generated program (Table 12.1).

However, long sample turnaround time, labor-intensive methodology, complicated data output, and the sensitivity to environmental disturbances (such as vibrations) are major limitations.

It was demonstrated that high maximum thrombin-induced platelet–fibrin clot strength (which is an indicator of "accelerated coagulability" or "hypercoagulability") and high ADP-induced platelet aggregation as measured by conventional aggregometry were risk factors for 6-month

Table 12.1 Thrombelastography-derived parameters.

Reaction time (R value) (minutes)	The time elapsed from the initiation of the test until the point where the onset of clotting provides enough resistance to produce a 2 mm amplitude reading on the TEG tracing
	It is most representative of the initiation phase of enzymatic clotting factors; this is the point at which all other platelet-poor plasma clotting assays are stopped (e.g., PT and aPTT)
K	A measurement of the time interval from the R time to the point where fibrin cross-linking provides enough clot resistance to produce a 20 mm amplitude reading
	It assesses the rapidity of fibrin cross-linking
∝ Angle	The angle formed by the slope of a tangent line traced from the R to the K time measured in degrees. K time and the ∝ angle denote the rate at which the clot strengthens
	It is most representative of thrombin's cleaving of the available fibrinogen into fibrin
Maximum amplitude (mm)	It indicates the point at which clot strength reaches its maximum measure in millimeters on the TEG tracing
	It reflects the end result of maximal platelet–fibrin interaction via the GPIIb/IIIa receptors
G (dynes/cm²)	It is a calculated measure of total clot strength derived from amplitude $(A) G = (5000 \times A)/(100 \times A)$
	Due to its exponential relationship with A, G is a more realistic representation of overall clot strength
	Since G is calculated from the progressive increase of amplitude (clot strength) as the TEG tracing develops, it is inclusive of both platelet and enzymatic contributions to overall clot strength
Delta (Δ)	It is calculated from the difference between R time and the time of initial split point (SP, minutes) of the TEG tracing (R–SP)
	It represents the time interval of greatest clot growth secondary to peak thrombin generation. A measure of enzymatic activity may permit identification of the contributions of platelet reactivity to hypercoagulability in patients who are hypercoagulable by G but with a normal delta
	Delta's linear correlation with TMRTG may allow for better identification of thrombin's contribution to the clot
Split point (SP)	The time elapsed from the initiation of the test until initial fibrin formation
MTRG	Maximum rate of thrombus generation
TMRTG	Time to maximum rate of thrombus generation

post-PCI ischemic events. In that study, high maximum platelet–fibrin clot strength was a better risk discriminator [3]. In the TEG platelet mapping assay, ADP-induced platelet–fibrin clot strength (MA_{ADP}) is used to assess response to $P2Y_{12}$ receptor inhibitors, and arachidonic acid-induced platelet–fibrin clot strength is used to assess response to aspirin (MA_{AA}). A relation between periprocedural MA_{ADP} and maximal thrombin-induced platelet–fibrin clot ($MA_{THROMBIN}$) strength and 3 years ischemic and bleeding event occurrences were also demonstrated [4]. Moreover, TEG-based transfusion algorithms have been demonstrated to reduce transfusion requirements in patients undergoing coronary artery bypass grafting [5, 6, 7]. The addition of $MA_{THROMBIN}$ to an existing risk-prediction model significantly improved the risk stratification for excessive blood loss in patients undergoing on-pump cardiac surgery [5, 6, 7]. The TARGET-CABG study suggested that delays in coronary artery bypass surgery in patients treated with clopidogrel may be reduced by preoperatively measuring MA_{ADP} and timing surgery according to the level of platelet function [8]. These results were corroborated by other studies [9, 10].

Novel techniques

Currently, there are other novel techniques under development that utilize hemodynamics, microfluidics, and nanotechnology principles.

CORA system

The CORA® (COagulation Resonance Analyzer®) instrument is a microfluidic cartridge-based device capable of performing all current TEG assays. It is a fully automated cartridge-based system with all reagents dried in place, replacing the cups and pins and reagent reconstitution of the TEG and thus eliminating potential user errors. In this assay, a disposable cartridge is inserted into the instrument, and blood samples are transferred into the cartridge using a disposable dropper or transfer pipette. There are up to four simultaneous channels per cartridge, and the system requires 280 µL of blood for the platelet mapping assay. Reconstitution of dried reagents within the cartridge is accomplished by moving the sample through reagent wells, under the control of microfluidic valves and bellows within the cartridge. After each sample has been mixed with reagent, it is delivered to a test cell where it can be monitored for changes due to hemostasis. The system performs an automatic electromechanical and pneumatic quality control.

T2 magnetic resonance (T2MR)

The T2 magnetic resonance (T2MR) (http://www.t2biosystems.com/index. asp) assays are in development. The assay is simple and rapid, requiring minimal or no sample preparation and a minimum amount of blood

(2–40 µL). T2MR provides real-time monitoring of platelet reactivity and an assessment of clotting time, fibrinolysis, anticoagulant effects, and hematocrit. During clot formation, the porous nature of the protein and cellular matrix in the clot influence the diffusion of water, and this influence on water diffusion is monitored. Multiple T2 signals arise from different compartments of water within the clotted sample. The T2MR system can be used for antiplatelet monitoring and anticoagulation therapy monitoring.

Shear-induced platelet aggregation assays

Shear-induced platelet aggregation (SIPA) plays a crucial role in the development of arterial thrombotic event occurrences [11]. Shear rates and flow patterns (fluid dynamics factors) affect platelet activation and aggregation. Computational fluid dynamic (CFD) can be used to assess flow-induced platelet activation. Digital particle image velocimetry (DPIV) is a planar optical measurement technique which can provide a means of measuring the velocity of platelets. These measurements can predict platelet activation potential and have correlated with platelet activation experiments conducted in a recirculation flow loop using the platelet activation state (PAS) assay (see succeeding text). It was demonstrated that the elevated flow shear stresses induced by model pathologies might carry platelets beyond their activation threshold, enhancing platelet aggregation and deposition. The DPIV is based on continuous real-time recording of the investigated field and can be used to calculate flow-induced platelet activation level (AL). Using CFD, platelet deposition in streamlined models of stenoses under steady flow can be measured, and numerical simulations to establish an AL parameter based on a summation of the instantaneous product of the shear stress level and exposure time along turbulent trajectories can be performed [12].

Flow-induced platelet activation was measured using the PAS assay, an innovative technique based on the modification of the prothrombinase method, in which acetylated prothrombin is used. The prothrombinase complex assembles on the activated platelet surface in the presence of factor Xa bound to the two essential cofactors provided by activated platelets: factor Va and anionic phospholipids. The thrombin, which is generated in the assay, is a powerful platelet agonist that reactivates the platelets in a positive feedback loop. The acetylated prothrombin reacts with the prothrombinase complex to produce a thrombin species that does not activate platelets. Removing the positive feedback activation results in easily measurable thrombin that accurately reflects the flow-induced procoagulant activity of the platelet. PAS measurements correlate with flow cytometric detection of negative phospholipid exposure measured by annexin V binding [13].

References

1 Gurbel, P.A., Becker, R.C., Mann, K.G., Steinhubl, S.R., and Michelson, A.D. (2007) Platelet function monitoring in patients with coronary artery disease. *Journal of the American College of Cardiology*, **50**, 1822–1834.

2 Hobson, A.R., Agarwala, R.A., Swallow, R.A., Dawkins, K.D., and Curzen, N.P. (2006) Thrombelastography: current clinical applications and its potential role in interventional cardiology. *Platelets*, **17**, 509–518.

3 Gurbel, P.A., Bliden, K.P., Guyer, K. *et al.* (2005) Platelet reactivity in patients and recurrent events post-stenting: results of the PREPARE POSTSTENTING Study. *Journal of the American College of Cardiology*, **46**, 1820–1826.

4 Gurbel, P.A., Bliden, K.P., Navickas, I.A. *et al.* (2010) Adenosine diphosphate-induced platelet-fibrin clot strength: a new thrombelastographic indicator of long-term poststenting ischemic events. American Heart Journal, **160**, 346–354.

5 Nuttall, G.A., Oliver, W.C., Santrach, P.J. *et al.* (2001) Efficacy of a simple intraoperative transfusion algorithm for nonerythrocyte component utilization after cardiopulmonary bypass. Anesthesiology, **94**, 773–781.

6 Shore-Lesserson, L., Manspeizer, H.E., DePerio, M., Francis, S., Vela-Cantos, F., and Ergin, M.A. (1999) Thromboelastography-guided transfusion algorithm reduces transfusions in complex cardiac surgery. *Anesthesia and Analgesia*, **88**, 312–319.

7 Wasowicz, M., McCluskey, S.A., Wijeysundera, D.N. *et al.* (2010) The incremental value of thrombelastography for prediction of excessive blood loss after cardiac surgery: an observational study. *Anesthesia and Analgesia*, **111**, 331–338.

8 Mahla, E., Suarez, T.A., Bliden, K.P. *et al.* (2012) Platelet function measurement-based strategy to reduce bleeding and waiting time in clopidogrel-treated patients undergoing coronary artery bypass graft surgery: the timing based on platelet function strategy to reduce clopidogrel-associated bleeding related to CABG (TARGET-CABG) study. *Circulation. Cardiovascular Interventions*, **5**, 261–269.

9 Chen, L., Bracey, A.W., Radovancevic, R. *et al.* (2004) Clopidogrel and bleeding in patients undergoing elective coronary artery bypass grafting. *Journal of Thoracic and Cardiovascular Surgery*, **128**, 425–431.

10 Kwak, Y.L., Kim, J.C., Choi, Y.S., Yoo, K.-J., Song, Y., and Shim, J.-K. (2010) Clopidogrel responsiveness regardless of the discontinuation date predicts increased blood loss and transfusion requirement after off-pump coronary artery bypass graft surgery. *Journal of the American College of Cardiology*, **56**, 1994–2002.

11 Kim, K., Bae, O.N., Lim, K.M. *et al.* (2012) Novel antiplatelet activity of protocatechuic acid through the inhibition of high shear stress-induced platelet aggregation. *Journal of Pharmacology and Experimental Therapeutics*, **343**, 704–711.

12 Raz, S., Einav, S., Alemu, Y., and Bluestein, D. (2007) DPIV prediction of flow induced platelet activation-comparison to numerical predictions. *Annals of Biomedical Engineering*, **35**, 493–504.

13 Jesty, J. and Bluestein, D. (1999) Acetylated prothrombin as a substrate in the measurement of the procoagulant activity of platelets: elimination of the feedback activation of platelets by thrombin. *Analytical Biochemistry*, **272**, 64–70.

Section III

Antiplatelet Pharmacology

13 Aspirin

Karsten Schrör and Thomas Hohlfeld

UniversitätsKlinikum, Heinrich-Heine Universität Düsseldorf, Düsseldorf, Germany

Aspirin is the first-choice antiplatelet agent in cardiocoronary prevention and an essential constituent of dual antiplatelet therapy. The reasons are its unique pharmacological mode of action; the long-lasting, more than 60 years, experience with its use as an antiplatelet agent; and the reliability of its pharmacological action in more than 95% of patients.

Mode of antiplatelet action

Aspirin, in contrast to most other antiplatelet drugs, is not a platelet-specific agent but exhibits a broad spectrum of biological activities on many cellular targets [1]. At low doses ($\leq$300 mg), aspirin inhibits platelet-dependent prostaglandin-endoperoxide (PGEP) formation via irreversible acetylation of COX-1. This results in downstream inhibition of thromboxane A_2 (TXA_2) formation, the only significant PGEP end product in platelets. This COX-1-mediated inhibition of prostaglandin formation is the generally accepted mode of antiplatelet action of aspirin [2, 3].

Consequently, measurement of platelet-dependent thromboxane formation, for example, by determining thromboxane-forming capacity in serum *ex vivo* or *in vitro*, is a simple and specific means to determine the pharmacological potency of aspirin as an antiplatelet drug on an individual basis. Because of the nonlinearity between thromboxane levels and thromboxane-related platelet stimulation, this inhibition has to be apparently complete, that is, >95% in terms of serum capacity, to become effective. This degree of inhibition is obtained in the vast majority of patients, while only 1–2% remain pharmacologically "resistant" against aspirin. Thus, the much more variable clinical efficacy of aspirin in preventing atherothrombotic cardiovascular events is due to variable environmental conditions of circulating platelets including platelet stimuli, which might or might not require platelet-dependent thromboxane formation as an amplifying event.

Antiplatelet Therapy in Cardiovascular Disease, First Edition. Edited by Ron Waksman, Paul A. Gurbel, and Michael A. Gaglia, Jr.
© 2014 John Wiley & Sons, Ltd. Published 2014 by John Wiley & Sons, Ltd.

Accordingly, the antiplatelet potency of aspirin *in vivo* is critically determined by the significance of thromboxane generation for platelet activation. This largely depends on the stimulus. Aspirin does not modify ADP-induced platelet aggregation and alpha-granule secretion in native blood. Nor does it prevent platelet aggregation induced by thrombin, shear stress, or other thromboxane-independent pathways of platelet activation.

The initial "explosion" of platelet-dependent thromboxane formation after appropriate stimuli starts platelet activation, secretion, and aggregate formation. However, the subcellular targets of thromboxane in platelets and their interactions are still not completely understood. At least theoretically, it is likely that thromboxane *per se* rather acts as a platelet-derived amplification factor for further platelet recruitment and activation than being a direct stimulus for platelet secretion [4, 5]. There is considerable clinical and experimental evidence for aspirin-sensitive, thromboxane-dependent thrombin formation, which occurs at the surface of activated platelets and connects platelet activation with the plasmatic clotting process [6, 7, 8, 9].

Time dependency of inhibition of platelet function by aspirin

If rapid inhibition of platelet function is required, that is, as an emergency first-line treatment in acute coronary syndromes, a loading dose of 250–500 mg soluble aspirin, for example, as lysine salt, can be administered IV. This results in sufficient (≥99%) inhibition of thromboxane formation within 5 min. For oral dosing of 500 mg, at least 40 min is required for a comparable effect [10] (Figure 13.1). After oral

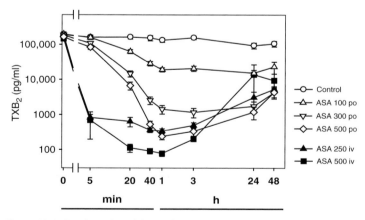

Figure 13.1 Time-dependent inhibition of thromboxane (TXB_2) formation by aspirin, depending on dose (mg) and route of administration. Data were obtained from 21 healthy subjects treated in a crossover design. Note that both axes are in logarithmic scale. (Source: Adapted from Schrör, K 2009 [1]. Reproduced with permission of John Wiley & Sons Ltd.)

administration, more time is necessary to obtain the required pharmacological effect. At least two to three daily doses (e.g., 75–325 mg) of standard aspirin are necessary to obtain sufficient inhibition of thromboxane formation. Once sufficient acetylation is obtained, only a maintenance dose of aspirin per day is necessary.

The inhibition of platelet COX-1 and platelet function by aspirin is functionally antagonized by the 10–15% fresh platelets that enter the circulation every day from the bone marrow. In certain clinical conditions with a more rapid platelet turnover rate, that is, diabetes or extracorporeal circulation, the efficacy and duration of the antiplatelet effect of aspirin might be reduced. A nearly complete recovery of (arachidonic acid-induced) platelet aggregation is seen about 3 days after aspirin withdrawal, but more than 10 days are required to fully restore plasma thromboxane levels [11]. This confirms that a small recovery, that is, 10–15%, even a small recovery of thromboxane formation is sufficient for a functionally significant thromboxane-induced platelet response.

Dose-dependent inhibition of platelet function by aspirin

No other issue in aspirin research has been discussed more intensively than the question of the optimal antithrombotic dose – frequently though not necessarily correct – considered to be equivalent with the antiplatelet dose. Oral single doses of 325, 162, and 75 mg aspirin result in peak plasma aspirin levels of 10.7, 6.8, and 0.3 μM, which are sufficient for inhibition of platelet function [12]. Currently, there is general agreement that daily doses of 100 mg aspirin are sufficient to inhibit platelet-dependent thromboxane formation in most patients. Somewhat higher doses may be required if enteric-coated preparations are used, possibly due to a lower systemic bioavailability of aspirin [13].

The large retrospective meta-analyses of randomized trials by the Antiplatelet Trialists suggest that daily aspirin doses between 75 and 325 mg will have a similar clinical potency with respect to secondary prevention of cardiovascular events. While this might be true, there are large disease-related differences between different groups of patients, and it is not finally established whether the full-spectrum antithrombotic activity of aspirin is seen at the same dose in all patients. It is also not known whether thromboxane-independent actions of aspirin contribute to the clinical outcome, such as inhibition of inflammatory cytokines [14], actions on endothelial function [15, 16], and endothelial NO synthesis [17]. Interestingly, high-dose aspirin (325 mg) in the CURRENT-OASIS 7 trial was associated with improved clinical outcome in dual antiplatelet treatment with clopidogrel [18], while the opposite was seen with ticagrelor and aspirin in the PLATO trial [19].

Negative interactions with other drugs

The platelet COX-1 inhibition by aspirin is initiated by reversible binding of the salicylate group inside the COX-1 channel, bringing the acetyl group in close neighborship to the serine, which has to become acetylated. Pretreatment with other lipophilic agents that can enter the COX channel as well, such as reversible COX-1 inhibitors, like ibuprofen or the analgesic dipyrone [20], will antagonize the antiplatelet effects of aspirin because of interfering with aspirin (salicylate) binding within the substrate channel of COX-1 [21, 22].

Platelets of patients at advanced stages of atherosclerosis bear an enhanced vascular risk, possibly due to the inflammatory conditions of the disease. In this situation, platelets are hyperreactive and might also become less sensitive to antiplatelet drugs. This "high on-treatment platelet reactivity" (HTPR) in case of aspirin might result from nonplatelet sources of PGEP, the immediate precursors of TXA_2, for example, an upregulated COX-2 in vascular endothelial or smooth muscle cells or leukocytes, such as monocytes/macrophages. This allows for transcellular precursor exchange and for platelet COX-1-independent thromboxane formation, which is less sensitive to aspirin [23]. Aspirin will also not antagonize the platelet stimulatory actions of isoprostanes, the nonenzymatic products of lipid peroxidation that bind to the platelet thromboxane receptor [24] and might act synergistically with enzymatically generated TXA_2. Thus, aspirin dosage recommendations, which are based solely on measuring platelet aggregate formation in whole blood assays or platelet-rich plasma of healthy volunteers *ex vivo*, may not apply directly to patients with atherosclerotic diseases and hyperreactive platelets *in vivo* [25].

Positive interactions with other drugs

Aspirin is the only antiplatelet agent in clinical use that solely acts by blocking thromboxane formation, having COX-1 as the molecular target. Therefore, aspirin will act synergistically with all other antiplatelet compounds, including P2Y12 ADP receptor antagonists and antithrombins, and is an essential constituent of treatment with GPIIb/IIIa receptor antagonists in order to block possible outside-in signaling by these compounds.

Positive interactions in terms of enhanced antithrombotic responses are also to be expected by cotreatment with anticoagulants. Because of the risk of bleeding, triple therapy of aspirin, ADP antagonists, and oral anticoagulants is usually restricted only to particular high-risk thrombotic situations, such as atrial fibrillation. The WOEST trial was the first prospective randomized study to show that aspirin can be withdrawn in those patients without elevated thrombotic risk but considerably reduced risk of bleeding [26]. Finally, many cardiovascular drugs that are given to patients with coronary vascular diseases also bear an antiplatelet potential. This includes nitrates, several Ca^{2+}-antagonists of the dihydropyridine group, as well as statins, most notably simvastatin and atorvastatin [27, 28].

Side effects of aspirin in antiplatelet doses

The most significant, mechanism-based side effect of aspirin at antiplatelet doses is a prolonged bleeding time and increased bleeding tendency, most notably in the gastrointestinal tract and CNS. This bleeding risk has to be balanced against the therapeutic benefit, that is, the antithrombotic effect, specifically in case of surgical interventions [1].

References

1 Schrör, K. (2009) Acetylsalicylic Acid. Wiley VCH, Weinheim.

2 Smith, J.B., and Willis, A.L. (1971) Aspirin selectively inhibits prostaglandin production in human platelets. *Nature: New Biology*, **231**, 235–237.

3 FitzGerald, G.A., Oates, J.A., Hawiger, J.A. *et al.* (1983) Endogenous biosynthesis of prostacyclin and thromboxane and platelet function during chronic administration of aspirin in man. *Journal of Clinical Investigation*, **71**, 676–688.

4 Djellas, Y., Antonakis, K., and Le Breton, G.C. (1998) A molecular mechanism for signaling between seven-transmembrane receptors: evidence for a redistribution of G-proteins. *Proceedings of the National Academy of Sciences of the United States of America*, **95**, 10944–10948.

5 Paul, B.Z.S., Jin, J., and Kunapuli, S.P. (1999) Molecular mechanism of thromboxane A_2-induced platelet aggregation. *Journal of Biological Chemistry*, **274**, 29108–29114.

6 Szczeklik, A., Krzanowski, M., Góra, P., and Radwan, J. (1992) Antiplatelet drugs and generation of thrombin in clotting blood. *Blood*, **80**, 2006–2011.

7 Yasu, T., Oshima, S., Imanishi, M. *et al.* (1993) Effects of aspirin on thrombin generation in unstable angina pectoris. *American Journal of Cardiology*, **71**, 1164–1168.

8 Undas, A., Brummel, K., Musial, J., Mann, K.G., and Szczeklik, A. (2001) Blood coagulation at the site of microvascular injury: effects of low-dose aspirin. *Blood*, **98**, 2423–2431.

9 Polzin, A., Rassaf, T., Böhm, A. *et al.* (2013) Aspirin inhibits release of platelet-derived sphingosine-1-phosphate in acute myocardial infarction. *International Journal of Cardiology* **62**, 1725–1726.

10 Nagelschmitz J., Blunk, M. Krätschmar J. *et al.* (2013) Pharmacokinetics and pharmacodynamics of acetylsalicylic acid after intravenous and oral administration to healthy volunteers, *Clinical Pharmacology*, **5**:1–9.

11 Li, C., Hirsh, J., Xie, C., Johnston, M.A., and Eikelboom, J.W. (2012) Reversal of the anti-platelet effect of aspirin and clopidogrel. *Journal of Thrombosis and Haemostasis*; **10** (4), 521–528.

12 Clarke, R., Mayo, G., Price, P., and FitzGerald, G.A. (1991) Suppression of thromboxane A_2 but not of systemic prostacyclin by controlled-release aspirin. *New England Journal of Medicine*, **325**, 1137–1141.

13 Cox, D., Maree, A.O., Dooley, M., Conroy, R., Byrne, M.F., and Fitzgerald, D.J. (2006) Effect of enteric coating on antiplatelet activity of low-dose aspirin in healthy volunteers. *Stroke*, **37**, 2153–2158.

14 Ikonomidis, I., Andreotti, F., Economou, E., Stefanadis, C., Toutouzas, P., and Nihoyannopoulos, P. (1999) Increased proinflammatory cytokines in patients with chronic stable angina and their reduction by aspirin. *Circulation*, **100**, 793–798.

15 Husain, S., Andrews, N.P., Mulcahy, D., Panza, J.A., and Quyyumi, A.A. (1998) Aspirin improves endothelial dysfunction in atherosclerosis. *Circulation*, **97**, 716–720.

16 Noon, J.P., Walker, B.R., Hand, M.F., and Webb, D.J. (1998) Impairment of forearm vasodilatation to acetylcholine in hypercholesterolemia is reversed by aspirin. *Cardiovascular Research*, **38**, 480–484.

17 Taubert, D., Berkels, R., Grosser, N., Schröder, H., Gründemann, D., and Schömig, E. (2004) Aspirin induces nitric oxide release from vascular endothelium: a novel mechanism of action. *British Journal of Pharmacology*, **143**, 159–165.

18 Mehta, S.R., Tanguay, J.F., Eikelboom, J.W. *et al.* (2010) Double-dose versus standard-dose clopidogrel and high-dose versus low-dose aspirin in individuals undergoing percutaneous coronary intervention for acute coronary syndromes (CURRENT-OASIS 7): a randomised factorial trial. *Lancet*, **376**, 1233–1243.

19 Mahaffey, K.W., Wojdyla, D.M., Becker, C.K. *et al.* (2011) Ticagrelor compared with clopidogrel by geographic region in the Platelet Inhibition and Patient Outcome (PLATO) trial. *Circulation*, **124**, 544–554.

20 Polzin, A., Zeus, T., and Schrör, K. (2013) Dipyrone (metamizole) can nullify the antiplatelet effect of aspirin in patients with coronary artery disease. *The Journal of the American College of Cardiology*, **62**, 1725–1726.

21 Catella-Lawson, F., Reilly, M.P., Kapoor, S.C. *et al.* (2001) Cyclooxygenase inhibitors and the antiplatelet effects of aspirin. *New England Journal of Medicine*, **345**, 1809–1817.

22 Hohlfeld, T., Saxena, A., and Schrör, K. (2013) HTPR against aspirin by NSAIDs – pharmacological mechanisms and clinical relevance. *Thrombosis and Haemostasis* , **109**, 825–833.

23 Weber, A.-A. (2004) Aspirin and activated platelets. In: P.B. Curtis-Prior (ed), The Eicosanoids, London. John Wiley and Sons, Ltd., pp. 373–385.

24 Audoly, L.P., Rocca, B., Fabre, J.E. *et al.* (2000) Cardiovascular responses to the isoprostanes iPF(2alpha)-III and iPE(2)-III are mediated via the thromboxane A(2) receptor in vivo. *Circulation*, **101**, 2833–2840.

25 Schrör, K., Huber, K., and Hohlfeld, T. (2011) Functional testing methods for the antiplatelet effect of aspirin. *Biomarkers in Medicine*, **5**, 31–42.

26 Dewilde, W.J., Oirbans, T., Verheugt, F.W. *et al.* (2013) Use of clopidogrel with or without aspirin in patients taking oral anticoagulant therapy and undergoing percutaneous coronary intervention: an open-label, randomised, controlled trial. *Lancet*, **381 (9872)**, 1107–1115.

27 Schrör, K., Löbel, P., and Steinhagen-Thiessen, E. (1989) Simvastatin reduces platelet thromboxane formation and restores normal platelet sensitivity against prostacyclin in type IIa hypercholesterolemia. *Eicosanoids*, **2**, 39–45.

28 Santos, M.T., Fuset, M.P., Ruano, M., Moscardó, A., and Valles, J. (2009) Effect of atorvastatin on platelet thromboxane A2 synthesis in aspirin-treated patients with acute myocardial infarction. *American Journal of Cardiology*, **104**,18–23.

14 Cilostazol

Seung-Whan Lee, Duk-Woo Park, and Seung-Jung Park
University of Ulsan College of Medicine, Asan Medical Center, Seoul,
Republic of Korea

Introduction

Cilostazol (6-[4-(1-cyclohexyl-1H-tetrazol-5-yl)butoxy]-3,4-dihydro-
2(1H)-quinolinone; OPC-13013) (Figure 14.1) is a selective reversible
inhibitor of phosphodiesterase 3 (PDE 3), resulting in increasing cyclic
adenosine monophosphate (cAMP). An increased level of cAMP results in
an elevation of the active form of protein kinase A (PKA), which is closely
related with an inhibition in platelet aggregation. PKA also prevents the
activation of an enzyme (myosin light-chain kinase) that is important in
the contraction of vascular smooth muscle cells, thereby exerting its
vasodilatory effect. This chapter reviews basic pharmacological actions of
cilostazol that might be related to clinical efficacy.

Mode of action of cilostazol

Cilostazol is a selective, reversible phosphodiesterase 3A (PDE 3A)
inhibitor with unique antithrombotic and vasodilatory properties.
Cilostazol is approved for the treatment of intermittent claudication by the
US Food and Drug Administration. The cilostazol does not affect other
types of phosphodiesterase (PDE). However, the local tissue levels of
cilostazol might be higher than the free concentration in plasma because
of the lipophilicity of the drug. Meanwhile, cilostazol does not have an
effect on PDE 1, 2, and 4 at comparable concentrations and only has a
minor effect on PDE 5. Because PDE 3 increases the breakdown of cAMP,
the inhibition of PDE 3 increases the level of cAMP. Since both platelets and
vascular smooth muscle cells contain PDE 3A, pharmacological actions of
cilostazol such as platelet inhibition and vasodilatory effects are associated
with the inhibition of PDE 3 [1]. Recently, the inhibition of adenosine
uptake has been reported to be another pharmacological action of
cilostazol. This leads to enhanced adenosine actions via A1 and A2
receptors. In platelets and vascular cells, A2-mediated increases in cAMP

Antiplatelet Therapy in Cardiovascular Disease, First Edition. Edited by Ron Waksman,
Paul A. Gurbel, and Michael A. Gaglia, Jr.
© 2014 John Wiley & Sons, Ltd. Published 2014 by John Wiley & Sons, Ltd.

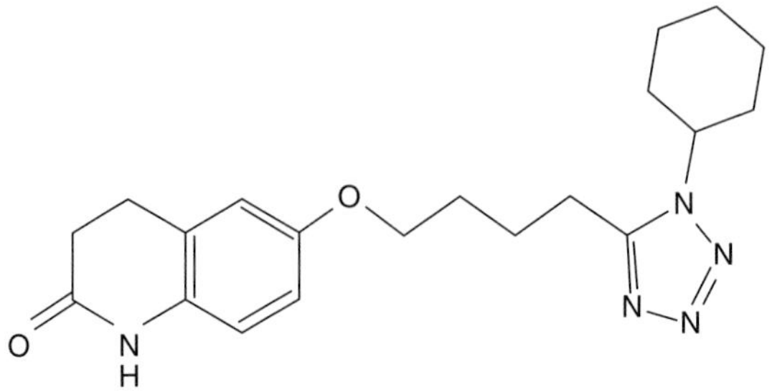

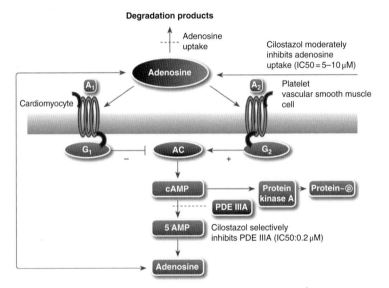

Figure 14.1 Chemical structure of cilostazol.

Figure 14.2 Mechanism of intracellular cAMP control by adenosine and PDE in platelets, vascular smooth muscle cells, and cardiomyocytes. The cAMP levels are controlled by degradation via PDE and by biosynthesis via adenylate cyclase (AC). AC activity in turn is controlled by stimulatory (Gs) and inhibitory (Gi) G-proteins. Adenosine, derived from either cellular metabolism or extracellular sources, activates Gs via A2 receptors and Gi via A1 receptors. This results in either amplification or inhibition of AC.

enhance the consequences of PDE inhibition, that is, result in additional increases in cAMP. In cardiocytes carrying the A1-receptor subtype, there will be a Gi-mediated inhibition of adenylate cyclase with subsequent reduction in cAMP (Figure 14.2). Moreover, cilostazol is a unique agent that operates through its action as endothelium-targeted antithrombotic therapy, achieving its effects by improving endothelial cell function and reducing the number of platelets partially activated by interacting with activated endothelial cells. According to current knowledge, the actions of cilostazol that are most important for its clinical efficacy involve effects on platelets and vascular cells.

Vascular smooth muscle cells

Cilostazol induces cAMP elevation in vascular smooth muscle cells via inhibition of PDE 3-dependent degradation and adenosine (A2)-induced stimulation of cAMP formation (Figure 14.2) [2]. An increased level of cAMP results in an increase in the active form of PKA, which is closely related with an inhibition in platelet aggregation. PKA also prevents the activation of an enzyme (myosin light-chain kinase) that is important in the contraction of vascular smooth muscle cells, thereby exerting its vasodilatory effect. Meanwhile, elevated cAMP inhibits calcium entry and migration, proliferation, and matrix synthesis in smooth muscle cells. Many downstream pathways have been suggested based on *in vitro* studies, including inhibition of [3H] thymidine incorporation into deoxyribonucleic acid (DNA), inhibition of interleukin-6 production, activation of cAMP-dependent PKA, induction of the p53 and p21 antioncogenes and apoptosis, downregulation of p27Kip1, and inhibition of expression of the E2F1, E2F2, and E2F4 proteins [3, 4]. After stent placement, cilostazol inhibits stent-induced P-selectin expression on platelets and upregulates leukocyte Mac-1, thereby inhibiting neointimal growth [5]. In the Cilostazol for REStenosis Trial (CREST), cilostazol showed reduced neointimal hyperplasia and restenosis rate after bare-metal stent implantation [6]. Cilostazol has also been shown to reduce the rate of ISR after drug-eluting stent (DES) implantation. In a group at risk of restenosis (diabetic patients, long-lesion patients), cilostazol was shown to reduce the rate of angiographic restenosis and target lesion revascularization without an increase in severe adverse effects after DES implantation [7, 8]. A recent meta-analysis of the effects of cilostazol in patients treated with both bare-metal stents and DES found that in 2809 patients pooled from 10 different randomized trials, cilostazol reduced late loss by a mean difference of 0.15 mm. Binary angiographic restenosis was also significantly lower in patients treated with cilostazol, regardless of the type of stent used [9].

Endothelial cells

Cilostazol induces elevation of endothelial cAMP via inhibition of PDE 3 degradation and A2-induced stimulation of cAMP formation in endothelial cells. Elevated cAMP stimulates endothelial cell proliferation, reduces expression of adhesion molecules (i.e., vascular cell adhesion molecule-1), inhibits cytokine release and action (monocyte chemoattractant protein-1, platelet-derived growth factor, tumor necrosis factor-α), and inhibits apoptosis; thereby, cilostazol improves endothelial cell function and reduces the number of platelets partially activated by interaction with activated endothelial cells [10, 11]. Furthermore, cilostazol induces nitric oxide (NO) production through endothelial nitric activation via a cAMP/PKA- and PI3K/Akt-dependent mechanism, and this effect is involved in capillary-like tube formation in human aortic endothelial cells [12]. Moreover, cilostazol has a potential anti-inflammatory effect on monocyte–endothelial interactions via upregulation of intracellular cAMP.

Platelets

Platelets exhibit predominant PDE 3 reaction, with subordinate PDE 2 and 5 reaction. Cilostazol elevates cAMP in human platelets via inhibition of PDE 3-dependent degradation at high concentrations. It also potentiates the cAMP-elevating and antiplatelet effects of adenylate cyclase-activating agents (prostaglandin E1 and I2) at a low concentration [3]. Increased cAMP levels facilitate the influx of free calcium ions back into storage granules in the platelets. The free calcium ions are needed for the formation of the glycoprotein IIb/IIIa complex, degranulation of the storage granules containing aggregating substances, and production of thromboxane A2 (Figure 14.3). In animal models, the antiplatelet effect of cilostazol is much stronger than that of aspirin [3]. Furthermore, platelet aggregation induced by adenosine 5′-diphosphate (ADP) or collagen is inhibited in dogs after oral administration of cilostazol [13]. Previous human studies have suggested that cilostazol has similar antiplatelet effects as ticlopidine or clopidogrel but fewer serious adverse side effects [14, 15]. The addition of cilostazol to aspirin and clopidogrel has been shown to provide additional inhibition of platelet activation after coronary stenting [16, 17, 18]. In addition, triple antiplatelet therapy, with aspirin, clopidogrel, and cilostazol, has been found to significantly reduce the rates of 1-month stent thrombosis ($p = 0.024$) after BMS implantation and 1-year stent thrombosis after DES implantation, without increasing the risk of bleeding complications [19, 20].

Heart

Pharmacological actions of cilostazol on the heart are usually related with side effects. PDE 3 inhibitors elevate the cAMP content in cardiocytes, thereby resulting in inotropic and chronotropic effects, but possibly also in arrhythmias. Milrinone, one of the inhibitors of PDE 3, has been reported to have fatal arrhythmias. However, there was no report regarding fatal arrhythmia of cilostazol. The inhibition of adenosine uptake by cilostazol might partly explain this difference. *In vitro*, cilostazol inhibited adenosine uptake into cardiac myocytes, coronary artery smooth muscle cells, and endothelial cells, with a median effective concentration of 10 mM, whereas milrinone was ineffective [21]. This might result from the stimulation of adenosine A1 receptors and might counteract the increase of cAMP via PDE inhibition (Figure 14.2).

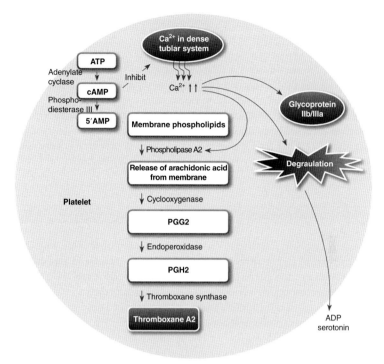

Figure 14.3 Action mechanism of cilostazol in platelets. When the action of PDE 3 in platelets is inhibited by cilostazol, there is an increase in the cAMP levels, which facilitates an influx of free calcium ions back into the storage granules in the platelets. ADP, adenosine diphosphate; ATP, adenosine triphosphate; cAMP, cyclic adenosine monophosphate; PDE 3, phosphodiesterase 3; PG, prostaglandin; PGG2, prostaglandin G2; PGH2, prostaglandin H2.

Brain cells

The antiplatelet and vasodilating effects of cilostazol are believed to underlie its preventive effect on recurrent stroke. In the Cilostazol Stroke Prevention Study in Japan, cilostazol was tested for its effect on secondary prevention of stroke in an extensive randomized, placebo-controlled, double-blind clinical trial of 1052 patients [22]. Cilostazol was found to significantly reduce the relative risk of recurrence of ischemic stroke (41.7%; confidence interval [CI], 9.2–62.5%). Meta-analysis of placebo-controlled trials of 5674 patients also showed similar efficacy of cilostazol for the prevention of stroke (42%; CI, 22–57%) [23]. It is also considered to be effective in promoting recovery from functional damage of the endothelium in cerebral penetrating arterioles. Cilostazol also promotes brain cell survival ascribed to maxi-K channel opening-coupled upregulation of creatinine kinase 2 phosphorylation and downregulation of PTEN phosphorylation, with a resultant increase in phosphorylation of Akt and CREB [24].

Lipid profiles

Cilostazol has also been shown to possess modest hypolipidemic action apart from the antithrombotic effect. Cilostazol reduced plasma triglycerides and raised plasma HDL cholesterol. A placebo-controlled clinical trial showed that after 12 weeks, as compared with placebo, cilostazol 100 mg bid produced a clinically significant reduction in triglycerides of 0.37 mmol/L (15%) and an increase in HDL cholesterol of 0.11 mmol/L (10%). Total cholesterol and LDL cholesterol levels were not significantly changed from baseline in either group at the end of treatment [25].

Pharmacokinetics

Cilostazol is slowly absorbed to reach peak concentration at 2–4 h with a 90% increase in maximum concentration and a 25% increase in area under the curve absorption after a high-fat meal. Therefore, cilostazol should be taken 30 min before or 2 h after meals. Cilostazol 50 mg daily to 100 mg twice daily significantly inhibits platelet aggregation in a dose-dependent fashion, with maximum effect occurring between 3 and 6 h after dosing. Cilostazol is highly plasma protein bound, mostly to albumin. Metabolism of the drug is extensive via the cytochrome P450 isoenzymes, primarily CYP3A4 and, to a lesser extent, CYP2C19. Elimination of cilostazol and its metabolites 3,4-dehydrocilostazol (OPC-13015) and 4′-trans-hydroxy-cilostazol (OPC-13213) depends on renal excretion, with a half-life of 11–13 h, although no dose adjustment is needed in patients with mild to moderate renal insufficiency. In patients with severe renal insufficiency (creatinine clearance < 25 mL/min), caution is necessary, although no dosing adjustment is recommended [26].

There was no difference in protein binding between those with hepatic impairment and healthy individuals (94.6% vs. 95.2%), but patients with hepatic dysfunction had reduced oral cilostazol clearance and total urinary metabolites compared with controls. Overall, however, the pharmacokinetics of cilostazol and its monohydroxy and dehydroxy metabolites were not substantially different in patients with mild to moderate hepatic disease from those measured in healthy individuals [27].

Conclusion

Cilostazol has cAMP-mediated unique pharmacological effects that mainly improve walking performance of patients with lower extremity intermittent claudication. Furthermore, cilostazol could be used for entire vascular therapy in patients with peripheral artery disease, coronary artery disease, and atherosclerotic ischemic stroke via vasodilatory, antiproliferative, hypolipidemic, and antiplatelet/antithrombotic action as well as improved endothelial function.

References

1 Ikeda, Y. (1999) Antiplatelet therapy using cilostazol, a specific PDE3 inhibitor. *Thrombosis and Haemostasis*, **82**, 435–438.

2 Takahashi, S., Oida, K., Fujiwara, R. *et al.* (1992) Effect of cilostazol, a cyclic AMP phosphodiesterase inhibitor, on the proliferation of rat aortic smooth muscle cells in culture. *Journal of Cardiovascular Pharmacology*, **20**, 900–906.

3 Okuda, Y.K.Y., and Yamashita, K. Cilostazol. (1993) *Cardiovascular Drug Reviews*, **11**, 451–465.

4 Lee, K.J., Yun, S.W., Kim, S.W., Kim, T.H., Kim, C.J., and Ryu, W.S. (2004) The effects of cilostazol on proliferation of vascular smooth muscle cells and expression of iNOS and p21. *Korean Circulation Journal*, **34**, 500–506.

5 Inoue, T., Uchida, T., Sakuma, M. *et al.* (2004) Cilostazol inhibits leukocyte integrin Mac-1, leading to a potential reduction in restenosis after coronary stent implantation. *Journal of the American College of Cardiology*, **44**, 1408–1414.

6 Douglas, J.S., Jr, Holmes, D.R., Jr, Kereiakes, D.J. *et al.* (2005) Coronary stent restenosis in patients treated with cilostazol. *Circulation*, **112**, 2826–2832.

7 Lee, S.W., Park, S.W., Kim, Y.H. *et al.* (2008) Drug-eluting stenting followed by cilostazol treatment reduces late restenosis in patients with diabetes mellitus: the DECLARE-DIABETES trial (A Randomized Comparison of Triple Antiplatelet Therapy with Dual Antiplatelet Therapy After Drug-Eluting Stent Implantation in Diabetic Patients). *Journal of the American College of Cardiology*, **51**, 1181–1187.

8 Lee, S.W., Park, S.W., Kim, Y.H. *et al.* (2007) Comparison of triple versus dual antiplatelet therapy after drug-eluting stent implantation (from the DECLARE-Long trial). *The American Journal of Cardiology*, **100**, 1103–1108.

9 Tamhane, U., Meier, P., Chetcuti, S. *et al.* (2009) Efficacy of cilostazol in reducing restenosis in patients undergoing contemporary stent based PCI: a meta-analysis of randomised controlled trials. *EuroIntervention*, **5**, 384–393.

10 Kim, M.J., Lee, J.H., Park, S.Y. *et al.* (2006) Protection from apoptotic cell death by cilostazol, phosphodiesterase type III inhibitor, via cAMP-dependent protein kinase activation. *Pharmacological Research*, **54**, 261–267.

11 Nishio, Y., Kashiwagi, A., Takahara, N., Hidaka, H., and Kikkawa, R. (1997) Cilostazol, a cAMP phosphodiesterase inhibitor, attenuates the production of monocyte chemoattractant protein-1 in response to tumor necrosis factor-alpha in vascular endothelial cells. *Hormone and Metabolic Research*, **29**, 491–495.

12 Hashimoto, A., Miyakoda, G., Hirose, Y., and Mori, T. (2006) Activation of endothelial nitric oxide synthase by cilostazol via a cAMP/protein kinase A- and phosphatidylinositol 3-kinase/Akt-dependent mechanism. *Atherosclerosis*, **189**, 350–357.

13 Kimura, Y., Tani, T., Kanbe, T., and Watanabe, K. (1985) Effect of cilostazol on platelet aggregation and experimental thrombosis. *Arzneimittel-Forschung*, **35**, 1144–1149.

14 Park, S.W., Lee, C.W., Kim, H.S., *et al.* (1999) Comparison of cilostazol versus ticlopidine therapy after stent implantation. *The American Journal of Cardiology*, **84**, 511–514.

15 Lee, S.W., Park, S.W., Hong, M.K. *et al.* (2005) Comparison of cilostazol and clopidogrel after successful coronary stenting. *The American Journal of Cardiology*, **95**, 859–862.

16 Ahn, J.C., Song, W.H., Kwon, J.A. *et al.* (2004) Effects of cilostazol on platelet activation in coronary stenting patients who already treated with aspirin and clopidogrel. *The Korean Journal of Internal Medicine*, **19**, 230–236.

17 Lee, B.K., Lee, S.W., Park, S.W. *et al.* (2007) Effects of triple antiplatelet therapy (aspirin, clopidogrel, and cilostazol) on platelet aggregation and P-selectin expression in patients undergoing coronary artery stent implantation. *The American Journal of Cardiology*, **100**, 610–614.

18 Angiolillo, D.J., Capranzano, P. and Goto, S. *et al.* (2008) A randomized study assessing the impact of cilostazol on platelet function profiles in patients with diabetes mellitus and coronary artery disease on dual antiplatelet therapy: results of the OPTIMUS-2 study. *European Heart Journal*, **29**, 2202–2211.

19 Lee, S.W., Park, S.W., Hong, M.K. *et al.* (2005) Triple versus dual antiplatelet therapy after coronary stenting: impact on stent thrombosis. *Journal of the American College of Cardiology*, **46**, 1833–1837.

20 Lee, S.W., Park, S.W., Yun, S.C. *et al.* (2010) Triple antiplatelet therapy reduces ischemic events after drug-eluting stent implantation: Drug-Eluting stenting followed by Cilostazol treatment REduces Adverse Serious cardiac Events (DECREASE registry). *American Heart Journal*, **159**, 284–291.

21 Cone, J., Wang, S., Tandon, N. *et al.* (1999) Comparison of the effects of cilostazol and milrinone on intracellular cAMP levels and cellular function in platelets and cardiac cells. *Journal of Cardiovascular Pharmacology*, **34**, 497–504.

22 Gotoh, F., Tohgi, H., Hirai, S. *et al.* (2000) Cilostazol Stroke Prevention Study: a placebo-controlled double-blind trial for secondary prevention of cerebral infarction. *Journal of Stroke and Cerebrovascular Diseases*, **9**, 147–157.

23 Uchiyama, S., Demaerschalk, B.M., Goto, S. *et al.* (2009) Stroke prevention by cilostazol in patients with atherothrombosis: meta-analysis of placebo-controlled randomized trials. *Journal of Stroke and Cerebrovascular Diseases*, **18**, 482–490.

24 Hong, K.W., Lee, J.H., Kima, K.Y., Park, S.Y., and Lee, W.S. (2006) Cilostazol: therapeutic potential against focal cerebral ischemic damage. *Current Pharmaceutical Design*, **12**, 565–573.

25 Elam, M.B., Heckman, J., Crouse, J.R. *et al.* (1998) Effect of the novel antiplatelet agent cilostazol on plasma lipoproteins in patients with intermittent claudication. *Arteriosclerosis, Thrombosis, and Vascular Biology*, **18**, 1942–1947.

26 Schror, K. The pharmacology of cilostazol. (2002) *Diabetes, Obesity & Metabolism*, **2**, S14–S19.

27 Bramer, S.L. and Forbes, W.P. (1999) Effect of hepatic impairment on the pharmacokinetics of a single dose of cilostazol. *Clinical Pharmacokinetics*, **37** (Suppl. 2), 25–32.

15 Abciximab

J. Emilio Exaire[1] and Jorge F. Saucedo[2]
[1]The University of Oklahoma Health Sciences Center, Oklahoma City, OK, USA
[2]NorthShore Medical Group, Evanston, IL, USA

The glycoprotein (GP)IIb/IIIa receptor is an integrin protein with binding domains on both the exterior of the cell and the cytoplasm; thus, its activation interacts with external adhesion ligands and cytoskeletal proteins. This receptor is highly expressed on the platelets (approximately 80,000 receptors per platelet) [1], making it a natural target for platelet inhibition. Platelet adhesion is started by active platelet surface receptors interacting with subendothelial proteins (e.g., von Willebrand factor and collagen). This initial interaction creates a layer of platelets that recruit additional platelets primarily by the activation of the GPIIb/IIIa receptor. This pivotal role mediating platelet–platelet interaction represents the final common pathway for platelet aggregation [2].

GP inhibitors block the binding of fibrinogen to GPIIb/IIIa receptors blocking the thrombus formation by preventing platelet aggregation. The chimeric 7E3 Fab half murine, half human fragment (abciximab) inhibits the clot formation by blocking platelet aggregation when 80% of receptor blockade is achieved [3, 4]. Abciximab has been used extensively in clinical trials establishing its efficacy, safety, and broad applicability as adjunct to percutaneous coronary intervention (PCI). The instrumentation of the coronary artery causes plaque rupture, vascular thrombosis, and platelet activation [5] potentially triggering thrombotic complications. The use of abciximab in PCI has helped reduce periprocedural ischemic complications and in some high-risk cohorts even mortality [6, 7]. However, most of the studies were performed in the era before the widespread use of prolonged oral dual antiplatelet therapy (DAPT), and therefore, the patterns of abciximab use have drastically changed in the current PCI era. Furthermore, cost concerns and the availability of powerful oral antiplatelet such as clopidogrel, prasugrel, or ticagrelor [8, 9] that offer robust platelet inhibition have limited abciximab and other GPIIb/IIIa inhibitor use. Nevertheless, the current ACC/AHA/SCAI Guidelines recommend the use of abciximab (either systemic or intracoronary) in patients with ST-segment-elevation myocardial infarction (STEMI) (class IIa and IIb, respectively) and in

Antiplatelet Therapy in Cardiovascular Disease, First Edition. Edited by Ron Waksman, Paul A. Gurbel, and Michael A. Gaglia, Jr.
© 2014 John Wiley & Sons, Ltd. Published 2014 by John Wiley & Sons, Ltd.

patients with unstable angina/non-ST-segment-elevation myocardial infarction (NSTEMI) with high-risk features (e.g., elevated troponins) with or without clopidogrel pretreatment (class I and IIa, respectively); in patients with stable CAD, it yields a class IIa indication for those patients not pretreated with clopidogrel and a IIb indication for patients pretreated with clopidogrel and unfractionated heparin.

Abciximab in PCI: The EPIC, EPILOG, and EPISTENT trials

The EPIC trial [10] tested the effect of abciximab in patients undergoing high-risk coronary angioplasty. The primary 30-day end point was a composite of death, nonfatal myocardial infarction (MI), unplanned surgical revascularization, unplanned repeat percutaneous procedure, unplanned implantation of a coronary stent, or insertion of an intra-aortic balloon pump for refractory ischemia. There was a 35% reduction in the primary end point (12.8% vs. 8.3%, $P = 0.008$) in patients randomized to the bolus plus infusion group and a 10% reduction in the bolus alone group (12.8% vs. 11.5%, $P = 0.43$). However, there was an increase in bleeding episodes and transfusions (7% vs. 14%, $p < 0.0001$). Most of the events were at the vascular access site, and they were deemed to be secondary to the lack of use of weight-adjusted heparin therapy. Thus, the follow-up to this study was the EPILOG trial [11] that randomly assigned patients undergoing urgent or elective PCI to receive abciximab with standard-dose, weight-adjusted heparin (bolus of 100 U/kg); abciximab with low-dose, weight-adjusted heparin (70 U/kg); or placebo with standard-dose, weight-adjusted heparin. The primary 30-day end point was a composite of death, MI, or urgent revascularization. The event rate was 11.7% versus 5.2% in the abciximab with low-dose heparin (HR, 0.43 [95% CI, 0.30–0.60; $P < 0.001$]) and 5.4% in the abciximab with standard-dose heparin (HR, 0.45 [95% CI, 0.32–0.63; $P < 0.001$]). There were no differences in the risk of major bleeding, although minor bleeding was more frequent among patients receiving abciximab with standard-dose heparin. The next large interventional trial with abciximab was the EPISTENT trial [12] that tested the contemporary use of bare metal stents in patients randomly assigned to stenting plus placebo, stenting plus abciximab, or balloon angioplasty plus abciximab. The primary 30-day composite end point included death, MI, or need for urgent revascularization. The primary end point occurred in 10.8% versus 5.3% of the abciximab group (HR, 0.48 [95% CI, 0.33–0.69; $p < 0.001$]) and 6.9% in the balloon plus abciximab group (HR, 0.63 [0.45–0.88]; $p = 0.007$). Major bleeding occurred in 2.2% of the placebo-assigned patients, 1.5% in stent plus abciximab group, and 1.4% in balloon angioplasty plus abciximab group ($p = 0.38$). These results validated the use of abciximab in a widespread group of patients with or without the use of stents in the era before the widespread use of ticlopidine or clopidogrel.

Abciximab in acute coronary syndromes: CAPTURE, RAPPORT, ADMIRAL, CADILLAC, and INFUSE-AMI trials

The CAPTURE trial [13] randomized patients with refractory unstable angina who were undergoing PCI to abciximab or placebo 18–24 h before PCI continuing until 1 h afterward. The trial was prematurely stopped due to the positive results. The primary 30-day end point was the occurrence of death, MI, or urgent intervention for recurrent ischemia. The primary end point occurred in 15.9% versus 11.3% of patients who received abciximab ($p = 0.012$). Major bleeding occurred more often with abciximab than with placebo (3.8% vs. 1.9%, $p = 0.043$). The RAPPORT trial [14] randomized patients with acute myocardial infarction (AMI) of <12 h to placebo or abciximab. The primary end point was death, reinfarction, or any target vessel revascularization (TVR) at 6 months. There was no difference in the incidence of the primary 6-month end point; however, abciximab significantly reduced the incidence of death, reinfarction, or urgent TVR at all time points assessed (9.9% vs. 3.3%, $P = 0.003$, at 7 days; 11.2% vs. 5.8%, $P = 0.03$, at 30 days; and 17.8% vs. 11.6%, $P = 0.05$, at 6 months). The need for unplanned stenting was reduced by 42% in the abciximab group. However, major bleeding occurred significantly more frequently in the abciximab group (16.6% vs. 9.5%, $P = 0.02$). The ADMIRAL trial [15] randomly assigned 300 patients with AMI to either abciximab plus stenting or placebo plus stenting before the angiography. At 30 days, the primary composite end point of death, reinfarction, or urgent revascularization occurred in 14.6% versus 6% ($P = 0.01$). The benefit was sustained at 6 months (15.9% vs. 7.4%, $P = 0.02$). More recently, the CADILLAC trial [16] randomly assigned 2082 patients with AMI to undergo PTCA alone, PTCA plus abciximab, stenting alone, or stenting plus abciximab. At 6 months, the primary combined end point was 20% in the PTCA group, 16.5% in the PTCA plus abciximab group, 11.5% after stenting, and 10.2% after stenting plus abciximab ($P < 0.001$). The difference in the incidence of the primary end point was due entirely to TVR. This study did not focus on 30-day outcomes, making it difficult to analyze the acute benefit of abciximab that had been seen in all previous studies.

Currently, abciximab has been tested in intracoronary infusion rather than systemic administration in the context of AMI. The INFUSE-AMI trial [17] tested two strategies to reduce distal embolization: intracoronary abciximab versus manual aspiration thrombectomy. Patients with anterior AMI within 4 h of presentation were randomized to either strategy. All patients received anticoagulation with bivalirudin. The primary end point (infarct size as measured per percentage of total left ventricular mass at 30 days) showed a significant reduction in infarct size in the abciximab-treated group (15.1% [IQR, 6.8–22.7%] vs. 17.9% [IQR, 10.3–25.4%], $P = 0.03$).

Head-to-head GPIIb/IIIa trial, noninferiority trials using abciximab versus bivalirudin, and the ISAR-REACT trials

The TARGET trial [18] remains the only well-powered head-to-head study comparing two GPIIb/IIIa inhibitors. It randomized patients in a double-blind, double-dummy fashion to either tirofiban or abciximab before undergoing PCI. The primary end point was a 30-day composite of death, nonfatal MI, or urgent TVR. The primary end point occurred more frequently among the patients in the tirofiban group (7.6% vs. 6.0% [HR, 1.26; one-sided 95% CI, 1.51], demonstrating lack of equivalence, and two-sided 95% CI of 1.01–1.57, demonstrating superiority of abciximab, $P = 0.038$). The relative benefit of abciximab was consistent regardless of age, sex, diabetes, or pretreatment with clopidogrel. There were no significant differences in the rates of major bleeding complications or transfusions, but tirofiban was associated with a lower rate of minor bleeding episodes and thrombocytopenia.

The use of bivalirudin with bailout GPIIb/IIIa if needed versus a strategy of abciximab plus heparin was tested in the REPLACE-2 trial [19]. This was a randomized, double-blind noninferiority trial in stable patients undergoing PCI. Patients were randomized to receive bivalirudin with provisional abciximab or eptifibatide or heparin with planned GPIIb/IIIa inhibition. Both groups received daily aspirin and a thienopyridine for at least 30 days after PCI. The primary composite end point was 30-day incidence of death, MI, urgent repeat revascularization, or inhospital major bleeding. The primary composite end point was 9.2% versus 10% (OR, 0.92; 95% CI, 0.77–1.09; $P = 0.32$). Inhospital major bleeding rates were significantly reduced by bivalirudin (2.4% vs. 4.1%, $P < 0.001$).

The ISAR-REACT study [20] tested the adjunct pretreatment with clopidogrel in elective PCI patients that received abciximab versus placebo. Patients were pretreated with a 600 mg dose of clopidogrel at least 2 h before the procedure. The 30-day composite primary end point included death, MI, and urgent TVR. The primary end point was identical in both groups (4% vs. 4% [RR, 1.05; 95% CI, 0.69–1.59; $P = 0.82$]). Thus, abciximab had no clinical benefit in low-to-intermediate risk patients undergoing PCI. However, the ISAR-REACT 2 [21] addressed the role of abciximab in a higher risk of ACS patients undergoing after pretreatment with 600 mg of clopidogrel. Patients were randomized to receive abciximab plus heparin or placebo plus heparin. The primary composite 30-day end point included death, MI, or urgent TVR. The primary end point was reached in 8.9% versus 11.9% favoring abciximab infusion (RR, 0.75 [95% CI, 0.58–0.97; $P = 0.03$]). This difference was more relevant in patients with elevated troponin levels. There were no significant differences regarding major bleeding. The ISAR-REACT 4 study [22] randomized NSTEMI patients to receive abciximab plus unfractionated heparin or bivalirudin. All patients received a 600 mg bolus of clopidogrel at least 2 h before the PCI. The primary 30-day composite end point (death, large recurrent MI, urgent vessel revascularization, or major bleeding) occurred in 10.9% versus 11% in the bivalirudin group ($P = 0.94$). Major bleeding occurred in 4.6% versus 2.6% in the bivalirudin group. Hence, the benefit of abciximab plus heparin appears to be less relevant after optimal pretreatment with clopidogrel in patients with NSTEMI treated with bivalirudin alone.

Conclusions

Despite the initial favorable data in the pre-DAPT, the use of abciximab has decreased with the appearance of powerful direct antithrombins and oral antiplatelet agents. The current indications supported by the Guidelines continue to encourage the use of abciximab and other GPIIb/IIIa inhibitors in the current PCI era.

References

1 Wagner, C.L., Mascelli, M.A., Neblock, D.S., Weisman, H.F., Coller, B.S., and Jordan, R.E. (1996) Analysis of GPIIb/IIIa receptor number by quantification of 7E3 binding to human platelets. *Blood*, **88 (3)**, 907–914.

2 Fernandez-Ortiz, A., Badimon, J.J., Falk, E. *et al.* (1994) Characterization of the relative thrombogenicity of atherosclerotic plaque components: implications for consequences of plaque rupture. *Journal of the American College of Cardiology*, **23 (7)**, 1562–1569.

3 Coller, B.S., Folts, J.D., Smith, S.R., Scudder, L.E., and Jordan, R. (1989) Abolition of in vivo platelet thrombus formation in primates with monoclonal antibodies to the platelet GPIIb/IIIa receptor. Correlation with bleeding time, platelet aggregation, and blockade of GPIIb/IIIa receptors. *Circulation*, **80 (6)**, 1766–1774.

4 Coller, B.S., Scudder, L.E., Beer, J. *et al.* (1991) Monoclonal antibodies to platelet glycoprotein IIb/IIIa as antithrombotic agents. *Annals of the New York Academy of Sciences*, **614**, 193–213.

5 Steele, P.M., Chesebro, J.H., Stanson, A.W. *et al.* (1985) Balloon angioplasty. *Natural history of the pathophysiological response to injury in a pig model.* *Circulation Research*, **57 (1)**, 105–112.

6 Winchester, D.E., Wen, X., Brearley, W.D., Park, K.E., David Anderson, R., and Bavry, A.A. (2011) Efficacy and safety of glycoprotein IIb/IIIa inhibitors during elective coronary revascularization: a meta-analysis of randomized trials performed in the era of stents and thienopyridines. *Journal of the American College of Cardiology*, **57 (10)**, 1190–1199.

7 De Luca, G., Suryapranata, H., Stone, G.W. *et al.* (2005) Abciximab as adjunctive therapy to reperfusion in acute ST-segment elevation myocardial infarction: a meta-analysis of randomized trials. *JAMA*, **293 (14)**, 1759–1765.

8 Wallentin, L., Becker, R.C., Budaj, A. *et al.* (2009) Ticagrelor versus clopidogrel in patients with acute coronary syndromes. *The New England Journal of Medicine*, **361 (11)**, 1045–1057.

9 Wiviott, S.D., Braunwald, E. *et al.* (2007) Prasugrel versus clopidogrel in patients with acute coronary syndromes. *The New England Journal of Medicine*, **357 (20)**, 2001–2015.

10 Anonymous (1994) Use of a monoclonal antibody directed against the platelet glycoprotein IIb/IIIa receptor in high-risk coronary angioplasty. The EPIC Investigation. *New England Journal of Medicine*, **330 (14)**, 956–961.

11 The EPILOG, I. (1997) Platelet glycoprotein IIb/IIIa receptor blockade and low-dose heparin during percutaneous coronary revascularization. *New England Journal of Medicine*, **336 (24)**, 1689–1696.

12 EPISTENT Investigators. (1998) Randomised placebo-controlled and balloon-angioplasty-controlled trial to assess safety of coronary stenting with use of platelet glycoprotein-IIb/IIIa blockade. *Lancet*, **352** (9122), 87–92.

13 Anonymous (1997) Randomised placebo-controlled trial of abciximab before and during coronary intervention in refractory unstable angina: the CAPTURE Study. *Lancet*, **349 (9063)**, 1429–1435.

14 Brener, S.J., Barr, L.A., Burchenal, J.E. *et al.* (1998) Randomized, placebo-controlled trial of platelet glycoprotein IIb/IIIa blockade with primary angioplasty for acute myocardial infarction. ReoPro and Primary PTCA Organization and Randomized Trial (RAPPORT) Investigators. *Circulation*, **98 (8)**, 734–741.

15 Montalescot, G., Barragan, P., Wittenberg, O. *et al.* (2001) Platelet glycoprotein IIb/IIIa inhibition with coronary stenting for acute myocardial infarction. *The New England Journal of Medicine*, **344 (25)**, 1895–1903.

16 Stone, G.W., Grines, C.L., Cox, D.A. *et al.* (2002) Comparison of angioplasty with stenting, with or without abciximab, in acute myocardial infarction. *The New England Journal of Medicine*, **346 (13)**, 957–966.

17 Stone, G.W., Maehara, A., Witzenbichler, B. *et al.* (2012) Intracoronary abciximab and aspiration thrombectomy in patients with large anterior myocardial infarction: the INFUSE-AMI randomized trial. *JAMA*, **307 (17)**, 1817–1826.

18 Topol, E.J., Moliterno, D.J., Herrmann, H.C. *et al.* (2001) Comparison of two platelet glycoprotein IIb/IIIa inhibitors, tirofiban and abciximab, for the prevention of ischemic events with percutaneous coronary revascularization. *The New England Journal of Medicine*, **344 (25)**, 1888–1894.

19 Lincoff, A.M., Bittl, J.A., Harrington, R.A. *et al.* (2003) Bivalirudin and provisional glycoprotein IIb/IIIa blockade compared with heparin and planned glycoprotein IIb/IIIa blockade during percutaneous coronary intervention: REPLACE-2 randomized trial. *JAMA*, **289 (7)**, 853–863.

20 Kastrati, A., Mehilli, J., Schühlen, H. *et al.* (2004) A clinical trial of abciximab in elective percutaneous coronary intervention after pretreatment with clopidogrel. *The New England Journal of Medicine*, **350 (3)**, 232–238.

21 Kastrati, A., Mehilli, J., Neumann, F.J. *et al.* (2006) Abciximab in patients with acute coronary syndromes undergoing percutaneous coronary intervention after clopidogrel pretreatment: the ISAR-REACT 2 randomized trial. *JAMA*, **295 (13)**, 1531–1538.

22 Kastrati, A., Neumann, F.J., Schulz, S. *et al.* (2011) Abciximab and heparin versus bivalirudin for non-ST-elevation myocardial infarction. *The New England Journal of Medicine*, **365 (21)**, 1980–1989.

16 Tirofiban

Marco Valgimigli[1], Arnoud W.J. van't Hof[2], and Christian Hamm[3]
[1] Thoraxcenter, Erasmus Medical Center, Rotterdam, The Netherlands
[2] Isala Academy, Isala Klinieken, Zwolle, The Netherlands
[3] Kerckhoff Heart and Thorax Center, Bad Nauheim, Germany

Introduction

Platelet reactivity plays a pivotal role in the pathogenesis of ischemic cardiovascular disorders. Among the proposed pharmacological targets for antiplatelet therapy, the glycoprotein IIb/IIIa (GPIIb/IIIa) continues to be a very attractive pathway as it represents the common final mechanism, which leads to platelet aggregation. The GPIIb/IIIa receptor binds several substrates, most notably fibrinogen, which forms a bridge between platelets, directly mediating aggregation. GPIIb/IIIa is the most abundant GP on the platelet surface; however, in the inactivated state, approximately 70% of GPIIb/IIIa complexes are distributed on the surface of the platelet, while the remaining receptors remain stealth [1]. Following platelet activation, the number of GPIIb/IIIa receptors on the cell surface increases exponentially. GPIIb/IIIa inhibitors, which include abciximab, tirofiban, and eptifibatide, selectively block the GPIIb/IIIa receptor on the surface of the platelet thus preventing the binding of fibrinogen to the receptor and have been regarded as the most potent inhibitors of platelet activity [2]. The first agent in this class introduced to clinical practice was abciximab, a chimeric human–murine monoclonal antibody Fab fragment (c7E3) [2].

Tirofiban

Tirofiban is a potent GPIIb/IIIa inhibitor that has been well studied and used clinically in a variety of settings including STEMI, non-ST-segment-elevation acute coronary syndromes (NSTE-ACS), and elective procedures. Similar to abciximab, tirofiban is a competitive GPIIb/IIIa inhibitor with high specificity and affinity for the GPIIb/IIIa receptor [3]. Unlike abciximab, tirofiban is a small-molecule, nonpeptide tyrosine derivative [4]. Tirofiban further differs from abciximab in that it dissociates from the GPIIb/IIIa receptor relatively rapidly and, with a half-life of 2–4 h, therefore is reversed within hours after the completion

Antiplatelet Therapy in Cardiovascular Disease, First Edition. Edited by Ron Waksman, Paul A. Gurbel, and Michael A. Gaglia, Jr.
© 2014 John Wiley & Sons, Ltd. Published 2014 by John Wiley & Sons, Ltd.

of the infusion [4]. Abciximab rather binds irreversibly to the IIb/IIIa receptor producing an effect that persists for the lifespan of the platelet [5]. Such reversibility may have significant implications with regard to bleeding, particularly in patients who require the need for emergent coronary artery bypass graft surgery.

Dosing of tirofiban

The dosing of tirofiban has evolved over time. It has been established that different dosing regimens may be required based on the patient's diagnosis and the timing of percutaneous coronary intervention (PCI). A regimen utilizing a loading infusion of 0.4 µg/kg/min run over 30 min followed by a 0.10 µg/kg/min maintenance infusion has proven quite effective in the management of patients with NSTE-ACS when administered at least 4 h prior to PCI [6, 7, 8]. Studies conducted in similar patient populations who rather than receiving tirofiban prior to PCI were administered immediately prior to PCI [9, 10] employed a dosing regimen including a bolus of 10 µg/kg administered over 3 min followed by an infusion of 0.15 µg/kg/min. Given the benefit seen with the upstream dosing regimen, one might assume that this dose would achieve adequate platelet inhibition even when administered immediately prior to initiation of PCI. Yet, results of such studies were not as favorable for tirofiban, revealing an increase in clinical events as compared to abciximab [10]. Follow-up studies have suggested that a higher incidence of myocardial infarction (MI) after PCI seen in these studies was likely due to suboptimal platelet inhibition from 15 to 60 min after onset of treatment [11]. These studies also indicated that this suboptimal platelet inhibition could be overcome by a regimen including a higher-dose bolus of tirofiban (25 µg/kg) and revealed that a high-dose bolus of tirofiban results in a level of platelet inhibition necessary for coronary intervention [12]. Therefore, a regimen using a 25 µg/kg bolus dose of tirofiban followed by a maintenance infusion of 0.15 µg/kg/min (high-dose bolus regimen) is considered more appropriate when administration immediately prior to PCI is warranted.

Likewise, a high-dose bolus regimen of tirofiban may potentially induce a potent effect on platelets as compared to abciximab. When platelet inhibition was compared in 112 STEMI patients who were either administered the standard dose of abciximab or one of two doses of tirofiban (10 µg/kg bolus or the regimen or the high-dose bolus regimen), mean periprocedural platelet inhibition exceeding 80% was seen only with the high-dose tirofiban regimen [13]. A separate study involving 66 patients with STEMI undergoing PCI provided comparable results [14]. The high-dose bolus regimen of tirofiban produced significantly higher levels of platelet inhibition than abciximab when measured immediately after PCI 30, 60, and 120 min. Given its similar effect on platelet function to abciximab, tirofiban administered using the high-dose bolus regimen may indeed be considered a beneficial cost-effective alternative for abciximab in patients suffering from thrombus-containing lesion undergoing PCI.

Tirofiban in STEMI

The utility of tirofiban in patients with STEMI has been investigated in several trials (Table 16.1). These studies have included assessment of both the 10 μg/kg bolus and high-dose bolus regimens. Furthermore, the effects of tirofiban were analyzed when administered early as well as immediately prior to primary PCI, in patients receiving or not receiving concomitant P2Y12 inhibition with clopidogrel or recently with prasugrel.

Early administration of tirofiban: High-dose bolus regimen

The Ongoing Tirofiban in Myocardial Infarction Evaluation (On-TIME) 2 trial [15], a placebo-controlled, multicenter, international randomized trial involving 984 patients with STEMI diagnosed in the ambulance or at a referral center, was the first study to determine the benefits of prehospital administration of tirofiban at the high-dose bolus regimen on top of dual antiplatelet therapy measured by ST-segment deviation resolution. Treatment was initiated in the ambulance or at the referral center. All patients received aspirin, high loading dose of clopidogrel (600 mg), heparin 5000 IU, and either tirofiban or placebo. Study drug was initiated at a median of 76 min after symptom onset and 55 min prior to angiography/PCI. Figure 16.1 summarizes the cumulative residual ST-segment deviation over the period of time from diagnosis until 60 min post PCI. At the time of arrival to the PCI center, patients treated with tirofiban had significantly lower cumulative residual ST-segment deviation as compared to those who received placebo (10.9 ± 9.2 mm vs. 12.1 ± 9.4 mm, $P = 0.028$) [15]. Moreover, ST-segment resolution prior to PCI occurred significantly more often in the tirofiban arm ($P = 0.041$ for trend). The cumulative residual ST deviation 1 h post PCI (primary end point) was 3.6 ± 4.6 mm for the tirofiban group versus 4.8 ± 6.3 mm in the no tirofiban (or placebo) group ($P = 0.003$). Additionally, the percentage of patients with more than 3 mm residual ST-segment deviation was significantly lower in the tirofiban versus the placebo arm (36.6% vs. 44.3%, $P = 0.026$). At 30 days, results demonstrated a significant benefit favoring tirofiban with regard to the combined incidence of death, recurrent MI, urgent target vessel revascularization (TVR), and thrombotic bailout (tirofiban 26.0% vs. placebo 32.9%, $P = 0.020$). Patients with less than 3 mm residual ST-segment deviation had a significantly lower mortality rate than those with greater than 3 mm (0.6% vs. 4.1%, $P < 0.001$). A recent angiographic analysis of the study showed that initial TIMI flow of the infarct related vessel improved as well. In addition, a significant interaction was found with time of administration of tirofiban. The effect on initial TIMI flow and on TIMI frame count after PCI was highest in patients who received the drug very early (<80 min) after the onset of symptoms (Figure 16.2).

Table 16.1 Summary of studies of tirofiban in patients with STEMI

Study	Period	Study design (number of patients)	Dose of tirofiban	Symptom duration (h)	Stent	Primary end points
Cutlip et al. [16]	2001–2002	Early (n = 28) versus late or no (n = 30) tirofiban	10 μg/kg bolus over 3 min/0.15 μg/kg/min infusion	<12	Yes	Preprocedural TIMI flow grade
Tiger-PA	1999–2001	Early (n = 50) versus late (n = 50) tirofiban	10 μg/kg bolus over 3 min/0.15 μg/kg/min infusion	<12	Yes	Preprocedural TIMI flow grade, cTFC, and TMPG
On-TIME	2001–2002	Early (n = 251) versus late (n = 256) tirofiban	10 μg/kg bolus over 3 min/0.15 μg/kg/min infusion	<6	Yes	Preprocedural TIMI flow grade
De Luca et al. [17]	1997–2002	Observational study of tirofiban (n = 481) versus no tirofiban (n = 1488)	10 μg/kg bolus over 3 min/0.15 μg/kg/min infusion	Yes	Yes	Postprocedural TIMI flow grade, distal embolization, TMPG
Emre et al. [18]	2002–2003	Early (n = 32) versus late (n = 34) tirofiban	10 μg/kg bolus over 3 min/0.15 μg/kg/min infusion	<6	Yes	Myocardial perfusion/ functional recovery at 30 days
Ernst et al. [13]	2002–2003	Comparison of platelet inhibition in 3 glycoprotein (GP)IIb/IIIa inhibitor regimens (N = 60)	10 μg/kg bolus regimen versus 25 μg/kg bolus regimen (both: 0.15 μg/kg/min infusion)	<6	Yes	Platelet inhibition at three different time points after percutaneous coronary intervention (PCI)
STRATEGY	2003–2004	Tirofiban + DES (n = 87) versus abciximab + BMS (n = 88)	25 μg/kg bolus over 3 min/0.15 μg/kg/min infusion	<12/12–24	Yes	Composite of death, nonfatal myocardial infarction (MI) stroke, or binary restenosis at 8 months
Danzi et al. [19]	2004	Tirofiban (n = 50) versus abciximab (n = 50)	25 μg/kg bolus over 3 min/0.15 μg/kg/min infusion	<6	Yes	Recovery of left ventricular function
Shen et al. [20]	2005–2006	Early (n = 57) versus late tirofiban (n = 57)	10 μg/kg bolus regimen and 25 μg/kg bolus regimen (both 0.15 μg/kg/min infusion)	<12	Yes	MACE at 30 days and 6 months

Study	Year	Description	Dosing	Time		Outcomes
Van Werkum et al. [14]	2005–2006	Comparison of platelet inhibition in 3 GPIIb/IIIa inhibitor regimens (N=60)	25 µg/kg bolus/0.15 µg/kg/min infusion	<6	Yes	Platelet inhibition at three different time points after PCI
Fu et al. [21]	2005–2007	Tirofiban (n=72) versus placebo (n=78)	10 µg/kg bolus over 3 min/ 0.15 µg/kg/min infusion	<12 h	Yes	Preprocedural/postprocedural TIMI flow grade, myocardial perfusion, platelet aggregation, CPK, CPK-MB, MACE at 6 months
MULTISTRATEGY	2004–2007	Tirofiban (n=372) versus abciximab (n=372)+either DES or BMS	25 µg/kg bolus over 3 min/0.15 µg/kg/min infusion	<12/12–24	Yes	≥50% ST-segment-elevation resolution at 90 min post PCI
On-TIME 2	2006–2007	Early tirofiban (n=491) versus placebo (n=493)	25 µg/kg bolus over 3 min/0.15 µg/kg/min infusion	<24	Yes	Residual ST-segment deviation 1 h after PCI
FABOLUS PRO	2010–2011	Tirofiban with or without prasugrel (N=48) versus prasugrel only therapy (N=52)	25 µg/kg bolus over 3 min/±0.15 µg/kg/min infusion	<24	Yes	Aggregometry after 20 µmol/L adenosine diphosphate (ADP) 30 min after the start of the treatment

CPK, creatine phosphokinase; CPK-MB, CPK isoenzyme-MB; cTFC, corrected TIMI frame counts; MACE, major adverse cardiac events; TMPG, TIMI myocardial perfusion grade.

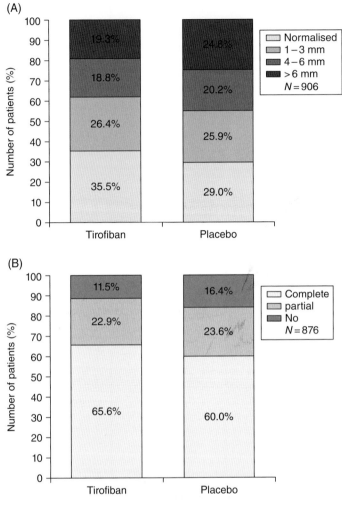

Figure 16.1 Myocardial reperfusion data for electrocardiography, according to treatment group. The percentages of patients are shown according to the degree of residual ST-segment deviation (A) or ST-segment resolution (B) on the electrocardiogram between 30 and 90 min after angiography or percutaneous coronary intervention (PCI).

Role of tirofiban with new P2Y12 inhibitors

More recently, the FABOLUS PRO study [22] was the first to assess the differential degree of platelet inhibition obtained after both adenosine diphosphate (ADP) and TRAP stimuli following prasugrel therapy and tirofiban therapy, administered as bolus only or bolus followed by 2 h infusion, or both treatments given simultaneously. This study showed that the degree of early platelet inhibition achieved after 60 mg loading dose of prasugrel is suboptimal at least for the first 2 h in STEMI patients undergoing primary PCI (Figure 16.3). Moreover, it showed that the administration of tirofiban, given as high bolus dose only, leads

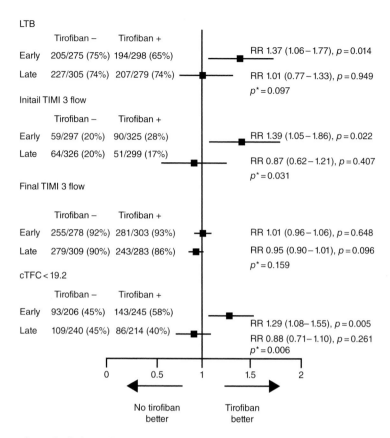

LTB

	Tirofiban −	Tirofiban +	
Early	205/275 (75%)	194/298 (65%)	RR 1.37 (1.06 – 1.77), $p = 0.014$
Late	227/305 (74%)	207/279 (74%)	RR 1.01 (0.77 – 1.33), $p = 0.949$
			$p^* = 0.097$

Initail TIMI 3 flow

	Tirofiban −	Tirofiban +	
Early	59/297 (20%)	90/325 (28%)	RR 1.39 (1.05 – 1.86), $p = 0.022$
Late	64/326 (20%)	51/299 (17%)	RR 0.87 (0.62 – 1.21), $p = 0.407$
			$p^* = 0.031$

Final TIMI 3 flow

	Tirofiban −	Tirofiban +	
Early	255/278 (92%)	281/303 (93%)	RR 1.01 (0.96 – 1.06), $p = 0.648$
Late	279/309 (90%)	243/283 (86%)	RR 0.95 (0.90 – 1.01), $p = 0.096$
			$p^* = 0.159$

cTFC < 19.2

	Tirofiban −	Tirofiban +	
Early	93/206 (45%)	143/245 (58%)	RR 1.29 (1.08 – 1.55), $p = 0.005$
Late	109/240 (45%)	86/214 (40%)	RR 0.88 (0.71 – 1.10), $p = 0.261$
			$p^* = 0.006$

0   0.5   1   1.5   2

← No tirofiban better   Tirofiban better →

$p^* = p$ value for interaction

Figure 16.2 Risk ratios of angiographic outcomes, as measured by quantitative coronary angiography analysis, in early versus late presenters. LTB 5 large thrombus burden. cTFC 5 corrected TIMI frame count.

to a high degree of platelet inhibition for at least 1 h on top of either clopidogrel or prasugrel loading dose. A 2 h postbolus tirofiban infusion allows to achieve a sustained degree of platelet inhibition for up to 6 h post bolus. Finally, the administration of high-dose bolus tirofiban and concomitant prasugrel allows to bridge the first hours in which prasugrel alone fails to provide complete platelet inhibition. Moreover, concomitant administration of tirofiban bolus only and prasugrel allows immediate, sustained, and consistent platelet inhibition throughout 24 h.

Head-to-head comparison of tirofiban high-dose bolus regimen and abciximab

As stated previously, smaller studies suggested similarities pertaining to inhibition of platelet reactivity between tirofiban, when administered at the high-dose bolus regimen, and abciximab [13, 14]. The Multicentre

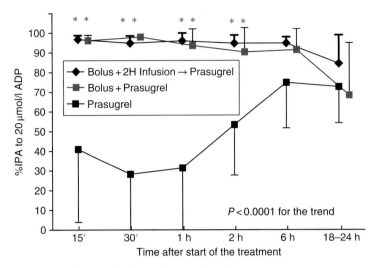

Figure 16.3 Kinetics of platelet inhibition over time after 20 μmol/L adenosine diphosphate (ADP) %IPA in patients treated with both tirofiban bolus with and without infusion versus prasugrel group alone. *p = 0.05 versus %IPA measured in the prasugrel alone group at *post hoc* analysis.

Evaluation of Single High-Dose Bolus Tirofiban versus Abciximab With Sirolimus-Eluting Stent or Bare Metal Stent in Acute Myocardial Infarction Study (MULTISTRATEGY) was the largest comparison of tirofiban to abciximab in the setting of primary PCI [23].

Utilizing a 2 × 2 factorial open-label design, MULTISTRATEGY compared tirofiban versus abciximab, BMS versus DES (in the form of a sirolimus stent), and the interaction between the two treatments (GPIIb/IIIa inhibitor and stent). Seven hundred and forty-five patients were enrolled from 16 centers and randomized to either tirofiban + sirolimus stent, tirofiban + BMS, abciximab + sirolimus stent, or abciximab + BMS. The majority of patients received triple antiplatelet therapy with aspirin and clopidogrel in addition to the GPIIb/IIIa inhibitor therapy.

Tirofiban was observed to be noninferior to abciximab with regard to the primary end point of ST-segment resolution at 90 min post procedure. At least 50% ST-segment resolution occurred in 85.3% and 83.6% of patients in the tirofiban and abciximab arms, respectively (RR 1.02, 95% CI 0.958–1.086, $P < 0.001$ for noninferiority).

Meta-analysis

Recently, an updated systematic review of randomized clinical trials comparing tirofiban versus placebo or any active control has been published [24]. The 31 studies included in the final analysis 20,006 randomized patients (average follow-up 5 months), 12,874 versus placebo, and 7,132 versus abciximab.

Tirofiban versus placebo or bivalirudin

Overall pooled effect estimate analysis showed a significant reduction in short-term (30-day) mortality (OR = 0.68 [0.54–0.86], $p = 0.001$), mortality or MI (OR = 0.69 [0.58–0.81], $p < 0.001$), MI alone (OR = 0.71 [0.56–0.90], $p = 0.004$), and the composite of death, MI, or TVR (OR = 0.73 [0.60–0.89], $p = 0.002$) in patients randomly allocated to receive tirofiban. According to an absolute risk reduction of 2.5%, the number needed to treat (NNT) is 40 to prevent 1 death or MI at 30 days, with an NNT of 100 to prevent 1 death.

To assess the effect of tirofiban when added to P2Y12 receptor blockers (i.e., ticlopidine or clopidogrel), studies where patients were adequately pretreated with clopidogrel ($n = 13$) or ticlopidine ($n = 1$) were selected, comprising 3424 patients. Consistent to previous analysis, tirofiban was associated with a significant decrease in mortality (OR = 0.56 [0.34, 0.93], $p = 0.02$) and the composite of death or MI (OR = 0.61 [0.48, 0.79], $p < 0.001$) at 30 days.

Tirofiban versus abciximab

Mortality (OR = 0.73 [0.36, 1.47]; $p = 0.38$, p for heterogeneity = 0.61, $I^2 = 0\%$), the composite of death or MI (OR = 0.87 [0.56, 1.35]; $p = 0.54$, p for heterogeneity = 0.58, $I^2 = 0\%$), or major adverse cardiac events (MACE) rate (OR = 0.87 [0.57, 1.32]; $p = 0.51$, p for heterogeneity = 0.63, $I^2 = 0\%$) were similar when tirofiban at high-dose bolus was compared to abciximab.

Tirofiban in ESC Guidelines

The ESC Guidelines for NSTE-ACS [25] as well as for STEMI [26] recently confirmed the role of tirofiban in ACS in addition to P2Y12 inhibitors. The NSTE guidelines recommend tirofiban or eptifibatide not only for high-risk patients (troponin positive, visible thrombus on angiography) (class 1 recommendation) but also as bridging alternative or in addition to P2Y12 loading in high-risk patients prior to urgent angiography. The STEMI guidelines, furthermore, recommend a GPIIb/IIIa inhibitor before or during primary PCI (recommendation IIa for high risk, as routine IIb) and do not differentiate between the different compounds, when the high bolus of tirofiban is used.

References

1 Phillips, D.R., Charo, I.F., Prise, L.V. & Fitzgerald, L.A. (1988) The platelet membrane glycoprotein IIb-IIIa complex. *Blood*, **71**, 831–843.
2 Tcheng, J.E., Ellis, S.G., George, B.S. *et al.* (1994) Pharmacodynamics of chimeric glycoprotein IIb/IIIa integrin antiplatelet antibody Fab 7E3 in high-risk coronary angioplasty. *Circulation*, **90 (4)**, 1757–1764.
3 Scarborough, R.M. & Kleiman, N.S. (1999) Phillips Platelet glycoprotein IIb/IIIa antagonists. What are the relevant issues concerning their pharmacology and clinical use? *Circulation*, **100**, 437–444.
4 Peerlinck, K., De Lepeleire, I., Goldberg, M. *et al.* (1993) MK-383 (L-700,462), a selective nonpeptide platelet glycoprotein IIb/IIIa antagonist, is active in man. *Circulation*, **88 (4 Pt 1)**, 1512–1517.

5 Mascelli, M.A., Lance, E.T., Damaraju, L., Wagner, C.L., Weisman, H.F. & Jordan, R.E. (1998) Pharmacodynamic profile of short-term abciximab treatment demonstrates prolonged platelet inhibition with gradual recovery from GP IIb/IIIa receptor blockade. *Circulation*, **97 (17)**, 1680–1688.

6 White, H. (1998) A comparison of aspirin plus tirofiban with aspirin plus heparin for unstable angina. Platelet Receptor Inhibition in Ischemic Syndrome Management (PRISM) Study Investigators. *The New England Journal of Medicine*, **338 (21)**, 1498–1505.

7 Théroux, P. (1998) Inhibition of the platelet glycoprotein IIb/IIIa receptor with tirofiban in unstable angina and non-Q-wave myocardial infarction. Platelet Receptor Inhibition in Ischemic Syndrome Management in Patients Limited by Unstable Signs and Symptoms (PRISM-PLUS) Study Investigators. *The New England Journal of Medicine*, **338 (21)**, 1488–1497.

8 Bolognese, L., Falsini, G., Liistro, F. *et al.* (2006) Randomized Comparison of Upstream versus downstream high bolus dose tirofiban or abciximab on tissue-level perfusion and troponin release in high-risk acute coronary syndromes treated with percutaneous coronary interventions: the EVEREST trial. *Journal of the American College of Cardiology*, **47**, 522–528.

9 King, S.B., III (1997) Effects of platelet glycoprotein IIb/IIIa blockade with tirofiban on adverse cardiac events in patients with unstable angina or acute myocardial infarction undergoing coronary angioplasty. *The RESTORE Investigators. Randomized Efficacy Study of Tirofiban for Outcomes and REstenosis. Circulation*, **96 (5)**, 1445–1453.

10 Topol, E.J., Moliterno, D.J., Herrmann, H.C. *et al.* (2001) Comparison of two platelet glycoprotein IIb/IIIa inhibitors, tirofiban and abciximab, for the prevention of ischemic events with percutaneous coronary revascularization. *The New England Journal of Medicine*, **344 (25)**, 1888–1894.

11 Kabbani, S.S., Aggarwal, A., Terrien, E.F. *et al.* (2002) Suboptimal early inhibition of platelets by treatment with tirofiban and implications for coronary interventions. *The American Journal of Cardiology*, **89 (5)**, 647–650.

12 Steinhubl, S.R., Talley, J.D., Braden, G.A. *et al.* (2001) Point-of-care measured platelet inhibition correlates with a reduced risk of an adverse cardiac event after percutaneous coronary intervention results of the GOLD (AU-Assessing Ultegra) multicenter study. *Circulation*, **103**, 2572–2578.

13 Ernst, N.M., Suryapranata, H., Miedema, K. *et al.* (2004) Achieved platelet aggregation inhibition after different antiplatelet regimens during percutaneous coronary intervention for ST-segment elevation myocardial infarction. *Journal of the American College of Cardiology*, **44**, 1187–1193.

14 van Werkum, J.W., Gerritsen, W.B.M., Kelder, J.C. *et al.* (2007) Inhibition of platelet function by abciximab or high-dose tirofiban in patients with STEMI undergoing primary PCI: a randomised trial. *The Netherlands Heart Journal*, **15 (11)**, 375–381.

15 van't Hof, A.W., Ten Berg, J., Heestermans, T. *et al.* (2008) Prehospital initiation of tirofiban in patients with ST-elevation myocardial infarction undergoing primary angioplasty (On-TIME) 2: a multicentre, double-blind, randomised controlled trial. *Lancet*, **372 (9638)**, 537–546.

16 Cutlip, D.E., Ricciardi, M.J., Ling, F.S. *et al.* (2003) Effect of tirofiban before primary angioplasty on initial coronary flow and early ST-segment resolution in patients with acute myocardial infarction. *American Journal of Cardiology*, **92 (8)**, 977–980.

17 De Luca, G., Suryapranata, H., de Boer, M.J. *et al.* (2007) Combination of electrocardiographic and angiographic markers of reperfusion in the prediction of infarct size in patients with ST-segment elevation myocardial infarction undergoing successful primary angioplasty. *International Journal of Cardiology*, **117 (2)**, 232–237.

18 Emre, A., Ucer, E., Yesilcimen, K. *et al.* (2006) Impact of early tirofiban administration on myocardial salvage in patients with acute myocardial infarction undergoing infarct-related artery stenting. *Cardiology*, **106 (4)**, 264–269.

19 Danzi, G.B., Sesana, M., Capuano, C. *et al.* (2004) Comparison in patients having primary coronary angioplasty of abciximab versus tirofiban on recovery of left ventricular function. *American Journal of Cardiology*, **94 (1)**, 35–39.

20 Shen, J., Zhang, Q., Zhang, R.Y., *et al.* (2008) Clinical benefits of adjunctive tirofiban therapy in patients with acute ST-segment elevation myocardial infarction undergoing primary percutaneous coronary intervention. *Coronary Artery Disease*, **19 (4)**, 271–277.

21 Fu, X.H., Hao, Q.Q., Jia, X.W., *et al.* (2008) Effect of tirofiban plus clopidogrel and aspirin on primary percutaneous coronary intervention via transradial approach in patients with acute myocardial infarction. *Chinese Medical Journal* **121 (6)**, 522–527.

22 Valgimigli, M., Tebaldi, M., Campo, G. *et al.* (2012) Prasugrel versus tirofiban bolus with or without short post-bolus infusion with or without concomitant prasugrel administration in patients with myocardial infarction undergoing coronary stenting: the FABOLUS PRO trial. *JACC. Cardiovascular Interventions*, **5 (3)**, 268–277.

23 Valgimigli, M., Campo, G., Percoco, G. *et al.* (2008) Comparison of angioplasty with infusion of tirofiban or abciximab and with implantation of sirolimus-eluting or uncoated stents for acute myocardial infarction: the MULTISTRATEGY randomized trial. *JAMA*, **299 (15)**, 1788–1799.

24 Valgimigli, M., Biondi-Zoccai, G., Tebaldi, M. *et al.* (2010) Tirofiban as adjunctive therapy for acute coronary syndromes and percutaneous coronary intervention: a meta-analysis of randomized trials. *European Heart Journal*, **31 (1)**, 35–49.

25 Hamm, C.W., Bassand, J.P., Agewall, S. *et al.* (2011) ESC Guidelines for the management of acute coronary syndromes in patients presenting without persistent ST-segment elevation: the Task Force for the management of acute coronary syndromes (ACS) in patients presenting without persistent ST-segment elevation of the European Society of Cardiology (ESC). *European Heart Journal*, **32 (23)**, 2999–3054.

26 Steg, P.G., James, S.K., Atar, D. *et al.* (2012) ESC Guidelines for the management of acute myocardial infarction in patients presenting with ST-segment elevation. *European Heart Journal*, **33 (20)**, 2569–2619.

17 Eptifibatide

Nevin C. Baker and Ron Waksman

MedStar Washington Hospital Center, Washington, DC, USA

Background

Glycoprotein (GP)IIb/IIIa inhibitors exert their antithrombotic effect by preventing the binding of fibrinogen to adjacent GPIIb/IIIa receptors, thus interfering with interplatelet bridging mediated by fibrinogen. Eptifibatide, abciximab, and tirofiban are the approved GPIIb/IIIa inhibitors for use during coronary interventions, with abciximab being the first approved. Similar to the other agents, eptifibatide blocks the final common pathway of platelet binding. These agents differ within their pharmacodynamics and pharmacokinetics.

Unlike abciximab (a monoclonal antibody), eptifibatide and tirofiban are small-molecule, competitive GPIIb/IIIa receptor inhibitors and share similar pharmacological profiles. Specifically, eptifibatide (Integrilin®) is a cyclic heptapeptide containing an amino acid mimetic sequence of RGD (Arg-Gly-Asp) that blocks the platelet GPIIb/IIIa receptor, the binding site for fibrinogen and von Willebrand factor [1]. Inhibition of binding at this final common receptor reversibly blocks platelet aggregation and prevents thrombosis. Eptifibatide has a longer free plasma half-life (hours vs. minutes) with a shorter platelet-bound half-life (seconds vs. hours) compared to abciximab [2]. Thus, eptifibatide is rapidly eliminated from the circulation, whereas platelet-bound abciximab can remain in the circulation for up to 1 week depending on the rate of platelet turnover. For this reason, the choice of GPIIb/IIIa inhibitor may become clinically important in certain situations. If surgery is required, the short half-life and reversibility of eptifibatide are advantageous and are not considered to confer an increased risk of perioperative bleeding [3].

Antiplatelet Therapy in Cardiovascular Disease, First Edition. Edited by Ron Waksman, Paul A. Gurbel, and Michael A. Gaglia, Jr.
© 2014 John Wiley & Sons, Ltd. Published 2014 by John Wiley & Sons, Ltd.

Dosing and efficacy

Eptifibatide is indicated as part of the antithrombotic therapy during acute coronary syndromes (ACS) in patients planned for either an invasive or a noninvasive approach. For ACS use, eptifibatide is given as a 180 mcg/kg intravenous bolus over 2 min followed immediately by a continuous infusion of 2 mcg/kg/min for 18–24 h. If percutaneous coronary intervention (PCI) is planned, a second bolus of 180 mcg/kg is given 10 min after the initial bolus. Unfractionated heparin (UFH) should also be coadministered during PCI to maintain an activated clotting time (ACT) of 200–250s.

While all GPIIb/IIIa inhibitors carry similar warnings regarding administration in patients with a history of bleeding diathesis or stroke, it is worth mentioning a few caveats, specifically between eptifibatide and abciximab. Eptifibatide is contraindicated in patients with recent stroke (30 days), while abciximab extends this contraindication out to a period of 2 years and includes patients with residual neurological deficits. While a relative contraindication for eptifibatide, thrombocytopenia (<100,000 cells/μL) or concurrent oral anticoagulant use within 7 days (unless prothrombin time $\leq$1.2$\times$ control) is a contraindication for abciximab. Eptifibatide requires dosing adjustment based on renal function and is contraindicated in dialysis patients, while abciximab does not require such adjustments.

The current dosing strategy of eptifibatide for ACS patients managed with or without PCI was refined in the late 1990s through a series of randomized controlled trials. The Integrilin to Minimize Platelet Aggregation and Prevent Coronary Thrombosis-II (IMPACT-II) trial failed to show a difference in 30-day event rates of either low-dose (135 mcg/kg bolus followed by 0.5 mcg/kg/min) or high-dose (135 mcg/kg bolus followed by 0.75 mcg/kg/min infusion) eptifibatide over placebo [4]. This dosing strategy only achieved 50–60% receptor inhibition, which was believed to be the mechanism of failure. An important pharmacological note to keep in mind is that GPIIb/IIIa inhibitors must maintain greater than 80% receptor occupancy to achieve sufficient therapeutic efficacy, and it was Tcheng *et al.* who provided evidence for both the safety and efficacy of the current high-dose eptifibatide during PCI to achieve this target [5, 6].

The double bolus recommendation was formulated based on the results of the Enhanced Suppression of the Platelet IIb/IIIa Receptor with Integrilin Therapy (ESPRIT) trial where 2064 stable patients undergoing PCI were randomized to either placebo or eptifibatide [7]. Of note, the trial was stopped prematurely after the eptifibatide group reduced the primary end point of death, myocardial infarction (MI), urgent revascularization, or the need for "bailout" GPIIb/IIIa use by 37% (6.6% vs. 10.5%, $p \leq 0.05$) compared with placebo. A list of randomized controlled trials evaluating eptifibatide under various clinical settings is found in Table 17.1.

Table 17.1 Major clinical trials of eptifibatide.

Acronym	Year	Study design (n, patients)	Population	Primary end point
IMPACT-II [4]	1997	Eptifibatide low-dose infusion (1349) versus high-dose infusion (1333) versus placebo (1328)	Elective, urgent, or emergent percutaneous transluminal coronary angioplasty (PTCA)	30-day death, myocardial infarction (MI), urgent revascularization
IMPACT-AMI [8]	1997	Eptifibatide at various bolus/infusion rates (125) versus placebo (55)	Acute myocardial infarction (AMI) treated with alteplase	Angiographic: Thrombolysis In Myocardial Infarction (TIMI)-3 flow at 90 min
PURSUIT [9]	1998	Eptifibatide (4722) versus placebo (4739)	High-risk unstable angina (UA), non-ST-segment-elevation MI (NSTEMI) ± percutaneous coronary intervention (PCI)	30-day death, MI
ESPRIT [7]	2000	Eptifibatide (1040) versus placebo (1024)	Stable, elective PCI	48-h death, MI, urgent target vessel revascularization (TVR), glycoprotein (GP) IIb/IIIa bailout
CLEAR-PLATELETS [10]	2005	Clopidogrel 300 mg with (30) or without (30) eptifibatide, clopidogrel 600 mg with (30) or without (30) eptifibatide	Stable angina, UA, NSTEMI with elective PCI	Platelet inhibition
PROTECT-TIMI-30 [11]	2006	Eptifibatide + unfractionated heparin (UFH) (298) versus eptifibatide + enoxaparin (275) versus bivalirudin (284)	High-risk acute coronary syndrome (ACS) undergoing PCI	Angiographic: myocardial perfusion
CLEAR-PLATELETS 2 [12]	2007	Bivalirudin (102) versus bivalirudin + eptifibatide (98)	Stable, enzyme-negative, elective PCI	Platelet inhibition and clot formation/strength
BRIEF-PCI [13]	2008	Abbreviated <2 h eptifibatide (312) versus standard 18 h eptifibatide infusion (312)	Nonemergent PCI	Periprocedural MI
EARLY ACS [14]	2009	Upstream eptifibatide (4722) versus provisional eptifibatide (4684)	High-risk NSTEMI undergoing PCI	96-h death, MI, urgent TVR, GPIIb/IIIa bailout
ASSIST [15]	2009	Eptifibatide + UFH (201) versus UFH alone (199)	STEMI with primary PCI	30-day death, MI, recurrent ischemia

AMI acute myocardial infarction, *MI* myocardial infarction, *NSTEMI* non-ST-segment-elevation MI, *PCI* percutaneous coronary intervention, *PTCA* percutaneous transluminal coronary angioplasty, *TIMI* Thrombolysis in Myocardial Infarction, *TVR* target vessel revascularization, *UA* unstable angina, *UFH* unfractionated heparin.

Eptifibatide use during non-ST-segment myocardial infarction

A few years before the results of the Acute Catheterization and Urgent Intervention Triage Strategy (ACUITY) trial were presented at the American College of Cardiology Annual Scientific Session, the Randomized Trial to Evaluate the Relative Protection Against Post-PCI Microvascular Dysfunction and Post-PCA Ischemia Among Antiplatelet and Anti-Thrombotic Agents (PROTECT-TIMI-30) was conducted, although both trial results were published in 2006. PROTECT-TIMI-30 [11] marks the first time eptifibatide plus an indirect thrombin inhibitor (UFH or enoxaparin) was paired against bivalirudin in high-risk ACS patients undergoing PCI. The primary end points were angiographic evidence of coronary flow reserve and myocardial perfusion as assessed by the corrected thrombolysis in myocardial infarction frame count (CTFC). Coronary flow reserve was higher in the bivalirudin group compared with eptifibatide (1.43 vs. 1.33, $p = 0.036$) when assessing "angiographically evaluable" patients (defined as patients with an open artery at the completion of PCI who did not sustain abrupt closure, emergent coronary artery bypass grafting needs, or thrombotic closure requiring GPIIb/IIIa bailout); however, this difference was no longer present upon intention to treat analysis. A trend toward lower events of death, MI, or ischemic events at 48 h was seen in the eptifibatide group (142% vs. 18.0%, $p = 0.15$). While Thrombolysis in Myocardial Infarction (TIMI) major bleeds were no different between eptifibatide and bivalirudin (0.7% vs. 0%), TIMI minor bleeds were higher with eptifibatide (2.5% vs. 0.4% $p = 0.03$). Criticism of this study includes the use of surrogate end points for clinical events rather than hard end points, such as death or MI, which were used for ACUITY.

The Platelet Glycoprotein IIb/IIIa in Unstable Angina: Receptor Suppression Using Integrilin Therapy (PURSUIT) trial [9] was the first look into the safety and efficacy of eptifibatide as a part of ACS therapy in combination with coronary stenting. As one of the largest, randomized controlled GPIIb/IIIa inhibitor trials to date, PURSUIT enrolled 10,948 ACS patients managed medically or with PCI [performed in ~50%, excluded ST-segment myocardial infarction (STEMI) patients] who were randomized to eptifibatide versus placebo. The result was a 1.5% absolute reduction in the primary end point of death or MI at 30 days (14.2% vs. 15.7%), a benefit seen as early as day four and present regardless of management strategy; however, the benefit of eptifibatide was greatest in the PCI group. Eptifibatide increased bleeding and the need for blood transfusions (11.6% vs. 9.2%; RR, 1.3; 95% CI, 1.1–1.4) compared to placebo.

Timing of eptifibatide administration

The only randomized controlled trial with a prespecified design to evaluate the optimal timing of GPIIb/IIIa inhibitor therapy in non-ST-segment myocardial infarction (NSTEMI) patients undergoing PCI is the

Early Glycoprotein IIb/IIIa Inhibition in Non-ST-Segment Elevation Acute Coronary Syndromes (EARLY ACS) trial where 9492 high-risk NSTEMI patients were given either early "upstream" or delayed "provisional" eptifibatide. The primary outcome of death, MI, urgent target vessel revascularization (TVR), or the need for GPIIb/IIIa inhibitor "bailout" occurred in 9.3% versus 10.0% of patients who received early versus delayed therapy (OR, 0.92; 95% CI, 0.80–1.06; $p = 0.23$). Similar findings were present at 30 days. TIMI major bleeding was increased with the upstream use of eptifibatide (2.6% vs. 1.8%, $p = 0.015$), as was Global Utilization of Streptokinase and TPA for Occluded Arteries (GUSTO) moderate or severe bleeding (7.6% vs. 5.1%, $p = 0.001$). Results from the EARLY ACS trial show that during the management of unstable angina (UA)/NSTEMI, eptifibatide administration ≥12 h before angiography is not superior to provisional use at the time of PCI and only offers higher rates of bleeding [14]. Timing of eptifibatide administration during STEMI will be discussed in the succeeding text.

Eptifibatide use during ST-segment myocardial infarction

Among patients undergoing primary PCI for acute STEMI, GPIIb/IIIa inhibitors given peripherally improve outcomes in patients, although the majority of this data comes from randomized controlled trials performed prior to the routine use of P2Y12 inhibitors as part of dual antiplatelet therapy [9, 16, 17]. Studies evaluating the efficacy of GPIIb/IIIa use during STEMI have preferentially evaluated abciximab over eptifibatide or tirofiban. While no large, randomized head-to-head comparisons of major adverse cardiovascular events (MACE) have been performed among these agents, observational studies and small randomized trials suggest equivalent efficacy [18, 19, 20, 21].

In the current era of duel antiplatelet therapy in combination with primary PCI for STEMI, only the Harmonizing Outcomes With Revascularization and Stents in Acute Myocardial Infarction (HORIZONS-AMI) study has evaluated eptifibatide plus UFH compared with bivalirudin alone. No difference in MACE at 30 days or at 1 year was seen between groups (5.4% vs. 5.5%, $p = 0.95$); however, there was a significant reduction in rates of major bleeding (5.9% vs. 9.6%, $p \leq 0.001$) between bivalirudin and the eptifibatide groups, respectively, which is a major limitation of eptifibatide use. An interesting finding was the increased rate of acute stent thrombosis (0.3% eptifibatide group compared to 1.3% with bivalirudin alone, HR: 5.93, $p < 0.001$) [8], postulated to be due to residual thrombin activity after the discontinuation of bivalirudin and before peak platelet inhibition with P2Y12 inhibitors. This theory has not been tested in a randomized trial.

Guidance for the use of eptifibatide upstream during treatment for patients presenting with STEMI and undergoing primary PCI comes from the A Safety and Efficacy Study of Integrilin-Facilitated Versus Primary PCI in STEMI (ASSIST) trial [15]. A total of 400 patients were given either eptifibatide prior to catheterization or at the time of angiography. There was no difference (6.5% vs. 5.5%, $p = 0.69$) in the 30-day outcome of death, MI, or recurrent ischemia between groups, upstream versus at time of angiography, respectively. Rates of major and minor bleeding were significantly higher with upstream eptifibatide compared with administration at time of angiography (22.4% vs. 14.6%, $p = 0.22$). Based on the findings of ASSIST, the routine precatheterization lab use of eptifibatide in the setting of STEMI on a background of aspirin and 600 mg of clopidogrel is not recommended.

Conclusions

With over fifteen years of clinical trial evidence speaking to the safety and clinical efficacy of eptifibatide, it remains one of the most studied agents for the management of ACS, with or without PCI. The integration of more potent and rapidly acting P2Y12 inhibitors for the treatment of acute MI in combination with primary PCI may challenge the current role of GPIIb/IIIa inhibitors. Still, eptifibatide remains a trusted agent for use during high-risk PCI in the setting of ACS, particularly STEMI.

References

1 Phillips, D.R. and Scarborough, R.M. (1997) Clinical pharmacology of eptifibatide. *The American Journal of Cardiology*, **80 (4A)**, 11B–20B.

2 Brown B. Glycoprotein IIb/IIIa inhibitors. S.D.Kristensen, R.Caterina, D.J.MoliternoTherapeutic strategies in thrombosis. 1Oxford Centre for Innovation, Clinical Publishing, Oxford; (2006).

3 Tardiff, B.E., Califf, R.M., Morris, D. *et al.* (1997) Coronary revascularization surgery after myocardial infarction: impact of bypass surgery on survival after thrombolysis GUSTO Investigators. Global Utilization of Streptokinase and Tissue Plasminogen Activator for Occluded Coronary Arteries. *Journal of the American College of Cardiology*, **29 (2)**, 240–249.

4 The, I.M.P.A.C.T.-I.I., and Investigators, T.I.-I. (1997) Randomised placebo-controlled trial of effect of eptifibatide on complications of percutaneous coronary intervention: IMPACT-II Integrilin to Minimise Platelet Aggregation and Coronary Thrombosis-II. *Lancet*, **349 (9063)**, 1422–1428.

5 Tcheng, J.E., Ellis, S.G., George, B.S. *et al.* (1994) Pharmacodynamics of chimeric glycoprotein IIb/IIIa integrin antiplatelet antibody Fab 7E3 in high-risk coronary angioplasty. *Circulation*, **90 (4)**, 1757–1764.

6 Tcheng, J.E., Talley, J.D., O'Shea, J.C. *et al.* (2001) Clinical pharmacology of higher dose eptifibatide in percutaneous coronary intervention (the PRIDE study). *The American Journal of Cardiology*, **88 (10)**, 1097–1102.

7 The, E.S.P.R.I.T. and Investigators, E. (2000) Novel dosing regimen of eptifibatide in planned coronary stent implantation (ESPRIT): a randomised, placebo-controlled trial. *Lancet*, **356 (9247)**, 2037–2044.

8 Stone, G.W., Witzenbichler, B., Guagliumi, G. *et al.* (2008) Bivalirudin during primary PCI in acute myocardial infarction. *The New England Journal of Medicine*, **358 (21)**, 2218–2230.

9 Anonymous (1998) Inhibition of platelet glycoprotein IIb/IIIa with eptifibatide in patients with acute coronary syndromes. The PURSUIT Trial Investigators. Platelet Glycoprotein IIb/IIIa in Unstable Angina: Receptor Suppression Using Integrilin Therapy. *The New England Journal of Medicine*, **339** (7), 436–443.

10 Gurbel, P.A., Bliden, K.P., Zaman, K.A., Yoho, J.A., Hayes, K.M., and Tantry, U.S. (2005) Clopidogrel loading with eptifibatide to arrest the reactivity of platelets: results of the Clopidogrel Loading with Eptifibatide to Arrest the Reactivity of Platelets (CLEAR PLATELETS) study. *Circulation*, **111** (9), 1153–1159.

11 Gibson, C.M., Morrow, D.A., Murphy, S.A. *et al.* (2006) A randomized trial to evaluate the relative protection against post-percutaneous coronary intervention microvascular dysfunction, ischemia, and inflammation among antiplatelet and antithrombotic agents: the PROTECT-TIMI-30 trial. *Journal of the American College of Cardiology*, **47** (12), 2364–2373.

12 Gurbel, P.A., Bliden, K.P., Saucedo, J.F. *et al.* (2009) Bivalirudin and clopidogrel with and without eptifibatide for elective stenting: effects on platelet function, thrombelastographic indexes, and their relation to periprocedural infarction results of the CLEAR PLATELETS-2 (Clopidogrel with Eptifibatide to Arrest the Reactivity of Platelets) study. *Journal of the American College of Cardiology*, **53** (8), 648–657.

13 Fung, A.Y., Saw, J., Starovoytov, A. *et al.* (2009) Abbreviated infusion of eptifibatide after successful coronary intervention The BRIEF-PCI (Brief Infusion of Eptifibatide Following Percutaneous Coronary Intervention) randomized trial. *Journal of the American College of Cardiology*, **53** (10), 837–845.

14 Giugliano, R.P., White, J.A., Bode, C. *et al.* (2009) Early versus delayed, provisional eptifibatide in acute coronary syndromes. *The New England Journal of Medicine*, **360** (21), 2176–2190.

15 Le May, M.R., Wells, G.A., Glover, C.A. *et al.* (2009) Primary percutaneous coronary angioplasty with and without eptifibatide in ST-segment elevation myocardial infarction: a safety and efficacy study of integrilin-facilitated versus primary percutaneous coronary intervention in ST-segment elevation myocardial infarction (ASSIST). *Circulation: Cardiovascular Interventions*, **2** (4), 330–338.

16 Sabatine, M.S. and Jang, I.K. (2000) The use of glycoprotein IIb/IIIa inhibitors in patients with coronary artery disease. *The American Journal of Medicine*, **109** (3), 224–237.

17 De Luca, G., Suryapranata, H., Stone, G.W. *et al.* (2005) Abciximab as adjunctive therapy to reperfusion in acute ST-segment elevation myocardial infarction: a meta-analysis of randomized trials. *JAMA*, **293** (14), 1759–1765.

18 Raveendran, G., Ting, H.H., Best, P.J. *et al.* (2007) Eptifibatide vs abciximab as adjunctive therapy during primary percutaneous coronary intervention for acute myocardial infarction. *Mayo Clinic Proceedings*, **82** (2), 196–202.

19 Zeymer, U., Margenet, A., Haude, M. *et al.* (2010) Randomized comparison of eptifibatide versus abciximab in primary percutaneous coronary intervention in patients with acute ST-segment elevation myocardial infarction: results of the EVA-AMI Trial. *Journal of the American College of Cardiology*, **56** (6), 463–469.

20 Gurm, H.S., Smith, D.E., Collins, J.S. *et al.* (2008) The relative safety and efficacy of abciximab and eptifibatide in patients undergoing primary

percutaneous coronary intervention: insights from a large regional registry of contemporary percutaneous coronary intervention. *Journal of the American College of Cardiology*, **51** (5), 529–535.

21 Akerblom, A., James, S.K., Koutouzis, M. *et al.* (2010) Eptifibatide is noninferior to abciximab in primary percutaneous coronary intervention: results from the SCAAR (Swedish Coronary Angiography and Angioplasty Registry). *Journal of the American College of Cardiology*, **56** (6), 470–475.

18 Ticlopidine

Fabiana Rollini, Francesco Franchi, Ana Muñiz-Lozano, and Dominick J. Angiolillo
University of Florida College of Medicine, Jacksonville, FL, USA

Dual antiplatelet therapy (DAPT) with aspirin and a $P2Y_{12}$ receptor inhibitor is the cornerstone of treatment to decrease ischemic events in patients with acute coronary syndrome (ACS) or undergoing percutaneous coronary intervention (PCI) [1]. Thienopyridines (ticlopidine, clopidogrel, and prasugrel) selectively and irreversibly inhibit the $P2Y_{12}$ receptor. However, these are prodrugs that require hepatic conversion into their active metabolite [2]. The first clinically available thienopyridine was ticlopidine, which was approved by the Food and Drug Administration for clinical use in the early 1990s and as adjunctive therapy to aspirin after stent implantation in 2001 [3]. Several studies have demonstrated the efficacy of ticlopidine as monotherapy in patients with cerebrovascular disease or with unstable angina [4, 5, 6]. The Canadian American Ticlopidine Study (CATS) trial showed a 30% reduction in the incidence of recurrent stroke, vascular death, and myocardial infarction (MI) in patients with recent thromboembolic stroke randomized to ticlopidine 500 mg/day (vs. placebo) [4]. The Ticlopidine Aspirin Stroke Study (TASS) trial compared ticlopidine with aspirin in patients with a history of transient ischemic attack, amaurosis fugax, or minor stroke showing a significant benefit with ticlopidine therapy [5]. Moreover, ticlopidine was previously considered the drug of choice for DAPT with aspirin in patients after coronary artery stenting to prevent stent thrombosis [7].

However, nowadays, the role of ticlopidine has become marginal due to its numerous and potentially severe side effects and the development of safer and more effective antiplatelet agents [8, 9]. This chapter will provide an overview on pharmacological properties and clinical development of ticlopidine.

Pharmacological properties

Ticlopidine [5-(2-chlorophenyl)methyl-4,5,6,7-tetrahydrothieno[3,2-c] pyridine], a first-generation thienopyridine, is an oral antagonist of the adenosine diphosphate (ADP) receptor, which acts by irreversible

Antiplatelet Therapy in Cardiovascular Disease, First Edition. Edited by Ron Waksman, Paul A. Gurbel, and Michael A. Gaglia, Jr.

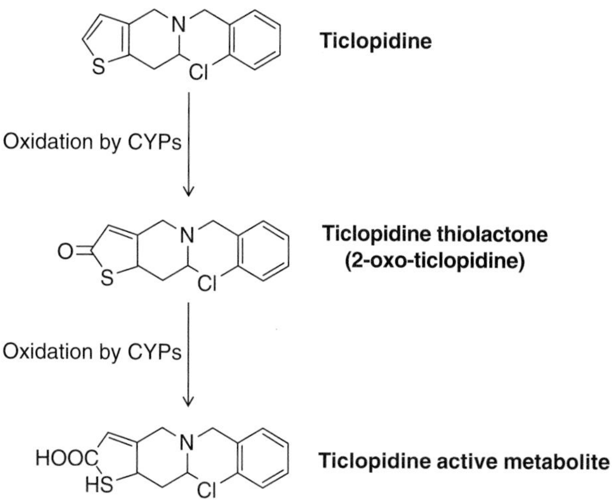

Figure 18.1 Ticlopidine metabolism. CYP, cytochrome P450.

blockade of the $P2Y_{12}$ platelet surface receptor [10]. Ticlopidine does not inhibit ADP-induced platelet aggregation *in vitro*, because it is a prodrug that requires hepatic biotransformation into an active metabolite [11]. Thirteen metabolites have been described and cytochrome P450 (CYP)2C19 and CYP2B6 are known to be involved in ticlopidine metabolism. However, the complete metabolic pathway producing the active thiolactone, which binds irreversibly the $P2Y_{12}$ receptor by generation of 2-oxo-ticolpidine, is still unclear (Figure 18.1) [12].

The *in vivo* onset of action after oral administration of ticlopidine (250 mg bid) occurs after 24–48 h, while about 5 days are required to reach maximal ADP-induced platelet inhibition. Approximately 85% of the drug is absorbed and the peak plasma concentration is reached after 2 h from drug intake. Bioavailability is increased by food and decreased by antacids. After repeated dosing, the clearance of ticlopidine decreases significantly, probably due to the inhibition on its own metabolism by inhibiting CYP2C19 and CYP2B6. Elimination of ticlopidine is 60% renal and 23% gastrointestinal. Platelet inhibitory effects are saturated at a dosage of 250 mg twice a day; a single 500 mg daily dose was also tested and showed a faster full inhibitory effect (4 days) but at the expense of more gastrointestinal side effects [7, 13, 14].

Pharmacodynamic profile

To date, few studies have been published on the pharmacodynamic (PD) effects of ticlopidine compared with other thienopyridines. Although platelet inhibition is dose dependent, the relation between the degree of platelet inhibition and plasma concentrations of active metabolites is still unclear [15]. Maximum platelet inhibition occurs 3–5 days after daily administration in healthy subjects, and the offset occurs 3–4 days after discontinuation of 250 mg daily doses and 11–13 days after 500 mg doses [14]. The addition of ticlopidine to aspirin allows reducing platelet reactivity more than what each single drug does [16], even in patients undergoing PCI (ADP (2 μM)-induced platelet aggregation: 36 ± 12 in aspirin plus ticlopidine versus 54 ± 12 in aspirin alone; $p < 0.0001$) [17]. Same results were found also using vasodilator-stimulated phosphoprotein (VASP), which is an assay specific to evaluate the $P2Y_{12}$ receptor signaling [18]. PD effects of ticlopidine were also evaluated in patients with chronic kidney disease, but no significant difference compared with healthy volunteers was shown; thus, no dose adjustment is required in patients with impaired renal function [19]. In a study on patients with stable angina scheduled for coronary angiography, the administration of a ticlopidine 1500 mg loading dose showed significantly higher platelet inhibition at 24 h compared to the modest antiplatelet effect achieved by the standard dosage (250 mg twice daily), as assessed by ADP-induced platelet fibrinogen binding. However, at 1 week, no difference was found between the two strategies [20].

Genetic considerations

It is well known that CYP2C19 polymorphisms reduce the antiplatelet effect of clopidogrel and increase the risk of ischemic cardiac events, such as stent thrombosis [21].Ticlopidine is a prodrug metabolized by multiple CYPs, including CYP2C19 as well [11]. However, *in vivo* production of ticlopidine active metabolites and pharmacokinetic properties do not depend mainly on CYP2C19 activity. Moreover, CYP2C19 polymorphisms did not show to reduce ticlopidine antiplatelet therapy [22]. Maeda *et al.* demonstrated that ADP (20 μmol/L)-induced platelet aggregation, evaluated by light transmittance aggregometry, was similar in extensive, intermediate, and poor metabolizers (PM), according to CYP2C19 genotypic status. Furthermore, platelet aggregation was significantly lower in PM patients on ticlopidine treatment group than on clopidogrel (33.8% vs. 19.1%; $P < 0.001$), and in clopidogrel PM that switched to ticlopidine, platelet aggregation was further suppressed (33.4% vs. 17.3%; $P < 0.01$) [23]. The role of ticlopidine in patients with pharmacological resistance to clopidogrel was tested in a case report series [24]. However, this was more adequately evaluated by Campo *et al.* who studied 143 patients undergoing PCI for stable coronary artery disease or ST-segment elevation MI [25]. The authors found that patients with resistance to clopidogrel (21%) were mainly responsive to ticlopidine and vice versa. In particular, 83% of patients who were clopidogrel nonresponders resulted to be responsive to ticlopidine, reaching a significant higher level of platelet inhibition (ADP (20 μmol/L)-induced platelet aggregation: 69 ± 15 vs. 44 ± 18; $P < 0.05$). Only 3.5% of patients (5 of 143) demonstrated both clopidogrel and ticlopidine resistance, suggesting a drug-specific mechanism, rather than a class effect, for thienopyridine resistance.

Clinical efficacy in patients undergoing PCI

Although some studies have assessed the role of ticlopidine in the other settings of vascular disease manifestations [4, 5], ticlopidine has been mostly acknowledged for its impact in the setting of patients undergoing PCI and stenting (Figure 18.2). In fact, despite the introduction of coronary stents in the late 1980s, the optimal antithrombotic treatment regimen to prevent stent thrombosis remained a challenge, hampering the clinical application of stent procedures. The combination of aspirin with anticoagulants was associated with high rates of thrombotic and bleeding complications. Therefore, an approach to achieve synergistic antiplatelet effects by blocking two key pathways, cyclooxygenase-1 with aspirin and the ADP receptor with ticlopidine, introducing the concept of "DAPT," was approached in four pivotal trials.

The Intracoronary Stenting and Antithrombotic Regimen (ISAR) trial evaluated the effect of ticlopidine after PCI and coronary stenting [26]. Patients ($n = 517$) were randomized to receive DAPT with aspirin (100 mg twice a day) plus ticlopidine (250 mg twice a day started immediately after the procedure and continued for 4 weeks) or conventional therapy with intravenous heparin, vitamin K antagonist (VKA), and aspirin. The primary cardiac end point was a composite of cardiovascular death, MI, aortocoronary bypass surgery, or repeated PCI of the stented vessel. At a 30-day follow-up, ticlopidine significantly reduced the incidence of the primary end point (1.6% vs. 6.2%; RR, 0.25; 95% CI, 0.06–0.77; $p = 0.01$) with an 82% reduction of MI. The rate of hemorrhagic events was also reduced in the ticlopidine group ($p < 0.001$).

In the Full Anticoagulation Versus Aspirin and Ticlopidine (FANTASTIC) study, patients ($n = 485$) undergoing stent implantation

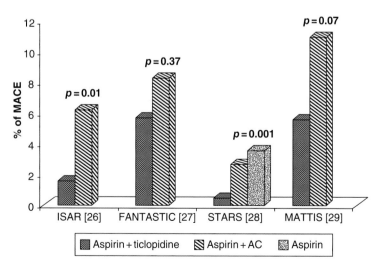

Figure 18.2 Rate of major adverse cardiac events (MACE) in the studies comparing ticlopidine plus aspirin to anticoagulant therapy plus aspirin. AC, anticoagulant therapy.

were randomized to receive DAPT with ticlopidine (500 mg loading dose administered immediately after procedure and then 250 mg bid for 6 weeks) plus aspirin (100–325 mg for life) or anticoagulant therapy (heparin and VKA) for 6 weeks plus aspirin [27]. The primary end point, the occurrence of any bleeding or peripheral vascular complications during the 6 weeks after stent implantation, was significantly reduced in the ticlopidine arm (13.5% vs. 21%; OR, 0.59; 95% CI, 0.39–0.98; $p = 0.03$). There was a lower overall cardiac event rate in the group randomized to antiplatelet therapy (5.7%) than in the group randomized to anticoagulation (8.3%), but the difference was not statistically significant ($p = 0.37$). Ticlopidine treatment was stopped because of side effects in 13 patients (5.2%).

The Stent Anticoagulation Restenosis Study (STARS) compared the efficacy and safety of three antithrombotic drug regimens (aspirin alone, aspirin and warfarin, and aspirin and ticlopidine) after coronary stenting in 1653 low-risk patients [28]. The primary end point (a composite of death from any cause, revascularization of the target lesion, angiographically evident thrombosis, or MI within 30 days) occurred in 3.6% of patients assigned to receive aspirin alone, 2.7% assigned to receive aspirin and warfarin, and 0.5% assigned to receive aspirin and ticlopidine ($p = 0.001$ for the comparison of all three groups; aspirin plus ticlopidine vs. aspirin alone (RR, 0.15; 95% CI, 0.05–0.43) and aspirin plus ticlopidine vs. aspirin plus warfarin (RR, 0.20; 95% CI, 0.07–0.61)). No significant difference was found in the risk of neutropenia or thrombocytopenia between the groups. However, the rate of hemorrhagic complications was 5.5% in the aspirin plus ticlopidine group, which was higher than aspirin alone (RR, 3.06; 95% CI, 1.57–5.97) but similar to aspirin plus warfarin (RR, 0.88; 95% CI, 0.55–1.43).

The Multicenter Aspirin and Ticlopidine Trial after Intracoronary Stenting (MATTIS) was the first to randomize procedural high-risk patients ($n = 350$) within 6 h after stent implantation to receive during 30 days either aspirin 250 mg plus ticlopidine 500 mg/day or aspirin 250 mg/day plus oral anticoagulation [29]. The primary efficacy end point, a composite of cardiovascular death, MI, or repeated revascularization at 30 days, was reduced in the ticlopidine group, without reaching statistical significance (5.6% vs. 11%; RR, 1.9; 95% CI, 0.9–4.1; $p = 0.07$). However, major vascular and bleeding complications were less frequent in the ticlopidine plus aspirin group (1.7%) than in the aspirin plus oral anticoagulant group (6.9%) (RR, 4.1; 95% CI, 1.2–14.3; $p = 0.02$). Asymptomatic neutropenia was noted in 1.7% of patients in ticlopidine arm; it occurred late (after the 30-day treatment period), did not lead to any clinical manifestation, and resolved spontaneously. All these trials evidenced that the benefit of ticlopidine therapy was greater than anticoagulant therapy but became evident after at least 24 h after the first dose [26, 27].

The major drawback of ticlopidine was the higher rate of nonbleeding side effects, as described in the following texts. This underscored the need for safer treatment alternatives, which was found in clopidogrel. Clopidogrel, a second-generation thienopyridine, is structurally similar to ticlopidine but with a better safety profile and comparable clinical efficacy [30, 31]. The Clopidogrel Aspirin Stent International Cooperative Study (CLASSICS) trial evaluated the safety of clopidogrel (75 mg/day with or without a 300 mg loading dose) in combination with aspirin (325 mg) compared to ticlopidine (250 mg/bid) in combination with aspirin in patients ($n = 1020$) who had undergone successful coronary stenting [32]. The primary end point, a composite of major peripheral or bleeding complications, neutropenia, thrombocytopenia, or early discontinuation of study drug as the result of a noncardiac adverse event during the 28-day study-drug treatment period, was significantly higher in the ticlopidine group than in the combined clopidogrel group (9.1% vs. 4.6%; RR, 0.50; 95% CI, 0.31–0.81; $p = 0.005$). This difference was primarily due to the higher incidence of skin, gastrointestinal, and allergic events. The 300 mg loading dose was well tolerated, with no increased risk of bleeding. Overall, there was a low incidence of major adverse cardiac events (MACE), without any significant difference between groups (0.9% with ticlopidine, 1.5% with 75 mg/day clopidogrel, 1.2% with the clopidogrel loading dose).

Bhatt *et al.* performed a meta-analysis on 13955 patients to compare ticlopidine plus aspirin to clopidogrel plus aspirin in the reduction of ischemic events in patients receiving coronary stents [33]. Combining data from 10 studies (three randomized trials and seven registries), clopidogrel showed a significant reduction in the rate of MACE at 30 days compared to ticlopidine (2.10% vs. 4.04%; OR, 0.72; 95% CI, 0.59–0.89; $p = 0.002$). Even all-cause mortality was reduced (0.48% vs. 1.09%; OR, 0.55; 95% CI, 0.37–0.82; $p = 0.003$). The authors concluded that clopidogrel, in addition to better safety, was at least as efficacious as ticlopidine, suggesting that the latter should be replaced by clopidogrel in DAPT. Interestingly, Mueller *et al.* found different results with a longer follow-up [34]. They randomized patients ($n = 700$) after stent implantation to receive either ticlopidine (250 bid) or clopidogrel (75 mg daily), administered immediately after stent implantation without loading dose, for 4 weeks. All patients received aspirin (100 mg daily) for life. The primary end point (cardiovascular death during the entire follow-up) was significantly reduced in the ticlopidine group (2.3% vs. 7.3%; HR, 0.30; 95% CI, 0.14–0.66; $p = 0.003$) after a median follow-up of 28 months. Ticlopidine significantly reduced also the secondary end point of cardiac death or nonfatal MI (5.5% vs. 11.3%; HR, 0.45; 95% CI, 0.25–0.80; $p = 0.005$). However, the study did not report any result on safety end points.

Ultimately, several randomized studies conducted in Asia also compared the efficacy of DAPT with aspirin plus ticlopidine to aspirin plus cilostazol after coronary stenting. In all these studies, cilostazol did not show significant differences in preventing MACE [35, 36, 37, 38]. However, the incidence of adverse side effects tended to be lower with cilostazol, which also showed greater inhibition of neointimal proliferation [36, 38]. However, the introduction of clopidogrel in Asian countries has also led to the replacement of cilostazol as part of the DAPT regimen of choice, although cilostazol is still broadly used as an adjunctive treatment ("triple antiplatelet therapy") in high-risk PCI settings.

Safety and side effects

Several and potentially severe side effects have been described with ticlopidine use. Gastrointestinal disorders, such as nausea, vomiting, and diarrhea, are common and occur in 30–50% of patients. Skin rash is also frequent (5%) [39]. Serious and potentially life-threatening hematological side effects are reported. Neutropenia (absolute neutrophil count of <1200/µL) occurs in about 2% of treated patients and severe neutropenia (<450/µL), which may be fatal, in 0.8–0.9% [40]. Thrombotic thrombocytopenic purpura is reported in 0.02% of cases with a mortality rate that exceeds 20% [41]. Even aplastic anemia has been described. Hematological complications may occur after few days with a peak of incidence of 3–6 weeks and, fortunately, are usually reversible with drug discontinuation. However, some cases appear to be irreversible and initially clinically silent. Full blood count monitoring is recommended every 2 weeks for the first 3 months of therapy [40]. Ticlopidine also showed to increase serum cholesterol by 8–10%, without an evident increase in cardiovascular mortality [5]. Compared to clopidogrel, the rate of skin or gastrointestinal side effects is higher, even though no statistically significant difference has been shown [32], whereas hematological disorders are significantly higher with ticlopidine plus aspirin compared to anticoagulant therapy [42].

Conclusions

Ticlopidine, the first thienopyridine clinically used, is approved in the settings of stroke and coronary stenting. Ticlopidine has been mostly acknowledged for its impact in the setting of patients undergoing coronary stenting, as it defined the optimal antithrombotic treatment regimen in addition to aspirin to prevent stent thrombosis by blocking two key pathways, cyclooxygenase-1 with aspirin and the ADP receptor with ticlopidine. This introduced the concept of DAPT and thus set the basis for almost two decades of investigation in the field with other thienopyridines (clopidogrel and prasugrel) and nonthienopyridine (ticagrelor) $P2Y_{12}$ receptor antagonists. However, the role of ticlopidine in modern day clinical practice is very limited due to its numerous side effects and the availability of other $P2Y_{12}$ receptor antagonists with a more favorable safety and efficacy profile.

References

1 Ferreiro, J.L. & Angiolillo, D.J. (2012) New directions in antiplatelet therapy. *Circulation: Cardiovascular Interventions*, **5**, 433–445.

2 Storey, R.F. (2006) Biology and pharmacology of the platelet P2Y12 receptor. *Current Pharmaceutical Design*, **12**, 1255–1259.

3 Food and Drug Administration (FDA) U.S. Food and Drug Administration's Approval Letter [internet]. Silver Spring: U.S. Food and Drug Administration; 2001.

4 Gent, M., Blakely, J.A., Easton, J.D. *et al.* (1989) The Canadian American Ticlopidine Study (CATS) in thromboembolic stroke. *Lancet*, **1**, 1215–1220.

5 Hass, W.K., Easton, J.D., Adams, H.P., Jr *et al.* (1989) A randomized trial comparing ticlopidine hydrochloride with aspirin for the prevention of stroke in high-risk patients. Ticlopidine Aspirin Stroke Study Group. *The New England Journal of Medicine*, **321**, 501–507.

6 Balsano, F., Rizzon, P., Violi, F. *et al.* (1990) Antiplatelet treatment with ticlopidine in unstable angina. A controlled multicenter clinical trial. The Studio della Ticlopidina nell'Angina Instabile Group. *Circulation*, **82**, 17–26.

7 Quinn, M.J. & Fitzgerald, D.J. (1999) Ticlopidine and clopidogrel. *Circulation*, **100**, 1667–1672.

8 Furie, K.L., Kasner, S.E., Adams, R.J. *et al.* (2011) Guidelines for the prevention of stroke in patients with stroke or transient ischemic attack: a guideline for healthcare professionals from the american heart association/american stroke association. *Stroke*, **42**, 227–276.

9 Levine, G.N., Bates, E.R., Blankenship, J.C. *et al.* (2011) ACCF/AHA/SCAI guideline for percutaneous coronary intervention: a report from the American College of Cardiology Foundation/American Heart Association Task Force on Practice Guidelines and the Society for Cardiovascular Angiography and Interventions. *Journal of the American College of Cardiology*, **58**, e44–e122.

10 Storey, F. (2001) The P2Y12 receptor as a therapeutic target in cardiovascular disease. *Platelets*, **12**, 197–209.

11 Di Minno, G., Cerbone, A.M., Mattioli, P.L., Turco, S., Iovine, C. & Mancini, M. (1985) Functionally thrombasthenic state in normal platelets following the administration of ticlopidine. *The Journal of Clinical Investigation*, **75**, 328–338.

12 Yoneda, K., Iwamura, R., Kishi, H., Mizukami, Y., Mogami, K. & Kobayashi, S. (2004) Identification of the active metabolite of ticlopidine from rat in vitro metabolites. *British Journal of Pharmacology*, **142**, 551–557.

13 Farid, N.A., Kurihara, A. & Wrighton, S.A. (2010) Metabolism and disposition of the thienopyridine antiplatelet drugs ticlopidine, clopidogrel, and prasugrel in humans. *The Journal of Clinical Pharmacology*, **50**, 126–142.

14 Kuzniar, J., Splawinska, B., Malinga, K., Mazurek, A.P. & Splawinski, J. (1996) Pharmacodynamics of ticlopidine: relation between dose and time of administration to platelet inhibition. *International Journal of Clinical Pharmacology and Therapeutics*, **34**, 357–361.

15 Di Perri, T., Pasini, F.L., Frigerio, C. *et al.* (1991) Pharmacodynamics of ticlopidine in man in relation to plasma and blood cell concentration. *European Journal of Clinical Pharmacology*, **41**, 429–434.

16 Altman, R., Scazziota, A., Rouvier, J. & Gonzalez, C. (1999) Effects of ticlopidine or ticlopidine plus aspirin on platelet aggregation and ATP release in normal volunteers: why aspirin improves ticlopidine antiplatelet activity. *Clinical and Applied Thrombosis/Hemostasis*, **5**, 243–246.

17 van de Loo, A., Nauck, M., Noory, E. *et al.* (1998) Enhancement of platelet inhibition of ticlopidine plus aspirin vs aspirin alone given prior to elective PTCA. *European Heart Journal*, **19**, 96–102.

18 Schwarz, U.R., Geiger, J., Walter, U. & Eigenthaler, M. (1999) Flow cytometry analysis of intracellular VASP phosphorylation for the assessment of activating and inhibitory signal transduction pathways in human platelets–definition and detection of ticlopidine/clopidogrel effects. *Journal of Thrombosis and Haemostasis*, **82**, 1145–1152.

19 Buur, T., Larsson, R., Berglund, U., Donat, F. & Tronquet, C. (1997) Pharmacokinetics and effect of ticlopidine on platelet aggregation in subjects with normal and impaired renal function. *Journal of Clinical Pharmacology*, **37**, 108–115.

20 Berglund, U. & Lindahl, T. (1998) Enhanced onset of platelet inhibition with a loading dose of ticlopidine in ASA-treated stable coronary patients. *International Journal of Cardiology*, **64**, 215–217.

21 Sofi, F., Giusti, B., Marcucci, R., Gori, A.M., Abbate, R. & Gensini, G.F. (2011) Cytochrome P450 2C19*2 polymorphism and cardiovascular recurrences in patients taking clopidogrel: a meta-analysis. *The Pharmacogenomics Journal*, **11**, 199–206.

22 Ieiri, I., Kimura, M., Irie, S., Urae, A., Otsubo, K. & Ishizaki, T. (2005) Interaction magnitude, pharmacokinetics and pharmacodynamics of ticlopidine in relation to CYP2C19 genotypic status. *Pharmacogenetics and Genomics*, **15**, 851–859.

23 Maeda, A., Ando, H., Asai, T. *et al.* (2011) Differential impacts of CYP2C19 gene polymorphisms on the antiplatelet effects of clopidogrel and ticlopidine. *Clinical Pharmacology and Therapeutics*, **89**, 229–233.

24 Aleil, B., Rochoux, G., Monassier, J.P., Cazenave, J.P. & Gachet, C. (2007) Ticlopidine could be an alternative therapy in the case of pharmacological resistance to clopidogrel: a report of three cases. *Journal of Thrombosis and Haemostasis*, **5**, 879–881.

25 Campo, G., Valgimigli, M., Gemmati, D. *et al.* (2007) Poor responsiveness to clopidogrel: drug-specific or class-effect mechanism? Evidence from a clopidogrel-to-ticlopidine crossover study. *Journal of the American College of Cardiology*, **50**, 1132–1137.

26 Schömig, A., Neumann, F.J., Kastrati, A. *et al.* (1996) A randomized comparison of antiplatelet and anticoagulant therapy after the placement of coronary-artery stents. *The New England Journal of Medicine*, **334**, 1084–1089.

27 Bertrand, M.E., Legrand, V., Boland, J. *et al.* (1998) Randomized multicenter comparison of conventional anticoagulation versus antiplatelet therapy in unplanned and elective coronary stenting. The full anticoagulation versus aspirin and ticlopidine (FANTASTIC) study. *Circulation*, **98**, 1597–1603.

28 Leon, M.B., Baim, D.S., Popma, J.J. *et al.* (1998) A clinical trial comparing three antithrombotic-drug regimens after coronary-artery stenting. Stent Anticoagulation Restenosis Study Investigators. *The New England Journal of Medicine*, **339**, 1665–1671.

29 Urban, P., Macaya, C., Rupprecht, H.J. *et al.* (1998) Randomized evaluation of anticoagulation versus antiplatelet therapy after coronary stent implantation in high-risk patients: the multicenter aspirin and ticlopidine trial after intracoronary stenting (MATTIS). *Circulation*, **98**, 2126–2132.

30 Herbert, J.M., Frehel, D., Vallee, E. *et al.* (1993) Clopidogrel, a novel antiplatelet and antithrombotic agent. *Cardiovascular Drug Reviews*, **11**, 180–198.

31 CAPRIE Steering Committee (1996) A randomised, blinded, trial of clopidogrel versus aspirin in patients at risk of ischaemic events (CAPRIE). *Lancet*, **348**, 1329–1339.

32 Bertrand, M.E., Rupprecht, H.J., Urban, P. & Gershlick, A.H. (2000) CLASSICS Investigators. Double-blind study of the safety of clopidogrel with and without a loading dose in combination with aspirin compared with

ticlopidine in combination with aspirin after coronary stenting: the clopidogrel aspirin stent international cooperative study (CLASSICS). *Circulation*, **102**, 624–629.

33 Bhatt, D.L., Bertrand, M.E., Berger, P.B. *et al.* (2002) Meta-analysis of randomized and registry comparisons of ticlopidine with clopidogrel after stenting. *Journal of the American College of Cardiology*, **39**, 9–14.

34 Mueller, C., Roskamm, H., Neumann, F.J. *et al.* (2003) A randomized comparison of clopidogrel and aspirin versus ticlopidine and aspirin after the placement of coronary artery stents. *Journal of the American College of Cardiology*, **41**, 969–973.

35 Yoon, Y., Shim, W.H., Lee, D.H. *et al.* (1999) Usefulness of cilostazol versus ticlopidine in coronary artery stenting. *The American Journal of Cardiology*, **84**, 1375–1380.

36 Sekiguchi, M., Hoshizaki, H., Adachi, H. *et al.* (2004) Effects of antiplatelet agents on subacute thrombosis and restenosis after successful coronary stenting: a randomized comparison of ticlopidine and cilostazol. *Circulation Journal*, **68**, 610–614.

37 Hashiguchi, M., Ohno, K., Nakazawa, R., Kishino, S., Mochizuki, M. & Shiga, T. (2004) Comparison of cilostazol and ticlopidine for one-month effectiveness and safety after elective coronary stenting. *Cardiovascular Drugs and Therapy*, **18**, 211–217.

38 Park, S.W., Lee, C.W., Kim, H.S. *et al.* (1999) Comparison of cilostazol versus ticlopidine therapy after stent implantation. *The American Journal of Cardiology*, **84**, 511–514.

39 McTavish, D., Faulds, D. & Goa, K.L. (1990) Ticlopidine: an updated review of its pharmacology and therapeutic use in platelet-dependent disorders. *Drugs*, **40**, 238–259.

40 Love, B., Biller, J. & Gent, M. (1998) Adverse haematological effects of ticlopidine: prevention, recognition and management. *Drug Safety*, **19**, 89–98.

41 Steinhubl, S.R., Tan, W.A., Foody, J.M. *et al.* (1999) Incidence and clinical course of thrombotic thrombocytopenic purpura due to ticlopidine following coronary stenting. EPISTENT Investigators. Evaluation of Platelet IIb/IIIa Inhibitor for Stenting. *The Journal of the American Medical Association*, **281**, 806–810.

42 Cosmi B, Rubboli A, Castelvetri C, Milandri, M. Ticlopidine versus oral anticoagulation for coronary stenting. *The Cochrane Database of Systematic Reviews* 2001; (4), Art. No.:CD002133.

19 Clopidogrel

Andrzej Budaj

Grochowski Hospital, Warsaw, Poland

Clopidogrel (CLP), since its first approval in 1997, has been the most prescribed and studied medication as percutaneous coronary intervention (PCI) became the dominant approach for myocardial revascularization.

Pharmacodynamic properties

Clopidogrel bisulfate, the thienopyridine, irreversibly inhibits the P2Y12 adenosine diphosphate platelet receptor.

Clopidogrel is metabolized in the liver via two competing pathways. In one, about 85% of absorbed CLP is hydrolyzed by carboxylesterase-1 to an inactive carboxylic acid metabolite. In the second, CLP is converted to the active metabolite (15%) in a two-step oxidative reaction catalyzed by cytochrome P450 (CYP450). In the first step, CLP is oxidized to the thiolactone derivative (2-oxo-clopidogrel) by CYP1A2, CYP2B6, and CYP2C19. Subsequently, from thiolactone, an active thiol metabolite is formed by a hydraulic cleavage of the γ-thiobutyrolactone ring. CYP2B6, CYP2C9, CYP2C19, and CYP3A4 are involved in this reaction [1]. Active metabolite is a highly labile compound that through a disulfate bridge binds irreversibly with cysteine on platelet P2Y12 receptor [2].

A recently published study has suggested that paraoxonase-1, a Ca+-dependent esterase that inhibits oxidative modification of LDL cholesterol, might play a role in the bioactivation of CLP [3]. However, subsequent studies have failed to reproduce this finding [4].

In the study with healthy volunteers, CLP in doses 300–400 mg produced a rapid onset of the pharmacodynamic action, with levels of platelet aggregation inhibition close to steady state reached within 2 h [5]. However, in a study of patients with stable coronary artery disease, only 16% of patients were observed to reach over 70% inhibition of platelet aggregation by 2 h after 600 mg of CLP loading dose (LD) [6]. Inhibition of platelet aggregation was higher with 600 and 900 mg than 300 mg LD [7]. These results suggest a variability of platelet response to CLP.

Antiplatelet Therapy in Cardiovascular Disease, First Edition. Edited by Ron Waksman, Paul A. Gurbel, and Michael A. Gaglia, Jr.
© 2014 John Wiley & Sons, Ltd. Published 2014 by John Wiley & Sons, Ltd.

Pharmacokinetic properties

About 50% of an orally administered dose of CLP is absorbed from the gastrointestinal tract. It has been demonstrated that CLP absorption in the intestine was diminished by active secretion via efflux pump P-glycoprotein (P-gp) encoded by the gene MDR1 (ABCB1) [8]. This mechanism is suggested as potentially diminishing the substrate for active metabolite of CLP [2].

The active metabolite of CLP is highly unstable and its pharmacokinetics have been only recently determined. Due to rapid and extensive metabolism in the liver, plasma concentrations of the parent compound are generally below the level of the detection beyond 2 h after administration of CLP 75 mg/day. Therefore, the pharmacokinetics of CLP have been characterized by evaluating the main circulating metabolite, the carboxylic acid derivative. In order to evaluate compliance to CLP therapy, it may be appropriate to measure the main inactive metabolite since it can be tracked for 24–48 h after cessation of therapy [9]. However, a number of analytical methods have been elaborated to measure the parent drug, CLP, and its active compound [10].

After an oral single-dose administration of CLP 75 mg to healthy volunteers, a mean peak plasma concentration (Cmax) of 2.8 mg/L for the carboxylic acid metabolite was achieved after 0.8 h [11]. The administration of various LDs in patients with stable CAD treated with PCI has been elaborated. Loading with 600 mg resulted in higher plasma concentrations of active metabolite, CLP, and carboxyl metabolite compared with loading with 300 mg. With administration of 900 mg, no further increase in plasma concentrations of active metabolite and CLP was achieved. Peak concentrations of each compound with administered LDs occurred within 40–60 min [7].

Both the parent and active metabolite are highly protein bound (>94%).

Following oral administration of ^{14}C-clopidogrel, approximately 50% and 46% of the drug was excreted in the urine and feces, respectively [12].

Therapeutic use

Clopidogrel has undergone extensive evaluation in several large, randomized, double-blind clinical trials that have, collectively, included over 100,000 patients. The studies have shown that CLP, either alone or added to aspirin (ASA), is superior to ASA monotherapy in reducing clinical end points (see Table 19.1 for efficacy results from selected major CLP trials). The CURE trial revealed a 20% relative risk reduction in the first coprimary end point and 14% relative risk reduction of the second coprimary end point (first primary end point or refractory ischemia). The benefits of CLP in preventing the first coprimary outcomes were evident at 30 days and were maintained to the end of the trial. Risk reduction in ischemic vascular events emerged within 24 h after starting treatment [13]. Subgroup analyses showed that the benefits of CLP were consistent in

Table 19.1 Efficacy of CLP in major trials with reperfusion therapy.

Trial	Treatments	Primary end points	Follow-up	Primary end point results % (p-value)
CURE [13] Acute coronary syndrome without ST-segment elevation (NSTE ACS) n = 12,562	CLP 300 mg LD, then 75 mg/day versus ASA alone	CV death, MI, or stroke	3–12 months	9.3 versus 11.4 (<0.001)
CREDO [14] Elective PCI n = 2,116	CLP 300 mg LD or PL before PCI. All patients received CLP 75 mg/day through day 29. From day 29 through 12 months, patients in the LD group received CLP 75 mg/day, and those in the control group received PL; both groups received ASA	Death, re-MI, or stroke in the ITT population	1 year	8.5 versus 11.5 (0.02)
		Death, MI, or urgent TVR in the per-protocol population	28 days	6.8 versus 8.3 (0.23)
CLARITY [15] STEMI plus fibrinolysis n = 3,491	CLP 300 mg LD, then 75 mg/day plus ASA 150–325 mg LD, then 75–162 mg/day versus ASA alone	Occluded infarct-related artery (IRA) (TIMI flow 0–1) on angiography, death, or re-MI before angiography	30 days	15.0 versus 21.7 (<0.001)
COMMIT [16] Acute MI n = 45,852	CLP 75 mg/day plus ASA versus ASA alone	Death, re-MI, or stroke	4 weeks	9.2 versus 10.1 (0.002)
		Death of any cause		7.5 versus 8.1 (0.03)
CURRENT-OASIS 7 [17] ACS plus intended PCI n = 25,086	CLP 600 mg LD, then 150 mg/day for 6 days, and 75 mg/day thereafter versus standard dose 300 mg LD and 75 mg/day thereafter	CV death, MI, or stroke	30 days	4.2 versus 4.4 (0.30)

ASA, aspirin; CLP, clopidogrel; IRA, infarct related artery; LD, loading dose; MI, myocardial infarction; NSTE ACS, acute coronary syndrome without ST-segment elevation; PCI, percutaneous coronary intervention; PL, placebo; re-MI, recurrent myocardial infarction; STEMI, myocardial infarction with ST-segment elevation; TIMI, Thrombolysis in Myocardial Infarction; TVR, target vessel revascularization.

low-, intermediate-, and high-risk groups according to the Thrombolysis in Myocardial Infarction (TIMI) Risk Score [18].

The PCI-CURE, a prospective study of patients undergoing PCI in the CURE trial, showed a significant reduction in primary end point (CV death, MI, or target vessel revascularization (TVR)): 4.5% in CLP group versus 6.4% in placebo (PL) group (relative risk 0.70 [95% CI 0.50–0.97]; $p = 0.03$) [19].

The CREDO study showed a significant benefit (26.9% relative risk reduction) of sustained dual antiplatelet therapy (CLP plus ASA) with pretreatment before PCI. The study demonstrated that patients who received an LD of CLP 6–24 h prior to PCI had a 38.6% relative reduction (95% CI 1.6, 62.9; $p = 0.051$) in the primary end point compared with those who received PL. The lack of benefit of pretreatment was revealed when the drug was administered within 6 h [14].

In the CLARITY-TIMI 28 trial in ST-segment-elevation myocardial infarction (STEMI) patients (≤75 years of age) presenting within 12 h treated with fibrinolytic therapy, a 36% relative risk reduction (odds ratio 0.64 [95% CI 0.53, 0.76]; $p < 0.001$) in primary end point in the CLP group was demonstrated. CLP improved angiographic measurements compared with PL: a 36% increase in the odds of achieving optimal epicardial flow (TIMI flow grade 3) [$p = 0.001$], a 21% increase in the odds of achieving optimal myocardial reperfusion (TIMI myocardial perfusion grade 3) [$p = 0.008$], and a 27% reduction in the odds of having an intracoronary thrombus ($p < 0.001$) [15].

The PCI-CLARITY, a prospectively planned analysis of patients who underwent PCI in the CLARITY-TIMI 28, showed that pretreatment with CLP prior to PCI significantly reduced the incidence of CV death, recurrent myocardial infarction (re-MI), or stroke both before and after PCI. Overall, the incidence of primary end point before and after PCI was significantly lower in the CLP group than in the PL group (7.5% vs. 12.0%; adjusted odds ratio 0.59 [95% CI 0.43, 0.81]; $p = 0.001$) [20].

In the COMMIT study of patients with suspected MI (93% STEMI), with no upper age limit, presenting within 24 h from the onset of symptoms, 54% received fibrinolytic therapy. A 7% relative risk reduction in all-cause mortality and 9% in composite of death, MI, or stroke was demonstrated in CLP group compared to PL. The benefits of CLP did not differ significantly in patients who did and did not receive fibrinolytic agents [16].

In the CURRENT-OASIS 7 trial, the primary end point did not differ between patients receiving high- and standard-dose CLP; however, in the prespecified large group of patients undergoing PCI, a significant advantage of high dose was revealed in primary end point. High-dose CLP also significantly reduced the incidence of stent thrombosis compared with standard dose (3.9% vs. 4.5%, HR 0.86 [95% CI 0.74, 0.99]; $p = 0.0390$) [17, 21].

Results of three multicenter trials (CURE, COMMIT, and CLARITY-TIMI 28) involving over 63,000 patients have led to the approved indications of CLP in patients with acute coronary syndromes. The studies with PCI-treated patients (PCI-CURE, CREDO, PCI-CLARITY, CURRENT-OASIS 7) and several others (e.g., CLASSICS, HORIZONS-AMI, ARMYDA-2, ALBION, ISAR-CHOICE) have established the indications and optimal doses of CLP in patients treated invasively.

References

1 Kazui, M., Nishiya, Y., Ishizuka, T. *et al.* (2010) Identification of the human cytochrome P450 enzymes involved in the two oxidative steps in the bioactivation of clopidogrel to its pharmacologically active metabolite. *Drug Metabolism and Disposition*, **38**, 92–99.

2 Karaźniewicz-Łada, M., Danielak, D., and Główka, F. (2012) Genetic and non-genetic factors affecting the response to clopidogrel therapy. *Expert Opinion on Pharmacotherapy*, **13**, 663–683.

3 Bouman, H.J., Schomig, E., van Werkum, J.W. *et al.* (2011) Paraoxonase-1 is a major determinant of clopidogrel efficacy. *Nature Medicine*, **17**, 110–116.

4 Reny, J.-L., Combescure, C., Daali, Y., Fontana, P., and PON1 Meta-Analysis Group (2012) Influence of the paraoxonase-1 Q192R genetic variant on clopidogrel responsiveness and recurrent cardiovascular events: a systematic review and meta-analysis. *Journal of Thrombosis and Haemostasis*, **10**, 1242–1251.

5 Savcic, M., Hauert, J., Bachmann, F., Wyld, P.J., Geudelin, B., and Cariou, R. (1999) Clopidogrel loading dose regimen: kinetic profile of pharmacodynamics response in healthy subjects. *Seminars in Thrombosis and Hemostasis*, **25**, 15–19.

6 Gurbel, P.A., Bliden, K.P., Butler, K. *et al.* (2009) Randomized double-blind assessment of the ONSET and OFFSET of the antiplatelet effects of ticagrelor versus clopidogrel in patients with stable coronary artery disease. The ONSET/OFFSET study. *Circulation*, **120**, 2577–2585.

7 Von Beckerath, N., Taubert, D., Pogatsa-Murray, G., Schömig, E., Kastrati, A., and Schömig, A. (2005) Absorption, metabolization, and antiplatelet effects of 300-, 600-, and 900-mg loading doses of clopidogrel. Results of the ISAR-CHOICE (Intracoronary Stenting and Antithrombotic Regimen: Choose Between 3 High Oral Doses for Immediate Clopidogrel Effect) trial. *Circulation*, **112**, 2946–2950.

8 Taubert, D., von Beckerath, N., Grimberg, G. *et al.* (2006) Impact of P-glycoprotein on clopidogrel absorption. *Clinical Pharmacology and Therapeutics*, **80**, 486–501.

9 Mani, H., Toennes, S.W., Linnemann, B. *et al.* (2008) Determination of clopidogrel main metabolite in plasma: a useful tool for monitoring therapy? *Therapeutic Drug Monitoring*, **30**, 84–89.

10 Mullangi, R. and Srinivas, N.R. (2009) Clopidogrel: review of bioanalytical methods, pharmacokinetics/pharmacodynamics, and update on recent trends in drug-drug interaction studies. *Biomedical Chromatography*, **23**, 26–41.

11 Caplain, H., Donat, F., Gaud, C., and Necciari, J. (1999) Pharmacokinetics of clopidogrel. *Seminars in Thrombosis and Hemostasis*, **25** (Suppl.2), 25–28.

12 Lins, R., Broekhuysen, J., Necciari, J., and Deroubaix, X. (1999) Pharmacokinetic profile of ^{14}C-labeled clopidogrel. *Seminars in Thrombosis and Hemostasis*, **25**, 29–33.

13 Yusuf, S., Zhao, F., Mehta, S.R. *et al.* (2001) Effects of clopidogrel in addition to aspirin in patients with acute coronary syndromes without ST-segment elevation. *The New England Journal of Medicine*, **345**, 494–502.

14 Steinhubl, S.R., Berger, P.B., Mann, J.T., 3rd *et al.* (2002) Early and sustained dual oral antiplatelet therapy following percutaneous coronary intervention: a randomized controlled trial. *The Journal of the American Medical Association*, **288**, 2411–2420.

15 Sabatine, M.S. and Cannon, C.P. (2005) CLARITY-TIMI 28 Investigators, *et al.* Addition of clopidogrel to aspirin and fibrinolytic therapy for myocardial infarction with ST-segment elevation. *The New England Journal of Medicine*, **352**, 1179–1189.

16 Chen, Z.M., Jiang, L.X., Chen, Y.P. *et al.* (2001) Addition of clopidogrel to aspirin and fibrinolytic therapy for myocardial infarction with ST-segment elevation. *The New England Journal of Medicine*, **345**, 494–502.

17 CURRENT-OASIS 7 Investigators, Mehta, S.R., Bassand, J.P. *et al.* (2010) Dose comparisons of clopidogrel and aspirin in acute coronary syndromes. *The New England Journal of Medicine*, **363**, 930–942.

18 Budaj, A., Yusuf, S., Mehta, S.R. *et al.* (2002) Benefit of clopidogrel in patients with acute coronary syndromes without ST-segment elevation in various risk groups. *Circulation*, **106**, 1622–6.

19 Mehta, S.R., Yusuf, S., Peters, R.J.G. *et al.* (2001) Effects of pretreatment with clopidogrel and aspirin followed by long-term therapy in patients undergoing percutaneous coronary intervention: the PCI-CURE study. The Clopidogrel in Unstable angina to prevent Recurrent Events trial (CURE) Investigators. *Lancet*, **358**, 527–533.

20 Sabatine, M.S., Cannon, C.P., Gibson, C.M. *et al.* (2005) Effect of clopidogrel pretreatment before percutaneous coronary intervention in patients with ST-elevation myocardial infarction treated with fibrinolytics: the PCI-CLARITY study. The Clopidogrel as adjunctive Reperfusion Therapy (CLARITY)-Thrombolysis in Myocardial Infarction (TIMI) 28 Investigators. *The Journal of the American Medical Association*, **294**, 1224–1232.

21 Mehta, S.R., Tanguay, J.F., Eikelboom, J.W. *et al.* (2010) Double-dose versus standard-dose clopidogrel and high-dose versus low-dose aspirin in individuals undergoing percutaneous coronary interventions for acute coronary syndromes (CURRENT-OASIS 7): a randomized factorial trial. *Lancet*, **376**, 1233–1243.

20 Prasugrel

Christoph Varenhorst[1,2], Anna Oskarsson[1], and Stefan James[1,2]
[1] Uppsala Clinical Research Center, Uppsala, Sweden
[2] Uppsala University Hospital, Uppsala, Sweden

Introduction

The thienopyridines (e.g., clopidogrel, prasugrel) are metabolized by cytochrome P450 (CYP450) in the liver to active metabolites that irreversibly bind to the P2Y12 receptor, causing inhibition of platelet activation. Clopidogrel efficacy is hampered by a number of factors and poor responsiveness to clopidogrel occurs in 20–30 % of patients [1]. This has prompted the development of antiplatelet drugs, such as prasugrel, that inhibit platelets more effectively.

Mechanism of action

Clopidogrel's and prasugrel's conversions to the active metabolite have some key differences. Clopidogrel is metabolized by two CYP-dependent pathways. Prasugrel, on the other hand, first undergoes a rapid de-esterification in the intestine to an intermediate metabolite, which then is converted to the active metabolite in one CYP-dependent step [2] (Figure 20.1). The simpler activation for prasugrel results in a more potent, faster acting, and less variable platelet inhibition compared to clopidogrel.

Interaction studies indicate that the conversion to the prasugrel active metabolite is not influenced by reduced function polymorphisms, whereas the active metabolite formation for clopidogrel is at least affected by CYP2C19 polymorphisms [3, 4]. Also, prasugrel does not seem to interact to any clinical relevant extent with other drugs, including those CYP450 isoenzymes involved in prasugrel metabolism (CYP3A4, CYP2C9, CYP2C19, and CYP2B6) [2, 5].

Antiplatelet Therapy in Cardiovascular Disease, First Edition. Edited by Ron Waksman, Paul A. Gurbel, and Michael A. Gaglia, Jr.

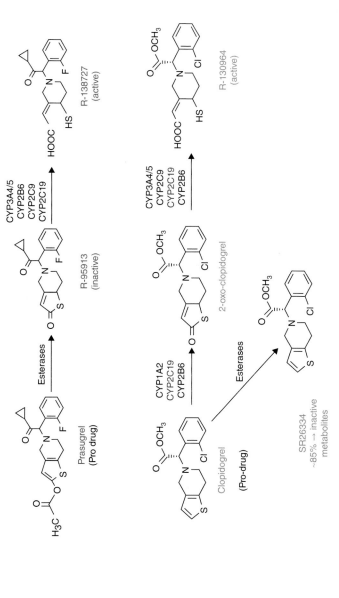

Figure 20.1 Prasugrel and clopidogrel metabolism. (Source: Adapted from Farid, N.A., Payne, C.D., Ernest, C.S. 2nd. et al. (2008) Prasugrel, a new thienopyridine antiplatelet drug, weakly inhibits cytochrome P450 2B6 in humans. *Journal of Clinical Pharmacology*, **48 (1)**, 53–59. Reproduced with permission of John Wiley & Sons Ltd.)

Prasugrel pharmacodynamics

Both the loading and maintenance doses of prasugrel result in a more rapid, consistent, and greater platelet inhibition than clopidogrel [1]. After a loading dose (LD) of 60 mg prasugrel, a maximum 60–70 % platelet inhibition is reached within 2–4 h in patients with stable coronary artery disease. Maintenance dosing with 10 mg prasugrel once daily achieves an average of 50 % platelet inhibition [6, 7]. However, in ST-segment elevation myocardial infarction (MI) patients undergoing primary PCI, the drug onset seems to be slower, with up to 4 h to achieve adequate platelet inhibition [8]. A possible explanation for the difference in time to drug-effect onset is altered gastrointestinal absorption in the acute phase of coronary syndromes. After the prasugrel treatment is discontinued, the platelet inhibition decreases to pretreatment levels within 7–10 days [9]. The SWAP (Switching Anti Platelet) study randomized patients who had received a run-in period of clopidogrel 75 mg once daily to a regimen of placebo LD/clopidogrel 75 mg maintenance dose (MD) or placebo LD/prasugrel 10 mg MD or prasugrel 60 mg LD/prasugrel 10 mg MD. Platelet reactivity was significantly lower with prasugrel maintenance dosing compared to clopidogrel maintenance dosing (41.1 % vs. 55.0 % inhibition of platelet aggregation (IPA); $p < 0.0001$) and prasugrel loading/maintenance dosing compared to clopidogrel maintenance dosing (41.0 % vs. 55.0 % IPA; $p < 0.0001$). The SWAP study confirmed that switching from clopidogrel to prasugrel leads to a further reduction in platelet reactivity by 1 week using prasugrel maintenance dosing or within 2 h with the administration of a prasugrel LD [10].

Clinical studies

The pivotal TRITON-TIMI (Trial to Assess Improvement in Therapeutic Outcomes by Optimizing Platelet Inhibition with Prasugrel – TIMI) 38 was the first mega trial assessing the hypothesis that higher and less variable P2Y12 platelet inhibition would prevent clinical ischemic events [11]. The trial was preceded by two phase II studies assessing the pharmacodynamics and safety of prasugrel. Although there was no significant difference in TIMI major and minor non-CABG-related bleeding in these studies, access site bleeding was more frequent with prasugrel compared to clopidogrel [12].

The TRITON-TIMI 38 enrolled 13,608 patients with moderate- and high-risk ACS and planned to PCI. Patients were randomized to prasugrel (60 mg LD and 10 mg daily MD) or clopidogrel (300 mg LD and 75 mg daily MD) for a median time of 14.5 months [11]. Prasugrel was associated with a significant reduction of the main efficacy end point (cardiovascular death, nonfatal MI, or nonfatal stroke), with an event rate of 12.1% in the clopidogrel group versus 9.9% in the prasugrel group ($p < 0.001$). This was mainly driven by a reduction in MI and stent thrombosis; no difference was observed in mortality. Study drugs were not given until the coronary anatomy was known. It has therefore been suggested that this design favored prasugrel over clopidogrel in preventing stent thrombosis by countervailing optimal upstream dosing.

The reduction of ischemic end points with prasugrel was accompanied by a higher incidence of major bleeding (TIMI major bleeding not related to CABG), occurring in 1.8% of the patients in the clopidogrel group versus 2.4% in the prasugrel group (HR 1.32; 95% CI 1.03–1.68; $P < 0.05$). *Post hoc* analyses showed that the highest bleeding risk was seen in the elderly (>75 years), in those with a low body weight (<60 kg), and in patients with previous stroke or transient ischemic attack in whom the net clinical benefit was neutral or in fact negative for the latter category of patients. The FDA has advised against prasugrel use in patients with active pathological bleeding, a history of TIA or stroke, or urgent need for CABG.

In the low-body-weight and elderly patients, an MD of prasugrel 5 mg has been recommended. Supporting this recommendation, Erlinge and colleagues recently showed, in two pharmacodynamic/pharmacokinetic studies, that prasugrel 5 mg in low body weight or elderly and prasugrel 10 mg in high body weight or nonelderly showed comparable reduction in platelet reactivity in patients with stable coronary artery disease [13, 14].

In the ST-elevation ACS subgroup from the TRITON-TIMI 38 ($n = 3534$) at 30 days, the primary composite end point of CV death, nonfatal MI, or nonfatal stroke occurred in 9.5 % of clopidogrel-treated patients compared to 6.5 % of prasugrel-treated patients ($p = 0.0017$) and the effect was seen to continue to 15 months [15]. No difference was seen in bleeding at 30 days or 15 months. In the secondary PCI group, the benefit of prasugrel was even more prominent. However, the incidence of bleeding complications in patients who had CABG surgery was fourfold higher in patients treated with prasugrel compared to clopidogrel (13.4 % vs. 3.2 %, HR 4.73; $p < 0.001$). The favorable bleeding risk in STEMI patients with prasugrel might be partly attributable to a lower risk of coronary artery bypass surgery in these patients.

Despite guideline recommendations in non-ST-elevation ACS, in real life, many patients (40–60% worldwide) are initially treated medically. The Targeted Platelet Inhibition to Clarify the Optimal Strategy to Medically Manage Acute Coronary Syndromes (TRILOGY ACS) trial compared aspirin coadministered with clopidogrel (300 mg LD, 75 mg MD) or prasugrel (30 mg LD, 5 or 10 mg MD (based upon weight and age)) in patients with unstable angina or non-ST-elevation ACS who were medically managed. There was no difference in the rate of the primary composite end point (death from cardiovascular causes, MI, or stroke) or its separate components between those who received prasugrel and those who received clopidogrel (13.9% vs. 16.0%, HR 0.91; 95% CI 0.79-1.00; $p = 0.04$ for the primary end point) [16]. Interestingly, the rates of severe and intracranial bleeds were similar in the two groups in all age groups. The 5 mg prasugrel dose appeared to be safe (which was not tested in the TRITON-TIMI 38) in patients aged 75 years and older and those under 60 kg.

The "A Comparison of Prasugrel at PCI or Time of Diagnosis of Non-ST Elevation Myocardial Infarction" (ACCOAST) trial assessed preloading with prasugrel at the time of diagnosis rather than after angioplasty in patients with non-ST-elevation ACS [17]. The trial's data and safety monitoring committee stopped enrolment at 4033 patients (designed to randomize 4100 patients) after noticing an increase in major and life-threatening bleeds and no reduction in cardiovascular events. Therefore, preloading with prasugrel in non-ST-ACS patients planned for PCI cannot be recommended.

The recently published ESC Guidelines for the management of ST-segment-elevation ACS patients give prasugrel and ticagrelor both class I indication (recommendation/level of evidence I b) whereas clopidogrel preferably only when prasugrel or ticagrelor is either not available or contraindicated (recommendation/level of evidence I c) [18]. For patients with non-ST-segment-elevation ACS, prasugrel is only recommended for P2Y12 inhibitor-naïve patients (especially diabetics) in whom coronary anatomy is known and who are proceeding to PCI unless there is a high risk of life-threatening bleeding or other contraindications (recommendation/level of evidence I b) [19].

In the American College of Cardiology Foundation/American Heart Association (ACCF/AHA) guidelines for ST-segment-elevation ACS, clopidogrel, prasugrel, and ticagrelor are given the same high level of recommendation (class I, level B) [20]. Also, for non-ST-segment-elevation ACS, the ACCF/AHA guidelines are not endorsing any of the three recommended P2Y12 receptor inhibitors over the other (prasugrel for PCI patients only) [21].

For patients undergoing CABG, the withdrawal period prior to surgery should be at least 7 days with prasugrel (recommendation/level of evidence IIa C).

Summary

As compared to clopidogrel, the novel antiplatelet drug prasugrel provides substantially improved outcome in patients with ACS treated with PCI. This is reflected in the updated ESC Guidelines where more potent P2Y12 receptor inhibitors are given priority over clopidogrel. Nonetheless, the better protection against ischemic events by a faster, greater, and less variable platelet inhibition with prasugrel is accompanied by an increased bleeding risk, especially in certain high-risk groups.

Reference

1 Wallentin, L. (2009) P2Y(12) inhibitors: differences in properties and mechanisms of action and potential consequences for clinical use. *European Heart Journal*, **30 (16)**, 1964–1977.
2 Farid, N.A., Smith, R.L., Gillespie, T.A. *et al* (2007) The disposition of prasugrel, a novel thienopyridine, in humans. *Drug Metabolism and Disposition: The Biological Fate of Chemicals*, **35 (7)**, 1096–1104.

3 Farid, N.A., Payne, C.D., Small, D.S. *et al.* (2007) Cytochrome P450 3A inhibition by ketoconazole affects prasugrel and clopidogrel pharmacokinetics and pharmacodynamics differently. *Clinical Pharmacology and Therapeutics*, **81 (5)**, 735–741.

4 Varenhorst, C., James, S., Erlinge, D. *et al.* (2009) Genetic variation of CYP2C19 affects both pharmacokinetic and pharmacodynamic responses to clopidogrel but not prasugrel in aspirin-treated patients with coronary artery disease. *European Heart Journal*, **30 (14)**, 1744–1752.

5 Dobesh, P.P. (2009) Pharmacokinetics and pharmacodynamics of prasugrel, a thienopyridine P2Y12 inhibitor. *Pharmacotherapy*, **29** (9), 1089–1102.

6 Jernberg, T., Payne, C.D., Winters, K.J. *et al.* (2006) Prasugrel achieves greater inhibition of platelet aggregation and a lower rate of non-responders compared with clopidogrel in aspirin-treated patients with stable coronary artery disease. *European Heart Journal*, **27 (10)**, 1166–1173.

7 Wallentin, L., Varenhorst, C., James, S. *et al.* (2008) Prasugrel achieves greater and faster P2Y12receptor-mediated platelet inhibition than clopidogrel due to more efficient generation of its active metabolite in aspirin-treated patients with coronary artery disease. *European Heart Journal*, **29 (1)**, 21–30.

8 Parodi, G., Valenti, R., Bellandi, B. *et al.* (2013) Comparison of Prasugrel and Ticagrelor loading doses in STEMI patients: The Rapid Activity of Platelet Inhibitor Drugs (RAPID) primary PCI Study. *Journal of the American College of Cardiology*, **61 (15)**, 1601–1606.

9 Jakubowski, J.A., Payne, C.D., Brandt, J.T. *et al.* (2006) The platelet inhibitory effects and pharmacokinetics of prasugrel after administration of loading and maintenance doses in healthy subjects. *Journal of Cardiovascular Pharmacology*, **47 (3)**, 377–384.

10 Angiolillo, D.J., Saucedo, J.F., Deraad, R. *et al.* (2010) Increased platelet inhibition after switching from maintenance clopidogrel to prasugrel in patients with acute coronary syndromes: results of the SWAP (SWitching Anti Platelet) study. *Journal of the American College of Cardiology*, **56** (13), 1017–1023.

11 Wiviott, S.D., Braunwald, E., McCabe, C.H. *et al.* (2007) Prasugrel versus clopidogrel in patients with acute coronary syndromes. *The New England Journal of Medicine*, **357 (20)**, 2001–2015.

12 Wiviott, S.D., Antman, E.M., Winters, K.J. *et al.* (2005) Randomized comparison of prasugrel (CS-747, LY640315), a novel thienopyridine P2Y12 antagonist, with clopidogrel in percutaneous coronary intervention: results of the Joint Utilization of Medications to Block Platelets Optimally (JUMBO)-TIMI 26 trial. *Circulation*, **111 (25)**, 3366–3373.

13 Erlinge, D., Ten Berg, J., Foley, D. *et al.* (2012) Reduction in platelet reactivity with prasugrel 5 mg in low-body-weight patients is noninferior to prasugrel 10 mg in higher-body-weight patients: results from the FEATHER trial. *Journal of the American College of Cardiology*, **60 (20)**, 2032–2040.

14 Erlinge, D., Gurbel, P., James, S. *et al.* (2012) Prasugrel 5 mg in the very elderly is non-inferior to prasugrel 10 mg in non-elderly patients: the generations trial, a pharmacodynamic (PD) study in stable CAD patients. http://spo.escardio.org/eslides/view.aspx?eevtid=54&fp=P3915 [accessed on February 18, 2014].

15 Montalescot, G., Wiviott, S.D., Braunwald, E. *et al.* (2009) Prasugrel compared with clopidogrel in patients undergoing percutaneous coronary intervention for ST-elevation myocardial infarction (TRITON-TIMI 38): double-blind, randomised controlled trial. *Lancet*, **373** (9665), 723–731.

16 Roe, M.T., Armstrong, P.W., Fox, K.A.A. *et al.* (2012) Prasugrel versus clopidogrel for acute coronary syndromes without revascularization. *The New England Journal of Medicine*, **367 (14)**, 1297–1309.

17 Montalescot, G., Bolognese, L., Dudek, D. *et al.* (2013) Pretreatment with prasugrel in non-ST-segment elevation acute coronary syndromes. *The New England Journal of Medicine*, **369**, 999–1010.

18 Steg, P.G., James, S.K., Atar, D. *et al.* (2012) ESC Guidelines for the management of acute myocardial infarction in patients presenting with ST-segment elevation: The Task Force on the management of ST-segment elevation acute myocardial infarction of the European Society of Cardiology (ESC). *European Heart Journal*, **33 (20)**, 2569–2619.

19 Hamm, C.W., Bassand, J.-P., Agewall, S. *et al.* (2011) ESC Guidelines for the management of acute coronary syndromes in patients presenting without persistent ST-segment elevation: The Task Force for the management of acute coronary syndromes (ACS) in patients presenting without persistent ST-segment elevation of the European Society of Cardiology (ESC). *European Heart Journal*, **32**, 2999–3054.

20 American College of Emergency Physicians, Society for Cardiovascular Angiography and Interventions, O'Gara, P.T. *et al.* (2013) ACCF/AHA guideline for the management of ST-elevation myocardial infarction: a report of the American College of Cardiology Foundation/American Heart Association Task Force on Practice Guidelines. *Journal of the American College of Cardiology*, **61(4)**:e78–e140.

21 Jneid, H., Anderson, J.L., Wright, R.S., Adams, C.D., Bridges, C.R. and Casey, D.E., Jr (2012) ACCF/AHA focused update of the guideline for the management of patients with unstable angina/non-ST-elevation myocardial infarction (updating the 2007 guideline and replacing the 2011 focused update): a report of the American College of Cardiology Foundation/American Heart Association Task Force on Practice Guidelines. *Journal of the American College of Cardiology*, **60 (7)**, 645–681.

21 Elinogrel

Matthew J. Chung[1,2] and Sunil V. Rao[1,2,3]
[1] Duke University Medical Center, Durham, NC, USA
[2] Durham Veterans Affairs Medical Center, Durham, NC, USA
[3] Duke Clinical Research Institute, Durham, NC, USA

Introduction

Antiplatelet therapy remains a cornerstone in the management of patients with coronary artery disease. Beginning with aspirin monotherapy, antiplatelet therapy has evolved to include the administration of $P2Y_{12}$ receptor inhibitors in addition to aspirin. This dual antiplatelet therapy provides greater platelet inhibition, which leads to a reduction in recurrent ischemic events, albeit at the cost of increased bleeding complications [1, 2, 3].

Shortcomings of current therapy

The thienopyridines (e.g., ticlopidine, clopidogrel, and prasugrel) irreversibly inhibit the $P2Y_{12}$ receptor. While all of these agents lead to a reduction in recurrent ischemic events, they each have their associated shortcomings. Ticlopidine suffers from association with hypercholesterolemia and, more seriously, hematological effects, including neutropenia, aplastic anemia, and thrombotic thrombocytopenic purpura [4]. Clopidogrel is plagued by its delayed onset of action, interindividual pharmacokinetic and pharmacodynamic variability, and drug–drug interactions [5]. Furthermore, the platelet inhibition induced by clopidogrel is irreversible and increases the risk of major bleeding [1] as well as leads to potential prolonged hospitalization if clopidogrel is administered before the decision is made to pursue coronary artery bypass surgery. Prasugrel has less interindividual variability and faster onset of action and provides more potent platelet inhibition; however, it also suffers from an increase in major bleeding and causes irreversible platelet inhibition [3]. Ticagrelor, a noncompetitive and reversible inhibitor of the $P2Y_{12}$ receptor, reduces mortality, but there are concerns about increased fatal intracranial bleeding and risks of patient noncompliance given the fast offset of the drug [6, 7].

Antiplatelet Therapy in Cardiovascular Disease, First Edition. Edited by Ron Waksman, Paul A. Gurbel, and Michael A. Gaglia, Jr.
© 2014 John Wiley & Sons, Ltd. Published 2014 by John Wiley & Sons, Ltd.

Pharmacological principles of elinogrel

Elinogrel, a novel, small-molecule, direct-acting, competitive, reversible, intravenous (IV) and oral quinazolinedione $P2Y_{12}$ receptor inhibitor (Portola Pharmaceuticals, San Francisco, CA, USA), has pharmacological properties that may address some of the limitations of current antiplatelet therapies. Elinogrel is synthesized from ethyl-5-chlorothiophen-2-ylsulfonylcarbamate and 3-(4-aminophenyl)-6-fluoro-7-(methylamino) quinazoline-2,4($1H$,$3H$)-dione [8]. Notably, it exists in both oral and IV preparations without interactions at the level of the $P2Y_{12}$ receptor, allowing for ease of transition from IV to oral formulations without interruption in platelet inhibition. Prior studies have shown a drug interaction between the intravenously administered cangrelor and the orally administered thienopyridines (e.g., clopidogrel and prasugrel) [9], which leads to an inability of thienopyridine-induced platelet inhibition because the $P2Y_{12}$ receptor is already bound by cangrelor. Since both the oral and IV forms of elinogrel do not have these interactions at the level of the $P2Y_{12}$ receptor, sustained platelet inhibition is feasible even when transitioning from IV to oral dosing. In addition, elinogrel has a direct-acting mechanism of action without the need to be metabolized into an active form. Thus, in contrast to clopidogrel and prasugrel, which are both prodrugs, elinogrel avoids potential drug–drug interactions that result from reliance on the cytochrome P450 (CYP) system.

The elimination half-life of elinogrel is 11–12 h, time to peak 20 min, and offset 24 h. Clearance is mainly via hepatic demethylation and renal excretion. Twice daily dosing is required to maintain stable plasma concentrations.

Phase I clinical studies

Table 21.1 summarizes the three phase I clinical studies investigating the tolerability and pharmacokinetic and pharmacodynamic properties of elinogrel.

The study by Lieu et al. showed tolerability of IV elinogrel and delineated its pharmacokinetic and pharmacodynamics properties [10].

The study by Conley et al. deserves additional comment due to seemingly discrepant results, based on the use of light transmission aggregometry (LTA) versus perfusion chamber assay (PCA), in regard to comparative efficacy of clopidogrel versus elinogrel in inducing platelet inhibition [11]. These observed differences in the pharmacodynamics of elinogrel suggest its unique ability to induce differential levels of platelet inhibition based on the concentration of adenosine diphosphate (ADP) present. Prior studies have shown that ADP concentrations are lower in thrombosis than in hemostasis [12]. Thus, elinogrel may be able to produce more platelet inhibition during arterial thrombosis in which there are low levels of ADP and less platelet inhibition during hemostasis in which there are high levels of ADP. This unique property derives from

Table 21.1 Phase I clinical studies of elinogrel.

Trial	Patient population	Intervention	Conclusions
Lieu et al. [10]	N=40. Healthy volunteers. Five groups of eight subjects (six active, two placebo)	Doses of IV elinogrel ranging from 1 mg to 40 mg given over 20 min	Maximum platelet inhibition was achieved at 20 min after stimuli ADP 10 μmol/L. A dose of 20 mg achieved 81% platelet inhibition. Single IV doses of elinogrel ≥10 mg achieved high levels of platelet inhibition, which was fully reversible within 8 h. Plasma concentrations were dose related and correlated well with the level of platelet inhibition
		Dose-escalation study with single oral doses of elinogrel (10, 30±aspirin, 100, 200, 400, and 800 mg) given	Dose-escalation study showed tolerance in all patients with no adverse events. LTA showed full inhibition of ADP-induced platelet aggregation in a dose-dependent manner and PCA revealed that elinogrel inhibited thrombus and destabilized thrombus starting at 30 mg. The addition of aspirin had a synergistic effect in the inhibition of collagen-induced platelet aggregation. A single dose of elinogrel 100 mg had the same effect as elinogrel 30 mg plus aspirin
Conley et al. [11]	N=24. Healthy volunteers. Each arm of the study had 12 subjects	Arm 1: oral elinogrel 100 mg twice daily Arm 2: clopidogrel 75 mg + aspirin 325 mg daily	LTA showed that clopidogrel induced higher platelet inhibition compared with elinogrel after 5 μmol/L (66 vs. 55%) and 20 μmol/L (52 vs. 33%) ADP stimuli. PCA showed that elinogrel was found to have more potent inhibition of thrombosis than clopidogrel (83 vs. 75%)
Gurbel et al. [7, 13]	N=45. Patients older than 18 years of age who had undergone previous coronary artery stenting and were treated with chronic daily 75 mg clopidogrel and 81 mg aspirin	Screened for HPR to ADP. Twenty subjects with HPR identified. Between 12 h and 16 h after the last dose of clopidogrel, a single oral dose of elinogrel 60 mg was given. All subjects continued maintenance aspirin and clopidogrel	In a majority of subjects, there was a significant reduction in maximum 5 μmol/L ADP-induced platelet aggregation at 4 h compared with baseline, and this returned to baseline within 24 h. Multiple different assays demonstrated that elinogrel was able to rapidly inhibit platelets and decrease thrombus size, which was reversible 24 h after treatment. Peak plasma concentrations of elinogrel and the observed pharmacodynamic inhibition correlated well using all assays The CYP2C19*2 allele was more common in subjects with HPR (77 vs. 16%, $P=0.0004$) during clopidogrel and aspirin therapy; however, a single 60 mg oral dose of elinogrel was able to effectively inhibit platelets despite the presence of the CYP2C19*2 allele. Elinogrel was tolerated by all subjects without adverse events

ADP, adenosine diphosphate; HPR, high platelet reactivity; IV, intravenous; LTA, light transmission aggregometry; and PCA, perfusion chamber assay.

elinogrel's reversible and competitive binding to the $P2Y_{12}$ receptor, which can be displaced by increased levels of ADP. Since LTA uses exogenous ADP, which competes with elinogrel for binding to the $P2Y_{12}$ receptor, this assay may underestimate the pharmacodynamic effect of elinogrel in a thrombotic state, whereas PCA indicates the concentration of $P2Y_{12}$ receptor inhibitor necessary to provide platelet inhibition under the low ADP concentrations seen in thrombosis. PCA simulates real-time platelet thrombus formation in a collagen-coated capillary tube under shear stress in the presence of Xa inhibitor and is felt to provide a theoretically more physiological model of thrombosis.

The study by Gurbel *et al.* found that certain CYP polymorphisms are associated with high platelet reactivity (HPR) in patients on standard dual antiplatelet therapy with aspirin and clopidogrel; however, elinogrel was able to effectively inhibit platelets in all patients, despite these CYP polymorphisms [13].

Phase II clinical studies

The Early Rapid ReversAl of platelet thromboSis with intravenous Elinogrel before PCI to optimize reperfusion in acute Myocardial Infarction (ERASE-MI) was a pilot, phase IIa, randomized, double-blind, placebo-controlled, dose-escalation study designed to evaluate the safety and tolerability of escalating doses of elinogrel administered as a single IV bolus compared with placebo in patients undergoing primary PCI for ST-elevation myocardial infarction (STEMI) [14]. In this study, elinogrel was administered just prior to primary PCI and was an adjunct to a 600 mg clopidogrel loading dose followed by a second 300 mg clopidogrel loading dose 4 h after PCI. This regimen was instituted because clopidogrel may in fact compete with oral elinogrel as well; thus, without a second oral load, there was the potential to have the patient "uncovered," that is, with no ADP inhibition. In-hospital bleeding, defined by the Thrombolysis in Myocardial Infarction (TIMI) and Global Use of Strategies to Open Occluded Coronary Arteries (GUSTO) bleeding scales, was the primary outcome. The study consisted of two parts – a dose-escalation study and a dose-confirmation study. In the dose-escalation study, 70 subjects were randomized to one of four doses of IV elinogrel (10, 20, 40, or 60 mg) or placebo prior to the start of the diagnostic angiogram preceding primary PCI. Results showed that the incidence of bleeding events was infrequent and appeared to be similar in all subjects irrespective of elinogrel dosage or placebo administration. In comparing elinogrel with placebo, there were no differences in serious adverse events, laboratory values, corrected TIMI frame count, or ST resolution. Although limited by a small study sample size, this pilot study suggested the feasibility and tolerability of escalating doses of elinogrel as an adjunctive therapy for primary PCI to treat STEMI.

The INtraveNous and Oral administration of elinogrel versus clopidogrel to eVAluate Tolerability and Efficacy in nonurgent Percutaneous Coronary

Interventions patients (INNOVATE-PCI) was a multicenter, phase IIb, randomized, double-blind, triple-dummy, clopidogrel-controlled study of IV and oral elinogrel compared with clopidogrel in patients undergoing nonurgent PCI [15]. After diagnostic angiography, subjects scheduled for nonurgent PCI were randomized to receive either 300 or 600 mg of clopidogrel pre-PCI followed by 75 mg daily or 80 or 120 mg of IV elinogrel

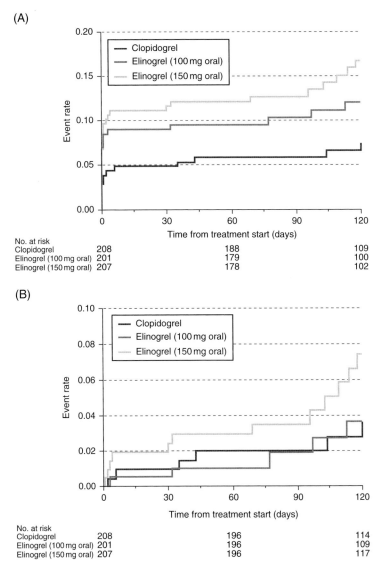

Figure 21.1 Kaplan–Meier curves of time to first bleeding event with adjudicated TIMI major, TIMI minor, and TIMI bleeding requiring medical attention (BRMA) (A) from treatment to day 120 or (B) from landmark analysis at 24 h or discharge (whichever occurred first) to 120 days (Source: Welsh RC et al., 2012 [15]. Reproduced with permission of Wolters Kluwer Health.)

followed by 50, 100, or 150 mg oral elinogrel twice daily. There was no prespecified primary end point; instead, the study was designed to assess numerous exploratory safety and efficacy outcomes. Combined TIMI major bleeding, minor bleeding, and bleeding requiring medical attention (BRMA) was increased with elinogrel, largely due to an increase in BRMA, which occurred primarily at the PCI access site. This occurred within the first 24 h after initiating IV elinogrel. There were no statistically significant differences in TIMI combined bleeding during the chronic (oral) phase of therapy (Figure 21.1). Importantly, there was no increase in TIMI major or minor bleeding during the acute (IV) or chronic (oral) phases of the study. Clinical efficacy end points and the incidence of periprocedural myocardial infarction were statistically similar; however, there was a nonsignificant trend towards higher frequency of periprocedural myocardial infarctions in the elinogrel arms. In terms of adverse events, there was a higher incidence of subjective dyspnea and elevations in liver transaminases in the elinogrel arms. The dyspnea was self-limited, the "transaminitis" was asymptomatic, and there were no cases of Hy's law or liver failure. There were no cases of heart block, bradycardia, or hypotension in the elinogrel arms. A substudy of the INNOVATE-PCI trial showed that compared with clopidogrel, the combination of IV and oral elinogrel achieved more rapid and enhanced antiplatelet effects that were sustained through the transition to oral elinogrel in the peri-PCI period, but these differences were not statistically significant during chronic dosing [16].

Conclusion

Elinogrel is a novel, direct-acting, competitive, reversible, IV and oral P2Y$_{12}$ receptor inhibitor. Although promising given its direct-acting and rapid onset and offset of action, potent antiplatelet activity, oral and IV formulations, and suggested tolerability and efficacy in phase II studies, definitive conclusions cannot be made until phase III studies are conducted.

References

1 Yusuf, S., Zhao, F., Mehta, S.R., Chrolavicius, S., Tognoni, G., and Fox, K.K. (2001) Effects of clopidogrel in addition to aspirin in patients with acute coronary syndromes without ST-segment elevation. *The New England Journal of Medicine*, **345**, 494–502.

2 Bertrand, M.E., Legrand, V., Boland, J. *et al.* (1998) Randomized multicenter comparison of conventional anticoagulation versus antiplatelet therapy in unplanned and elective coronary stenting. The full anticoagulation versus aspirin and ticlopidine (fantastic) study. *Circulation*, **98**, 1597–1603.

3 Wiviott, S.D., Braunwald, E., McCabe, C.H. *et al.* (2007) Prasugrel versus clopidogrel in patients with acute coronary syndromes. *The New England Journal of Medicine*, **357**, 2001–2015.

4 Myat, A.G.T. (2010) The contemporary use of antiplatelet therapy in interventional cardiology. In: S.C.N. Redwood and M. Thomas (eds), Oxford Textbook of Interventional Cardiology. 1st. Oxford University Press Inc., New York.

5 Leonardi, S., Rao, S.V., Harrington, R.A. *et al.* (2010) Rationale and design of the randomized, double-blind trial testing INtraveNous and Oral administration of elinogrel, a selective and reversible P2Y(12)-receptor inhibitor, versus clopidogrel to eVAluate Tolerability and Efficacy in nonurgent Percutaneous Coronary Interventions patients (INNOVATE-PCI). *American Heart Journal*, **160**, 65–72.

6 Cannon, C.P., Harrington, R.A., James, S. *et al.* (2010) Comparison of ticagrelor with clopidogrel in patients with a planned invasive strategy for acute coronary syndromes (PLATO): a randomised double-blind study. *Lancet*, **375**, 283–293.

7 Gurbel, P.A., Bliden, K.P., Butler, K. *et al.* (2009) Randomized double-blind assessment of the ONSET and OFFSET of the antiplatelet effects of ticagrelor versus clopidogrel in patients with stable coronary artery disease: the ONSET/OFFSET study. *Circulation*, **120**, 2577–2585.

8 Oestreich, J.H. (2010) Elinogrel, a reversible P2Y12 receptor antagonist for the treatment of acute coronary syndrome and prevention of secondary thrombotic events. *Current Opinion in Investigational Drugs*, **11**, 340–348.

9 Dovlatova, N.L., Jakubowski, J.A., Sugidachi, A., and Heptinstall, S. (2008) The reversible P2Y antagonist cangrelor influences the ability of the active metabolites of clopidogrel and prasugrel to produce irreversible inhibition of platelet function. *Journal of Thrombosis and Haemostasis*, **6**, 1153–1159.

10 Lieu, H.D., Conley, P.B., Andre, P. *et al.* (2007) Initial intravenous experience with PRT 060128, an orally available, direct acting, and reversible $P2Y_{12}$ inhibitor. *Journal of Thrombosis and Haemostasis*, **5 (2)**, P-T-292.

11 Conley, P.B., Andre, P., Stephens, G. *et al.* (2009) ADP-mediated aggregation as a pharmacodynamic assay underestimates the antithrombotic activity of elinogrel, a competitive, reversible P2Y12 inhibitor, relative to clopidogrel. *J Thromb Haemost*, **7** (Suppl 2Abstract PP-TH-027).

12 Folie, B.J. and McIntire, L.V. (1989) Mathematical analysis of mural thrombogenesis. Concentration profiles of platelet-activating agents and effects of viscous shear flow. *Biophysical Journal*, **56**, 1121–1141.

13 Gurbel, P.A., Bliden, K.P., Antonio, M.J. *et al.* (2010) The effect of elinogrel on high platelet reactivity during dual antiplatelet therapy and the relation to CYP 2C19*2 genotype: first experience in patients. *Journal of Thrombosis and Haemostasis*, **8**, 43–53.

14 Berger, J.S., Roe, M.T., Gibson, C.M. *et al.* (2009) Safety and feasibility of adjunctive antiplatelet therapy with intravenous elinogrel, a direct-acting and reversible P2Y12 ADP-receptor antagonist, before primary percutaneous intervention in patients with ST-elevation myocardial infarction: the Early Rapid ReversAl of platelet thromboSis with intravenous Elinogrel before PCI to optimize reperfusion in acute Myocardial Infarction (ERASE MI) pilot trial. *American Heart Journal*, **158**, 998.e1–1004.e1.

15 Welsh, R.C., Rao, S.V., Zeymer, U. *et al.* (2012) A randomized, double-blind, active-controlled phase 2 trial to evaluate a novel selective and reversible intravenous and oral P2Y12 inhibitor elinogrel versus clopidogrel in patients undergoing nonurgent percutaneous coronary intervention: the INNOVATE-PCI trial. *Circulation. Cardiovascular Interventions*, **5**, 336–346.

16 Angiolillo, D.J., Welsh, R.C., Trenk, D. *et al.* (2012) Pharmacokinetic and pharmacodynamic effects of elinogrel: results of the platelet function substudy from the intravenous and oral administration of elinogrel to evaluate tolerability and efficacy in nonurgent percutaneous coronary intervention patients (INNOVATE-PCI) trial. *Circulation. Cardiovascular Interventions*, **5**, 347–356.

22 Cangrelor

Francesco Franchi, Fabiana Rollini, Ana Muñiz-Lozano, and Dominick J. Angiolillo
University of Florida College of Medicine, Jacksonville, FL, USA

Oral adenosine diphosphate (ADP) $P2Y_{12}$ receptor inhibitors have consistently demonstrated to reduce the risk of thrombotic events in patients with acute coronary syndrome (ACS) and undergoing percutaneous coronary intervention (PCI) [1, 2, 3]. However, oral $P2Y_{12}$ receptor inhibitors mostly utilized in clinical practice (clopidogrel, prasugrel, and ticagrelor) have several limitations. Clopidogrel is a prodrug characterized by high variability in absorption, delayed onset of action, drug–drug interactions, incomplete $P2Y_{12}$ receptor inhibition, and broad interindividual response variability [4]. Prasugrel is, like clopidogrel, a thienopyridine but with faster and more potent $P2Y_{12}$ receptor inhibition [5]. Ticagrelor, a direct-acting reversible $P2Y_{12}$ inhibitor, also has faster and more potent platelet inhibitory effects compared with clopidogrel [6]. However, both prasugrel and ticagrelor have delayed and suboptimal platelet inhibition in the first 2 h following drug administration in patients with ST-elevation myocardial infarction (STEMI), a setting where immediate and potent platelet inhibitory effects are needed [7, 8]. In addition, clopidogrel and prasugrel are irreversible platelet inhibitors, with duration of effects of 7–10 days [9], while ticagrelor, even if it is a reversible inhibitor, should be stopped at least 5 days before surgery [6]. Therefore, many physicians refrain from administering $P2Y_{12}$ inhibitors before angiography, since irreversible platelet blockade increases the risk of coronary artery bypass grafting (CABG)-related bleeding [2, 3].

In addition to the concerns raised on the limitations of oral $P2Y_{12}$ receptor inhibitors, about 5–20% of patients need to undergo some kind of surgery within the year after stent implant or ACS diagnosis. The risk of perioperative cardiac ischemic events, particularly stent thrombosis (ST), is high in these patients, because surgery has a prothrombotic effect and antiplatelet therapy is often withdrawn in order to avoid bleeding [10]. Several antithrombotic approaches have been proposed for bridging strategies. However, heparin and low-molecular-weight heparin are generally not recommended, because they do not have antiplatelet effects (unfractionated heparin can actually increase platelet reactivity). Small-molecule glycoprotein IIb/IIIa inhibitors (GPIs), such as tirofiban and

Antiplatelet Therapy in Cardiovascular Disease, First Edition. Edited by Ron Waksman, Paul A. Gurbel, and Michael A. Gaglia, Jr.
© 2014 John Wiley & Sons, Ltd. Published 2014 by John Wiley & Sons, Ltd.

eptifibatide, have been tested in small studies because of their rapid onset of action and consistent platelet inhibitory effects [11]. However, they have a relatively slow offset of action (~4–6 h), and their prolonged administration in the setting of bridging can increase the risk of bleeding [12].

Ultimately, current $P2Y_{12}$ inhibitors are only available orally and cannot provide reliable inhibition in patients who are unable to swallow or rapidly absorb medications taken orally, such as patients who are sedated, intubated, or in shock or those with nausea or vomiting [13]. Overall, these findings underscore the need for a $P2Y_{12}$ inhibiting agent available for intravenous use with a prompt and potent onset of action, limited interindividual variability, and fast offset of action.

Cangrelor is an intravenous adenosine triphosphate (ATP) analog which directly inhibits, without being metabolized, the $P2Y_{12}$ receptor in a reversible manner; it has a rapid onset and offset mechanism of action and achieves high degrees of platelet inhibition [14]. This chapter provides an overview of the current status of knowledge on cangrelor, focusing on its pharmacological properties and clinical development.

Pharmacological properties

ATP targets mainly the $P2Y_1$ receptor, which is involved in platelet shape change and helps amplify platelet responses mediated by other agonists [15]. It has less affinity to the $P2Y_1$ and $P2Y_{12}$ receptors because it is rapidly metabolized by ectonucleotidases [16]. The final therapeutic compound of cangrelor (2-trifluoropropylthio, N-(2-(methylthio)ethyl)-β,γ-dichloromethylene ATP) was modified from ATP to confer higher affinity, longer half-life, and higher antagonistic property with a potency increased by six times [14]. These structural changes resulted in unique pharmacological advantages. Cangrelor has high affinity for the $P2Y_{12}$ receptor, has a higher resistance to ectonucleotidases [16], does not require hepatic conversion, and is directly active. Cangrelor has a linear dose-dependent pharmacokinetic profile, with predictable plasma levels, and reaches steady-state concentrations within minutes, providing stable pharmacodynamic effects. Moreover, it has a very short half-life (2–5 min) leading to a fast offset of action (30–60 min) [17].

Preclinical studies and early phase clinical investigations

Cangrelor inhibited thrombus formation and ADP-induced platelet aggregation in animal models and showed lower increase in bleeding time when compared to GPIs [18]. Infusion in a range of 0.1–4 μg/kg/min showed a dose-dependent effect on platelet inhibition. The steady-state plasmatic concentrations were achieved rapidly and platelet inhibition reversed after 20 min of infusion discontinuation [19]. Greater inhibition of ADP-induced platelet aggregation and less response variability with cangrelor than with clopidogrel were also demonstrated, and cangrelor was able to essentially abolish ADP-induced platelet aggregation in clopidogrel-treated patients [20, 21].

The safety and preliminary efficacy results of cangrelor have been evaluated in several phase II clinical investigations. In ACS patients, cangrelor showed a mean half-life of less than 5 min, a small volume of distribution, and a dose-dependent effect. The steady-state level of inhibition was achieved within 30 min, and the proportions of patients with 100% inhibition of maximal platelet aggregation induced by ADP at 24 h were 77% with 2 µg/kg/min and 86% with 4 µg/kg/min. All patients had greater than 80% inhibition of aggregation, and 60% of the baseline platelet aggregation was recovered within 1 h after stopping infusion. Minor bleedings were observed in 56% patients, with no major bleeding and a poor correlation between bleeding time and drug plasmatic concentrations [22].

Another study on STEMI patients demonstrated no difference between full dose of alteplase and combination of half-dose of alteplase along with cangrelor in Thrombolysis in Myocardial Infarction (TIMI)-3 flow at 60 min, while cangrelor alone was significantly inferior. However, a trend toward improvement in ST-segment recovery was observed in patients receiving combination therapy. Bleeding events and major adverse clinical events were similar among groups [23]. Among patients undergoing PCI, cangrelor demonstrated similar 30-day incidence of cardiac adverse events compared with abciximab (7.6 vs. 5.3%; $P = $ ns). Platelet inhibition was similar during the steady-state phase, but 12–24 h after terminating infusion, it persisted in the abciximab group while returned to baseline in cangrelor-treated patients. No significant difference in rates of bleeding was found comparing cangrelor either with placebo or abciximab [24].

Since diabetes mellitus (DM) is known to be associated with impaired response to antiplatelet therapies [25], the pharmacodynamic effect of cangrelor was compared in clopidogrel-naïve coronary artery disease patients ($n = 103$) with and without DM. After *in vitro* incubation with 500 nmol/L of cangrelor, a significant reduction in vasodilator-stimulated phosphoprotein $P2Y_{12}$ reactivity index (VASP-PRI) was observed in the overall population (80.6 ± 14.0% relative reduction in PRI). Interestingly, this reduction was consistent in DM and non-DM patients ($P < 0.0001$ for both comparisons), with no difference in PRI values between groups (16.1 ± 12.3 vs. 16.8 ± 11.3; $P = 0.346$). Moreover, the dose-dependent effect of cangrelor was not influenced by DM status [26].

Drug interactions

A study on healthy volunteers randomized to receive clopidogrel (600 mg loading dose) either simultaneously or immediately after cangrelor administration (bolus of 30 µg/kg and 1-h infusion of 4 µg/kg/min) showed a competitive interaction between the two drugs. The very high affinity of cangrelor to $P2Y_{12}$ receptor prevents the active metabolite of clopidogrel to bind to the receptor during infusion. Therefore, clopidogrel-induced platelet inhibition is precluded if the $P2Y_{12}$ receptor is already inhibited by cangrelor [27]. The same effect was demonstrated also on prasugrel ability to inhibit platelet aggregation. In contrast, addition of cangrelor after preincubation with active metabolites of clopidogrel or prasugrel led to a sustained platelet inhibition [28]. Instead, no significant pharmacodynamic interaction was observed between cangrelor and the direct-acting $P2Y_{12}$ receptor antagonist ticagrelor using an *ex vivo* canine model [29]. Overall, these observations underline the need of an appropriate transitioning strategy from cangrelor to oral $P2Y_{12}$ receptor inhibitors. Thus far, transitioning studies have only been performed from cangrelor to clopidogrel in which clopidogrel should be administered only after cangrelor infusion discontinuation [30, 31, 32, 33]. Transitioning studies from cangrelor to prasugrel or ticagrelor have yet to be reported.

Cangrelor in patients undergoing PCI: phase III studies

The efficacy of cangrelor in patients undergoing PCI predominantly with ACS was first studied in two parallel large phase III trials, the Platelet Inhibition with Cangrelor in Patients Undergoing PCI (CHAMPION-PCI) trial [30] and the Intravenous Platelet Blockade with Cangrelor during PCI (CHAMPION-PLATFORM) trial [31]. The primary end point for both studies was a composite of death from any cause, myocardial infarction (MI), and ischemia-driven revascularization (IDR) at 48 h post randomization.

In CHAMPION-PCI, patients were randomized to receive a 30-µg/kg bolus dose of cangrelor followed by a 4-µg/kg/min infusion (administered within 30 min of the PCI start and continued for a minimum of 2 h and no longer than 4 h) plus 600-mg loading dose of clopidogrel at the end of infusion or a 600-mg loading dose of clopidogrel prior to the start of PCI. In CHAMPION-PLATFORM, patients were randomized to receive cangrelor bolus of 30 µg/kg and infusion 4 µg/kg/min or a matching placebo bolus and infusion. Patients in the placebo group received a loading dose of 600 mg of clopidogrel at the end of the PCI, while patients in the cangrelor group at the end of infusion (Figure 22.1). In both trials, patients randomized to cangrelor received their loading dose of clopidogrel after infusion discontinuation, in order to avoid interaction between clopidogrel and cangrelor. Patients with STEMI and on prior clopidogrel therapy were eligible for CHAMPION-PCI but excluded from CHAMPION-PLATFORM. However, enrollment was terminated early for low likelihood of achieving the primary end point (98% of patients enrolled in CHAMPION-PCI and 84% in CHAMPION-PLATFORM), and both trials failed to demonstrate the superiority of adjunctive cangrelor therapy for the primary end point (7.5% vs. 7.1%; OR 1.05; 95% CI, 0.88–1.24; $P=0.59$ and 7% vs. 8%; OR 0.87; 95% CI, 0.71–1.07; $P=0.17$, respectively). Of note, a benefit with cangrelor was shown in

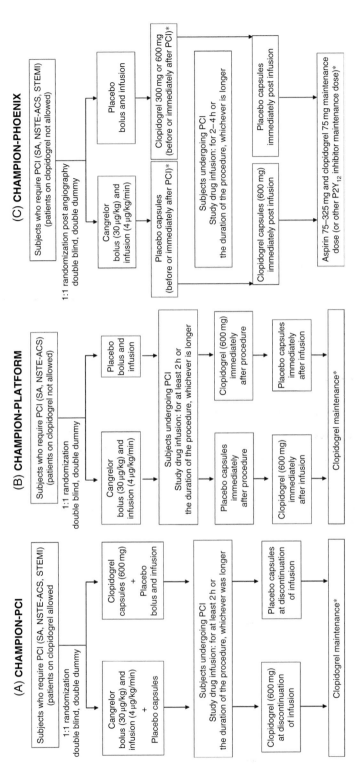

Figure 22.1 Study designs of the CHAMPION trials [30, 31, 31, 33]. (A) CHAMPION-PCI. (B) CHAMPION-PLATFORM. (C) CHAMPION PHOENIX. NSTE-ACS, non-ST-segment elevation acute coronary syndrome; PCI, percutaneous coronary intervention; SA, stable angina; STEMI, ST-segment elevation myocardial infarction; *, at the discretion of the physician.

prespecified secondary end points not dependent on cardiac biomarkers and, overall, in the rate of ST. In addition, the time from randomization to PCI was very short, making difficult the assessment of PCI-related MI. Interestingly, the rate of major bleeding was higher with cangrelor according to Acute Catheterization and Urgent Intervention Triage Strategy (ACUITY) criteria but not with other bleeding scores.

A predefined prospectively designed platelet function substudy of CHAMPION trials was also performed in a selected cohort of patients ($n = 234$) to provide insight into the pharmacodynamic effects of cangrelor, particularly exploring if cangrelor therapy may interfere with the inhibitory effects of clopidogrel [32]. Pharmacodynamic assays included $P2Y_{12}$ reaction units (PRU) assessed by VerifyNow $P2Y_{12}$ testing, as well as other assays. The difference in the percent of patients who reached the primary end point (percentage of patients who achieved <20% change in PRU between baseline and 10 h after PCI) in the cangrelor arm (38.1%) compared to the clopidogrel arm (25.3%) was not statistically significant (difference: 12.79%; 95% CI: −1.18%, 26.77%; $P = 0.076$). During infusion, cangrelor patients achieved a significant lower platelet aggregation (median PRU: 93.5 vs. 277.0; $P < 0.001$). Moreover, cangrelor treatment significantly reduces the prevalence of patients with high on-treatment platelet reactivity ($P < 0.01$), defined as PRU greater than 235. However, the value of platelet reactivity measured after infusion discontinuation was not significantly different between groups, suggesting that the pharmacodynamic effects of clopidogrel were not attenuated by cangrelor and confirming the rapid recovery of platelet function after discontinuation of infusion.

In both CHAMPION trials, the primary end point was driven by the occurrence of MI. However, MI is difficult to evaluate post-PCI particularly when cardiac biomarkers are elevated before the procedure and when the time from hospital admission to PCI is short as in the CHAMPION trials (6.3 (interquartile range 2.6–23.7 h) in PCI and 7.9 (interquartile range 3.3–24.1 h) in PLATFORM). In fact, a benefit with cangrelor was observed in prespecified secondary end points not dependent on cardiac biomarkers and in the CHAMPION-PLATFORM subgroup of patients without elevated troponin levels at baseline. Considering all these issues, a prespecified pooled analysis of data from CHAMPION trials utilizing the universal definition to define MI was performed [34]. The universal definition of MI defined MI associated with PCI as elevation of biomarkers greater than 3 times the 99th percentile upper limit of normal [35]. Moreover, if biomarkers are elevated before the procedure and not stable, biomarker criteria for the diagnosis of periprocedural MI are not recommended. Applying the universal definition of MI, 59.5% of events were removed from the analysis, and the authors showed that at 48 h cangrelor significantly reduced the primary end point (3.1% vs. 3.8; OR 0.82; 95% CI, 0.68–0.99; $P = 0.037$). At 30 days, the absolute difference in the primary end point was similar (0.6% vs. 0.7%) but was no longer statistically significant ($P = 0.10$).

Given these data, the Cangrelor versus standard therapy to acHieve optimal Management of Platelet InhibitiON (CHAMPION) PHOENIX trial was designed to compare cangrelor to clopidogrel standard of care in clopidogrel-naïve patients undergoing PCI (for stable angina (SA), non-ST-segment elevation acute coronary syndrome (NSTE-ACS), and STEMI) [33]. After angiography, patients ($n = 11,145$) were randomized to receive either cangrelor bolus (30 µg/kg) followed by infusion (4 µg/kg per minute) or clopidogrel loading dose (300 or 600 mg as per institutional standard) (Figure 22.1). The infusion had to be continued for at least 2 h or until the conclusion of the index PCI, whichever was longer. At the discretion of the physician, patients received either the loading dose of clopidogrel or matching placebo before or at the end of the procedure. The primary efficacy end point was a composite of death from any cause, MI (determined using the universal definition), IDR, and ST assessed at 48 h defined on a modified intention-to-treat basis (patients needed to be assigned to study treatment and undergo PCI). The key secondary end point was the incidence of ST at 48 h (including definite ST and intraprocedural ST). The primary safety end point was severe bleeding not related to CABG, according to the Global Use of Strategies to Open Occluded Coronary Arteries (GUSTO) criteria, at 48 h. Cangrelor significantly reduced the primary efficacy end point (4.7% in the cangrelor group vs. 5.9% in the clopidogrel group; adjusted OR with cangrelor, 0.78; 95% CI, 0.66–0.93; $P = 0.005$), with a number needed to treat to prevent one primary end point event of 84 (95% CI, 49–285). The efficacy of cangrelor was primarily driven by a reduction in the rate of MI (3.8% vs. 4.7%; OR, 0.80; 95% CI 0.67–0.97; $P = 0.02$), but also ST was significantly reduced in the cangrelor arm (0.8% vs. 1.4%; OR 0.62; 95% CI, 0.43–0.90; $P = 0.01$) (Table 22.1). These results were persistent at 30 days, and the benefit with respect to the primary end point was consistent across multiple prespecified subgroups. In particular, the benefit with cangrelor was irrespective of clopidogrel dosing and similar among patients presenting with STEMI and NSTE-ACS and those presenting with SA. Importantly, the rate of severe bleeding was not significantly increased by cangrelor with GUSTO criteria (0.16% vs. 0.11%; OR 1.50; 95% CI, 0.53–4.22; $P = 0.44$), as well as with other definitions of bleeding (Table 22.1). The occurrence of adverse events was low in both groups. The rate of transient dyspnea was low but significantly higher in patients treated with cangrelor (1.2% vs. 0.3%; $P < 0.001$), but the rate of discontinuation of the study drug due to adverse events was similar between groups (0.5% vs. 0.4%).

Cangrelor in patients undergoing surgery

Small-molecule GPIs have been tested in small studies and have been proposed for bridging to surgery patients on dual antiplatelet therapy. However, they have many limitations such as a relatively slow offset of action and an increased risk of bleeding. On the other hand, cangrelor

Table 22.1 Efficacy and safety major end point in CHAMPION PHOENIX trial

	Cangrelor	Clopidogrel	Odds ratio (95% CI)	P value
Efficacy end point				
No. of patients*	5472	5470		
Primary end point: all-cause death, MI, IDR, ST	257 (4.7%)	322 (5.9%)	0.78 (0.66–0.93)	0.005
ST	46 (0.8%)	74 (1.4%)	0.62 (0.43–0.90)	0.01
MI	207 (3.8%)	255 (4.7%)	0.80 (0.67–0.97)	0.02
Cardiovascular death	18 (0.3%)	18 (0.3%)	1.00 (0.52–1.92)	>0.999
Safety end point (non-CABG-related bleeding)				
No. of patients†	5529	5527		
GUSTO severe or life threatening	9 (0.2%)	6 (0.1%)	1.50 (0.53–4.22)	0.44
GUSTO moderate	22 (0.4%)	13 (0.2%)	1.69 (0.85–3.37)	0.13
GUSTO severe or moderate	31 (0.6%)	19 (0.3%)	1.63 (0.92–2.90)	0.09
TIMI major	5 (0.1%)	5 (0.1%)	1.00 (0.29–3.45)	>0.999
Net adverse clinical events				
Death, MI, IDR, ST, or GUSTO severe bleeding	264 (4.8%)	327 (6.0%)	0.80 (0.68–0.94)	0.008

CABG, coronary artery bypass graft; GUSTO, Global Use of Strategies to Open Occluded Coronary Arteries; IDR, ischemia-driven revascularization; MI, myocardial infarction; ST, stent thrombosis; TIMI, Thrombolysis in Myocardial Infarction.

*Modified intention-to-treat population defined as patients receiving study treatment and undergoing PCI.

†Safety population defined as patients exposed to study medication.

Table 22.2 Pharmacological differences between GPIs and cangrelor as bridging strategy.

	GPIs	Cangrelor
Fast onset (min)	Yes	Yes
Potent platelet inhibition	Yes	Yes
Rapid offset (<1 h)	No	Yes
P2Y$_{12}$ specific (Natural Bridge)	No	Yes
"Targeted" inhibition (thienopyridine-like)	No	Yes

GPIs, small-molecule glycoprotein IIb/IIIa inhibitors (tirofiban, eptifibatide).

with its fast onset/offset and high antiplatelet effect may be considered an ideal bridging antiplatelet drug (Table 22.2).

The role of cangrelor in patients on dual antiplatelet therapy undergoing cardiac surgery was recently investigated in the bridging antiplatelet therapy with cangrelor in patients undergoing cardiac surgery (BRIDGE) trial [36]. This double-blind, placebo-controlled, multicenter trial enrolled 210 patients with ACS or treated with a coronary stent, receiving a thienopyridine (ticlopidine, clopidogrel, or prasugrel) within at least 72 h prior to randomization and awaiting CABG surgery. After a dose-finding phase in which escalating doses of drug were tested, enrolled patients were randomized to receive cangrelor infusion (0.75 mg/kg/min) plus standard of care or placebo infusion plus standard of care after thienopyridine discontinuation. Infusion was continued throughout the preoperative period up to 1–6 h before surgical incision. CABG surgery had to occur no sooner than 48 h but no longer than 7 days from randomization, at discretion of the investigator. The primary efficacy end point was the proportion of patients with platelet reactivity of less than 240 PRU (measured by VerifyNow P2Y$_{12}$ testing) for all samples assessed during infusion prior to surgery. The main safety end point was excessive CABG surgery-related bleeding. The primary end point was significantly higher in the cangrelor group than in the placebo group (98.8% vs. 19.0%; RR: 5.2 (95% CI, 3.3–8.1); $P < 0.001$). After discontinuation of infusion prior to surgical incision, PRU levels ($P = 0.21$) and the percentage of patients with platelet reactivity lower than 240 PRU ($P = 0.31$) were similar between groups. Study-defined excessive CABG surgery-related bleeding was not significantly different between groups (11.8% vs. 10.4%; $P = 0.76$) (Figure 22.2). Significant pre-CABG surgery major bleeding events were rare and similar between treatment groups, although there were more minor bleedings with cangrelor, which was used up to 7 days of infusion, largely attributed to ecchymosis at the site of venous punctures. Ischemic end points prior to surgery were low, 2.8% in cangrelor and 4.0% in placebo, even if the trial was not powered to assess these differences. Importantly, the rate of adverse events was similar in both groups. In particular, the incidence of dyspnea was low (1.9% with cangrelor and

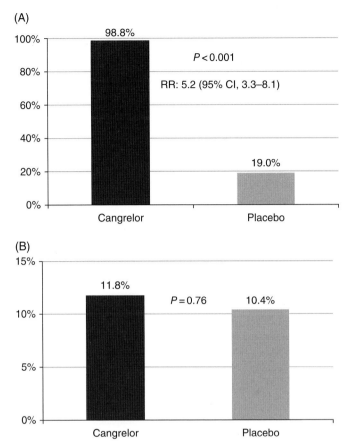

(A)

(B)

Figure 22.2 Primary efficacy and safety end point of the BRIDGE trial. (A) Percent of patients with PRU lower than 240 for all on-treatment samples. (B) Excessive CABG surgery-related bleeding [36].

1% with placebo) as well as the occurrence of liver function test abnormalities (2.3% vs. 3.8%), despite prolonged duration of cangrelor infusion. The authors concluded that intravenous cangrelor is a feasible strategy in patients waiting for cardiac surgery who require prolonged $P2Y_{12}$ inhibition after thienopyridine discontinuation.

Conclusion

Cangrelor is an intravenous antagonist of the $P2Y_{12}$ receptor characterized by rapid, potent, predictable, and reversible platelet inhibition with rapid offset. These pharmacological properties make cangrelor a desirable agent for bridging therapies in patients requiring surgery but also need to maintain adequate platelet blockade, as demonstrated in the BRIDGE trial. In addition, cangrelor is an attractive strategy in patients requiring PCI who have not been pretreated with an oral $P2Y_{12}$ inhibitor, as shown by the clinical benefits in the CHAMPION PHOENIX trial. Ultimately cangrelor may result as a treatment option for patients requiring $P2Y_{12}$ receptor blockade but not able to assume oral medications. Ongoing studies will better determine how to optimally transition from cangrelor to the novel oral $P2Y_{12}$ receptor inhibitors (prasugrel, ticagrelor). Although cangrelor is still not approved for clinical use, this is being evaluated by drug regulating agencies in the USA and Europe.

References

1 Yusuf, S., Zhao, F., Mehta, S.R. *et al.* (2001) Effects of clopidogrel in addition to aspirin in patients with acute coronary syndromes without ST-segment elevation. *The New England Journal of Medicine*, **345**, 494–502.

2 Wiviott, S.D., Braunwald, E., McCabe, C.H. *et al.* (2007) Prasugrel versus clopidogrel in patients with acute coronary syndromes. *The New England Journal of Medicine*, **357**, 2001–2015.

3 Wallentin, L., Becker, R.C., Budaj, A. *et al.* (2009) Ticagrelor versus clopidogrel in patients with acute coronary syndromes. *The New England Journal of Medicine*, **361**, 1045–1057.

4 Angiolillo, D.J. (2012) The evolution of antiplatelet therapy in the treatment of acute coronary syndromes: from aspirin to the present day. *Drugs*, **72**, 2087–2116.

5 Angiolillo, D.J., Saucedo, J.F., Deraad, R. *et al.* (2010) Increased platelet inhibition after switching from maintenance clopidogrel to prasugrel in patients with acute coronary syndromes: results of the SWAP (SWitching Anti Platelet) study. *Journal of the American College of Cardiology*, **56**, 1017–1023.

6 Gurbel, P.A., Bliden, K.P., Butler, K. *et al.* (2009) Randomized double-blind assessment of the ONSET and OFFSET of the antiplatelet effects of ticagrelor versus clopidogrel in patients with stable coronary artery disease: the ONSET/OFFSET study. *Circulation*, **120**, 2577–2585.

7 Alexopoulos, D., Xanthopoulou, I., Gkizas, V. *et al.* (2012) Randomized assessment of ticagrelor versus prasugrel antiplatelet effects in patients with ST-segment-elevation myocardial infarction. *Circulation. Cardiovascular Interventions*, **5**, 797–804.

8 Parodi, G., Valenti, R., Bellandi, B. *et al.* (2013) Comparison of Prasugrel and Ticagrelor loading doses in STEMI patients: the Rapid Activity of Platelet Inhibitor Drugs (RAPID) primary PCI Study. *Journal of the American College of Cardiology*, **61**, 1601–1606.

9 Price, M.J., Walder, J.S., Baker, B.A. *et al.* (2012) Recovery of platelet function after discontinuation of prasugrel or clopidogrel maintenance dosing in aspirin-treated patients with stable coronary disease: the recovery trial. *Journal of the American College of Cardiology*, **59**, 2338–2343.

10 Brilakis, E.S., Banerjee, S. and Berger, P.B. (2007) Perioperative management of patients with coronary stents. *Journal of the American College of Cardiology*, **49**, 2145–2150.

11 Savonitto, S., Caracciolo, M., Cattaneo, M., and De Servi, S. (2011) Management of patients with recently implanted coronary stents on dual antiplatelet therapy who need to undergo major surgery. *Journal of Thrombosis and Haemostasis*, **9**, 2133–2142.

12 Bhatt, D.L. and Topol, E.J. (2000) Current role of platelet glycoprotein IIb/IIIa inhibitors in acute coronary syndromes. *JAMA*, **284**, 1549–1558.

13 Osmancik, P., Jirmar, R., Hulikova, K. *et al.* (2010) A comparison of the VASP index between patients with hemodynamically complicated and uncomplicated acute myocardial infarction. *Catheterization and Cardiovascular Interventions*, **75**, 158–166.

14 Ueno, M., Ferreiro, J.L., and Angiolillo, D.J. (2010) Update on the clinical development of cangrelor. *Expert Review of Cardiovascular Therapy*, **8**, 1069–1077.

15 Dorsam, R.T. and Kunapuli, S.P. (2004) Central role of the $P2Y_{12}$ receptor in platelet activation. *The Journal of Clinical Investigation*, **113**, 340–345.

16 Ingall, A.H., Dixon, J., Bailey, A. *et al.* (1999) Antagonists of the platelet P2T receptor: a novel approach to antithrombotic therapy. *Journal of Medicinal Chemistry*, **42**, 213–220.

17 Angiolillo, D.J., Bhatt, D.L., Gurbel, P.A., and Jennings, L.K. (2009) Advances in antiplatelet therapy: agents in clinical development. *The American Journal of Cardiology*, **103**, 40A–51A.

18 van Giezen, J.J. and Humphries, R.G. (2005) Preclinical and clinical studies with selective reversible direct $P2Y_{12}$ antagonists. *Seminars in Thrombosis and Hemostasis*, **31**, 195–204.

19 Nassim, M.A., Sanderson, J.B., Clarke, C. *et al.* (1999) Investigation of the novel P2T receptor antagonist AR-C69931MX on ex vivo adenosine diphosphate-induced platelet aggregation and bleeding time in healthy volunteers. *Journal of the American College of Cardiology*, **33** (2 Suppl A), A255.

20 Javis, G.E., Nassim, M.A., Humphries, R.G. *et al.* (1999) The P2Y antagonist AR-C69931MX is a more effective inhibitor of ADP-induced platelet aggregation than clopidogrel. *Blood*, **94** (Suppl. 1), A22.

21 Aleil, B., Ravanat, C., Cazenave, J.P., Rochoux, G., Heitz, A. and Gachet, C. (2005) Flow cytometric analysis of intraplatelet VASP phosphorylation for the detection of clopidogrel resistance in patients with ischemic cardiovascular diseases. *Journal of Thrombosis and Haemostasis*, **3**, 85–92.

22 Storey, R.F., Oldroyd, K.G., and Wilcox, R.G. (2001) Open multicentre study of the P2T receptor antagonist AR-C69931MX assessing safety, tolerability and activity in patients with acute coronary syndrome. *Thrombosis and Haemostasis*, **85**, 401–407.

23 Greenbaum, A.B., Ohman, E.M., Gibson, C.M. *et al.* (2007) Preliminary experience with intravenous $P2Y_{12}$ platelet receptor inhibition as an adjunct to reduced-dose alteplase during acute myocardial infarction: results of the Safety, Tolerability and Effect on Patency in Acute Myocardial Infarction (STEP-AMI) angiographic trial. *American Heart Journal*, **154**, 702–709.

24 Greenbaum, A.B., Grines, C.L., Bittl, J.A. *et al.* (2006) Initial experience with an intravenous P2Y12 platelet receptor antagonist in patients undergoing percutaneous coronary intervention: results from a 2-part, phase II, multicenter, randomized, placebo- and active-controlled trial. *American Heart Journal*, **151**, 689.e1–689.e10.

25 Ferreiro, J.L. and Angiolillo, D.J. (2011) Diabetes and antiplatelet therapy in acute coronary syndrome. *Circulation*, **123**, 798–813.

26 Ferreiro, J.L., Ueno, M., Tello-Montoliu, A. *et al.* (2013) Effects of cangrelor in coronary artery disease patients with and without diabetes mellitus: an in vitro pharmacodynamic investigation. *Journal of Thrombosis and Thrombolysis*, **35**, 155–164.

27 Steinhubl, S.R., Oh, J.J., Oestreich, J.H., Ferraris, S., Charnigo, R., and Akers, W.S. (2008) Transitioning patients from cangrelor to clopidogrel:

pharmacodynamic evidence of a competitive effect. *Thrombosis Research*, **121**, 527–534.

28 Dovlatova, N.L., Jakubowski, J.A., Sugidachi, A., and Heptinstall, S. (2008) The reversible P2Y antagonist cangrelor influences the ability of the active metabolites of clopidogrel and prasugrel to produce irreversible inhibition of platelet function. *Journal of Thrombosis and Haemostasis*, **6**, 1153–1159.

29 Ravnefjord, A., Weilitz, J., Emanuelsson, B.M., and van Giezen, J.J. (2012) Evaluation of ticagrelor pharmacodynamic interactions with reversibly binding or non-reversibly binding $P2Y_{12}$ antagonists in an ex-vivo canine model. *Thrombosis Research*, **130**, 622–628.

30 Harrington, R.A., Stone, G.W., McNulty, S. *et al.* (2009) Platelet inhibition with cangrelor in patients undergoing PCI. *The New England Journal of Medicine*, **361**, 2318–2329.

31 Bhatt, D.L., Lincoff, M., Gibson, M. *et al.* (2009) Intravenous platelet blockade with cangrelor during PCI. *The New England Journal of Medicine*, **361**, 2330–2341.

32 Angiolillo, D.J., Schneider, D.J., Bhatt, D.L. *et al.* (2012) Pharmacodynamic effects of cangrelor and clopidogrel: the platelet function substudy from the cangrelor versus standard therapy to achieve optimal management of platelet inhibition (CHAMPION) trials. *Journal of Thrombosis and Thrombolysis*, **34**, 44–55.

33 Bhatt, D.L., Stone, G.W., Mahaffey, K.W. *et al.* (2013) Effect of platelet inhibition with cangrelor during PCI on ischemic events. *The New England Journal of Medicine*, **368**, 1303–1313.

34 White, H.D., Chew, D.P., Dauerman, H.L. *et al.* (2012) Reduced immediate ischemic events with cangrelor in PCI: a pooled analysis of the CHAMPION trials using the universal definition of myocardial infarction. *American Heart Journal*, **163**, 182.e4–190.e4.

35 Thygesen, K., Alpert, J.S., White, H.D. *et al.* (2007) Universal definition of myocardial infarction. *Circulation*, **116**, 2634–2653.

36 Angiolillo, D.J., Firstenberg, M.S., Price, M.J. *et al.* (2012) Bridging antiplatelet therapy with cangrelor in patients undergoing cardiac surgery: a randomized controlled trial. *JAMA*, **307**, 265–274.

23 Ticagrelor

Anna Oskarsson[1], Christoph Varenhorst[1,2], and Stefan James[1,2]

[1] Uppsala Clinical Research Center, Uppsala, Sweden
[2] Uppsala University Hospital, Uppsala, Sweden

Introduction

Ticagrelor is a high affinity reversible $P2Y_{12}$ receptor inhibitor belonging to a new group of agents called cyclopentyltriazolopyrimidines. Because it is a direct-acting compound, further activation is not required unlike the irreversible $P2Y_{12}$ receptor inhibitor clopidogrel. Ticagrelor therefore results in consistent and fast onset platelet inhibition, while about 15–40% of individuals have high on-treatment platelet reactivity on clopidogrel [1, 2].

Mechanisms of action

Following oral administration, ticagrelor is rapidly absorbed and then directly inhibits the $P2Y_{12}$ receptor in a reversible manner. It undergoes enzymatic degradation mainly by CYP3A4 to one pivotal active metabolite, which has the same pharmacokinetics as the parent compound and a systemic exposure of 30–40% out of the parent compound. Ticagrelor's direct inhibition of the $P2Y_{12}$ receptor makes it more potent and faster acting than clopidogrel [2].

Ticagrelor treatment resulted in a lower incidence of cardiovascular deaths, myocardial infarction (MI), and stroke compared with clopidogrel treatment, irrespective of polymorphism of CYP2C19 and ABCB1 in a genetic substudy of the multicenter phase 3 trial PLATelet inhibition and patient Outcomes (PLATO). This indicates less influence of CYP polymorphism upon ticagrelor treatment than on clopidogrel treatment [1].

Pharmacodynamics

Treatment with ticagrelor results in significant faster, greater, and more consistent platelet inhibition than treatment with clopidogrel. In a substudy of the phase 2b dose-guiding Dose confirmation Study assessing

Antiplatelet Therapy in Cardiovascular Disease, First Edition. Edited by Ron Waksman, Paul A. Gurbel, and Michael A. Gaglia, Jr.
© 2014 John Wiley & Sons, Ltd. Published 2014 by John Wiley & Sons, Ltd.

anti-Platelet Effects of AZD6140 vs. clopidogRel in non-ST-segment Elevation myocardial infarction (DISPERSE)-2 trial, a loading dose (LD) of 180 mg ticagrelor resulted in a maximum of 50–60% inhibition of platelet aggregation within 2–4 h. This degree of inhibition was sustained during maintenance therapy with 90 mg twice a day (bid). The most consistent response was seen in the group taking ticagrelor 180 mg bid. Further platelet inhibition was gained when patients switched from clopidogrel to ticagrelor treatment regardless of high or low platelet inhibition response while on clopidogrel [3].

Ticagrelor and its active metabolite are primarily excreted in feces (57.8%) and to a minor extent in urine (26.5%) [4]. Compared to healthy individuals, the exposure to ticagrelor and its main metabolite is higher in patients with renal impairment (glomerular filtration rate <30 mL/min) and in those with mild hepatic impairment. This seems to lack clinical importance since the unbound fraction and the fraction of platelet aggregation inhibition are the same as in control populations [5, 6].

Clinical studies

Clinical benefit and special patient groups

In the PLATO trial, the primary end point – death from vascular causes, MI, or stroke – was evaluated in 18,624 acute coronary syndrome (ACS) patients receiving ticagrelor (180 mg LD, thereafter 90 mg bid) or clopidogrel (300–600 mg LD, thereafter 75 mg daily) in addition to aspirin. At 12 months, the primary end point was significantly lower in the ticagrelor group 9.8% compared to the clopidogrel group 11.7% (hazard ratio (HR) 0.84; 95% confidence interval (CI), 0.77–0.92; $p < 0.001$) as well as total mortality (4.5% vs. 5.9%; $P < 0.001$) [7]. The results were consistent in patients with ST-elevation acute coronary syndrome (STE-ACS) at admission planned for percutaneous coronary intervention (PCI), patients planned for invasive strategy independent of ST elevation or non-ST elevation (NSTE) on electrocardiogram (ECG), as well as for those initially intended for noninvasive management [8, 9, 10]. Patients with diabetes mellitus had the same benefit of ticagrelor as the rest of the trial population, while patients with chronic kidney disease tended to derive a greater benefit [11, 12]. The rate of primary end point was lower without any increase in bleeding rate in ticagrelor-treated patients with a prior history of ischemic stroke or transient ischemic attack (TIA) compared to clopidogrel [13]. Patients undergoing coronary artery bypass grafting (CABG), within 7 days after stopping ticagrelor treatment, had a considerably greater relative reduction of the primary outcome when treated with ticagrelor compared to clopidogrel [14].

Adverse events

In the PLATO trial, rates of total major bleeding (defined by the PLATO criteria) were similar in the ticagrelor and clopidogrel groups (11.6% vs. 11.2%, $P = 0.43$). However, major bleeding not related to CABG was found to be significantly higher in the ticagrelor group (4.5% vs. 3.8%, $P = 0.02$), primarily after 30 days on study drug. Ticagrelor- and clopidogrel-treated patients had in total similar rates of fatal bleeding and transfusions [15].

The DISPERSE-2 trial compared safety and initial efficacy of ticagrelor in NSTE-ACS patients. 990 patients were randomized to ticagrelor 90 mg bid, ticagrelor 180 mg bid, or clopidogrel 300 mg LD and thereafter 75 mg once daily for 12 weeks. Concerning bleeding at 4 weeks, no difference was seen comparing the groups: clopidogrel 8.1%, ticagrelor 90 mg 9.8%, and ticagrelor 180 mg 8.0% ($p = 0.43$ and $p = 0.96$, respectively, vs. clopidogrel). The rates of major bleeding at 4 weeks were similar for clopidogrel 6.9% and the two ticagrelor groups, 7.1% and 5.1%, respectively, while minor bleeding at 4 weeks was more common in the 180 mg ticagrelor group (3.8%) than in the 90 mg ticagrelor group (2.7%) and the clopidogrel group (1.3%) ($p = 0.05$ and $p = 0.18$ vs. clopidogrel, respectively) [16].

In the DISPERSE-2 and PLATO trials, ticagrelor-treated patients reported higher frequencies of dyspnea compared to clopidogrel-treated patients, although in both studies dyspnea was classified as nonserious and resulted in few treatment discontinuations [16, 17]. The clinical benefit of ticagrelor was similar or in fact greater in patients reporting dyspnea. At 1 week with cECG recording, ventricular pauses greater than 3 s occurred more often in ticagrelor-treated patients than in patients treated with clopidogrel (5.8% vs. 3.6%; relative risk 1.61; $p = 0.006$). Yet at 1 month, there were no divergency between the two groups (2.1% vs. 1.7%, ticagrelor and clopidogrel, respectively), and no apparent clinical consequences were seen [18]. A transient increase from baseline in serum uric acid and serum creatinine at 12 month was noted in patients receiving ticagrelor without clinical consequences [8, 15].

Current recommendations

Ticagrelor and prasugrel both have class I indication (recommendation/level of evidence IB) in the management of STE-ACS with PCI according to European Society of Cardiology (ESC) Guidelines. In acute, subacute, and long-term phase of STE-ACS, either ticagrelor or prasugrel in combination with aspirin is recommended (recommendation/level of evidence IA) over clopidogrel with aspirin [19]. All patients with NSTE-ACS and moderate to high risk of ischemic events are recommended to have ticagrelor (recommendation/level of evidence IB). Before nonemergent major surgery, including CABG, patients are recommended to stop ticagrelor treatment 3 days before surgery (recommendation/level of evidence IIa C) [19, 20].

According to the American College of Cardiology Foundation/American Heart Association (ACCF/AHA) Guidelines, clopidogrel, prasugrel, and ticagrelor have the same level of recommendation in the management of STE-ACS (class I, level B) and clopidogrel and ticagrelor in the management of NSTE-ACS [21, 22].

Summary

Ticagrelor compared with clopidogrel has faster, greater, more consistent, and less variable platelet inhibition. Ticagrelor treatment gives a higher grade of prevention against death from vascular causes, MI, and stroke as well as total mortality, among ACS patients. There is an increased risk for nonprocedural major bleeding and transient dyspnea with ticagrelor treatment in comparison with clopidogrel treatment.

References

1 Wallentin, L., James, S., Storey, R.F. *et al.* (2010) Effect of CYP2C19 and ABCB1 single nucleotide polymorphisms on outcomes of treatment with ticagrelor versus clopidogrel for acute coronary syndromes: a genetic substudy of the PLATO trial. *The Lancet*, **376 (9749)**, 1320–1328.

2 Wallentin, L. (2009) P2Y(12) inhibitors: differences in properties and mechanisms of action and potential consequences for clinical use. *European Heart Journal*, **30 (16)**, 1964–1977.

3 Storey, R.F., Husted, S., Harrington, R.A. *et al.* (2007) Inhibition of platelet aggregation by AZD6140, a reversible oral P2Y12 receptor antagonist, compared with clopidogrel in patients with acute coronary syndromes. *Journal of the American College of Cardiology*, **50 (19)**, 1852–1856.

4 Teng, R., Oliver, S., Hayes, M.A. and Butler, K. (2010) Absorption, distribution, metabolism, and excretion of ticagrelor in healthy subjects. *Drug Metabolism and Disposition*, **38 (9)**, 1514–1521.

5 Butler, K. and Teng, R. (2012) Pharmacokinetics, pharmacodynamics, and safety of ticagrelor in volunteers with severe renal impairment. *The Journal of Clinical Pharmacology*, **52 (9)**, 1388–1398.

6 Butler, K. and Teng, R. (2011) Pharmacokinetics, pharmacodynamics, and safety of ticagrelor in volunteers with mild hepatic impairment. *The Journal of Clinical Pharmacology*, **51 (7)**, 978–987.

7 Wallentin, L., Becker, R.C., Budaj, A. *et al.* (2009) Ticagrelor versus clopidogrel in patients with acute coronary syndromes. *New England Journal of Medicine*, **361 (11)**, 1045–1057.

8 Steg, P.G., James, S., Harrington, R.A. *et al.* (2010) Ticagrelor versus clopidogrel in patients with ST-elevation acute coronary syndromes intended for reperfusion with primary percutaneous coronary intervention: a platelet inhibition and patient outcomes (PLATO) trial subgroup analysis. *Circulation*, **122 (21)**, 2131–2141.

9 Cannon, C.P., Harrington, R.A., James, S. *et al.* (2010) Comparison of ticagrelor with clopidogrel in patients with a planned invasive strategy for acute coronary syndromes (PLATO): a randomised double-blind study. *The Lancet*, **375 (9711)**, 283–293.

10 James, S.K., Roe, M.T., Cannon, C.P. *et al.* (2011) Ticagrelor versus clopidogrel in patients with acute coronary syndromes intended for non-invasive management: sub study from prospective randomised PLATelet inhibition and patient Outcomes (PLATO) trial. *BMJ*, **342** (Jun17 1), d3527.

11 James, S., Angiolillo, D.J., Cornel, J.H. *et al.* (2010) Ticagrelor vs. clopidogrel in patients with acute coronary syndromes and diabetes: a substudy from the PLATelet inhibition and patient Outcomes (PLATO) trial. *European Heart Journal*, **31 (24)**, 3006–3016.

12 James, S., Budaj, A., Aylward, P. *et al.* (2010) Ticagrelor versus clopidogrel in acute coronary syndromes in relation to renal function: results from the platelet inhibition and patient outcomes (PLATO) trial. *Circulation*, **122 (11)**, 1056–1067.

13 James, S.K., Storey, R.F., Khurmi, N.S. *et al.* (2012) Ticagrelor versus clopidogrel in patients with acute coronary syndromes and a history of stroke or transient ischemic attack. *Circulation*, **125 (23)**, 2914–2921.

14 Held, C., Åsenblad, N., Bassand, J.P. *et al.* (2011) Ticagrelor versus clopidogrel in patients with acute coronary syndromes undergoing coronary artery bypass surgery. *Journal of the American College of Cardiology*, **57 (6)**, 672–684.

15 Becker, R.C., Bassand, J.P., Budaj, A. *et al.* (2011) Bleeding complications with the P2Y12 receptor antagonists clopidogrel and ticagrelor in the PLATelet inhibition and patient Outcomes (PLATO) trial. *European Heart Journal*, **32 (23)**, 2933–2944.

16 Cannon, C.P., Husted, S., Harrington, R.A. *et al.* (2007) Safety, tolerability, and initial efficacy of AZD6140, the first reversible oral adenosine diphosphate receptor antagonist, compared with clopidogrel, in patients with non–ST-segment elevation acute coronary syndrome. *Journal of the American College of Cardiology*, **50 (19)**, 1844–1851.

17 Storey, R.F., Becker, R.C., Harrington, R.A. *et al.* (2011) Characterization of dyspnoea in PLATO study patients treated with ticagrelor or clopidogrel and its association with clinical outcomes. *European Heart Journal*, **32 (23)**, 2945–2953.

18 Scirica, B.M., Cannon, C.P., Emanuelsson, H. *et al.* (2011) The incidence of bradyarrhythmias and clinical bradyarrhythmic events in patients with acute coronary syndromes treated with ticagrelor or clopidogrel in the PLATO (Platelet Inhibition and Patient Outcomes) trial. *Journal of the American College of Cardiology*, **57 (19)**, 1908–1916.

19 Authors/Task Force Members, Steg, P.G., James, S.K. *et al.* (2012) ESC guidelines for the management of acute myocardial infarction in patients presenting with ST-segment elevation: The Task Force on the management of ST-segment elevation acute myocardial infarction of the European Society of Cardiology (ESC). *European Heart Journal*, **33 (20)**, 2569–2619.

20 Authors/Task Force Members, Hamm, C.W., Bassand, J.-P. *et al.* (2011) ESC guidelines for the management of acute coronary syndromes in patients presenting without persistent ST-segment elevation: The Task Force for the management of acute coronary syndromes (ACS) in patients presenting without persistent ST-segment elevation of the European Society of Cardiology (ESC). *European Heart Journal*, **32 (23)**, 2999–3054.

21 O'Gara, P.T., Kushner, F.G., Ascheim, D.D. *et al.* (2013) 2013 ACCF/AHA guideline for the management of ST-elevation myocardial infarction. *Journal of the American College of Cardiology*, **61 (4)**, e78–e140.

22 Jneid, H., Anderson, J.L., Wright, R.S. *et al.* (2012) 2012 ACCF/AHA focused update of the guideline for the management of patients with unstable angina/non–ST-elevation myocardial infarction (Updating the 2007 Guideline and Replacing the 2011 Focused Update). *Journal of the American College of Cardiology*, **60 (7)**, 645–681.

24 Thrombin Receptor Antagonists

Flávio de Souza Brito and Pierluigi Tricoci
Duke University Medical Center, Duke Clinical Research Institute, Durham, NC, USA

Introduction

Secondary prevention strategies in patients with coronary artery disease are centered upon the use of antiplatelet therapies. Currently recommended agents are aspirin and P2Y12 receptor antagonists. Their use in combination reduces the risk of ischemic events in patients presenting with acute coronary syndromes (ACS) and is pivotal in the management of patients undergoing percutaneous coronary intervention (PCI) [1, 2]. Dual antiplatelet therapy also increased risk of bleeding, and in addition to this, occurrence of ischemic events continues to occur at a significant rate [3, 4]. Therefore, additional and alternative mechanisms to modulate platelet function have been investigated. Thrombin is known to be a potent platelet activator, and continued increased thrombin generation has been demonstrated in patients treated with dual antiplatelet therapy [5]. Antagonists of platelets' thrombin receptor have been developed. In this chapter, we will describe the mode of action of thrombin receptor on platelets and pharmacological strategies to antagonize thrombin-mediated platelet activation, with particular emphasis on vorapaxar, to date the most studied thrombin receptor antagonist.

Protease-activated receptors (PARs) and thrombin-induced platelet activation

Thrombin, a serine protease, is the main effector protease of the coagulation cascade and the most potent platelet activator [6, 7]. The action of thrombin on platelets is mediated by the platelet protease-activated receptors (PARs), which are G protein-coupled receptors members of the seven-transmembrane domain receptor superfamily. Thrombin activates PARs by cleaving a peptide bond (Arg41-Ser42) in the receptor's extracellular domain that discloses a new N-terminus of

Antiplatelet Therapy in Cardiovascular Disease, First Edition. Edited by Ron Waksman, Paul A. Gurbel, and Michael A. Gaglia, Jr.
© 2014 John Wiley & Sons, Ltd. Published 2014 by John Wiley & Sons, Ltd.

the receptor, referred to as a tethered ligand [8, 9]. This new "tail" of the receptor interacts with a distinct domain of the cleaved receptor and causes its activation. To date, four subtypes of PARs were described: PAR-1, PAR-2, PAR-3, and PAR-4 [10]. Among them, only PAR-1 and PAR-4 were identified on human platelets [11]. PARs are not only located on platelets, but they are elsewhere including smooth muscle cells, endothelial cells, fibroblasts, and the brain [12]. The PAR-1 is recognized to be the main platelet thrombin receptor in light of the very high affinity to thrombin, while the role of PAR-4 in humans (which requires higher thrombin concentration) is not completely understood. A pivotal concept behind the development of thrombin receptor antagonist was that thrombin-mediated platelet activation was not essential to normal hemostasis, and therefore, blocking PAR-1 would not increase the risk of clinically significant bleeding. This concept derives from studies in mice, which showed that PAR-4 −/− mice (PAR-4 in mice is equivalent to PAR-1 in humans) were totally unresponsive to thrombin-mediated platelet activation, and despite so, they had normal platelet shape, they did not have increased tendency to bleed, and females could tolerate a pregnancy [13]. Preliminary investigations have also suggested that platelet activation by thrombin is necessary for platelet thrombus propagation, but not for initial platelet thrombus formation in injured vessels [14].

Thrombin receptor antagonists: pharmacokinetics and pharmacodynamics

Two PAR-1 antagonists have been developed and tested in clinical studies: a synthetic derivative of natural himbacine (vorapaxar) and a synthetic compound based on the bicyclic amidine motif (atopaxar).

Vorapaxar

Vorapaxar is a potent, selective PAR-1 inhibitor. It is rapidly absorbed after oral administration with a slow elimination with a half-life of up to 311 h. After a single loading dose of vorapaxar, platelet function recovers (returns to >50% of baseline) within 2–3 weeks. Vorapaxar is extensively metabolized by the liver, particularly the CYP3A4 enzyme. The routes of elimination are mainly via feces and secondarily by renal clearance (<5%). In patients with end-stage renal disease, a performed study showed similar overall exposure and bioavailability compared with normal subjects. Dialysis did not appear to affect elimination [15]. Hepatic impairment did not change the pharmacokinetics of vorapaxar [16]. In Folts thrombosis models, an intravenous vorapaxar analog (SCH 602539) alone or in combination with P2Y12 inhibitor cangrelor showed synergistic effect on inhibition of thrombosis, while there was no increase in surgical bleeding in cynomolgus monkeys [17].

Clinical trials of vorapaxar

The first large experience of vorapaxar in clinical trials was a phase II clinical trial among 1030 patients undergoing angiography and intent to perform PCI. Before coronary angiography, patients were randomized 3:1 to one of three loading doses (10, 20, or 40 mg) or matching placebo, in addition to standard of care. Patients who actually received PCI (56% of all patients), defined as the primary cohort, were further randomized to a 60-day maintenance treatment of 0.5, 1, or 2.5 mg/day of vorapaxar, or matching placebo. The primary end point of Thrombolysis in Myocardial Infarction (TIMI) major or minor bleeding was not different between aggregated vorapaxar and placebo groups. A trend toward reduced myocardial rates was observed with the highest vorapaxar loading dose [18].

Vorapaxar was evaluated in two large phase III trials: Thrombin Receptor Antagonist for Clinical Event Reduction in Acute Coronary Syndrome (TRACER) and Thrombin Receptor Antagonist in Secondary Prevention of Atherothrombotic Ischemic Events (TRA 2P)-TIMI 50, totaling nearly 40,000 patients enrolled.

The TRACER trial was an international, multicenter, double-blind, randomized trial that compared vorapaxar against placebo on top of standard of care in 12,944 patients who presented with ACS without ST-segment elevation. Patients were randomly assigned in a 1:1 ratio to receive vorapaxar 40 mg, followed by 2.5 mg daily maintenance dose or placebo. Nearly 90% of patients were treated with dual antiplatelet therapy (aspirin and clopidogrel); therefore, TRACER largely tested vorapaxar in the context of "triple" antiplatelet therapy. The trial was prematurely discontinued by the Data Safety Monitoring Board (DSMB) during follow-up phase (5 months prior to planned end) after a target number of events had been achieved and in view of increase risk of bleeding. After a median follow-up of 502 days, the primary end point (a composite of death from cardiovascular (CV) causes, myocardial infarction (MI), stroke, recurrent ischemia with rehospitalization, or urgent coronary revascularization) occurred 18.5% of vorapaxar versus 19.9% of placebo patients (hazard ratio (HR), 0.92; CI 95%, 0.85–1.01; $P=0.07$); thus, the superiority of vorapaxar on the primary end point was not achieved (Table 24.1). However, there was a nominally statistically significant reduction of the key secondary end point, a composite of death from CV causes, MI, or stroke (14.7% and 16.4%, respectively; HR, 0.89; 95% CI, 0.81–0.98; $P=0.02$), which suggested modest efficacy of vorapaxar when softer end points are excluded. The effect of vorapaxar was mostly due to a 12% reduction of MI (HR, 0.88; CI 95%, 0.79–0.98; $P=0.007$), with most marked effect noted in spontaneous (Type 1) MIs. Vorapaxar, when added on top standard of care with high use of dual antiplatelet therapy, significantly increased the risk of bleeding. The rate of GUSTO moderate or severe bleeding was increased from 5.2% to 7.2% (HR, 1.35; 95% CI, 1.16–1.58; $P<0.001$). There was also a significant increase in the occurrence of intracranial hemorrhage with vorapaxar (1.1% vs. 0.2%; HR, 3.39; 95% CI, 1.78–6.45; $P<0.001$) [19].

Table 24.1 Phase III studies testing vorapaxar – bleeding and efficacy end points.

	TRACER			TRA 2P-TIMI 50		
	Placebo	Vorapaxar	P value	Placebo	Vorapaxar	P value
	N: 6441	N: 6446		N: 13224	N: 13225	
CV death, MI, stroke, recurrent ischemia with rehospitalization, or urgent coronary revascularization*	1102 (17.0%)	1031 (15.9%)	0.07	NA	NA	NA
CV death, MI, stroke†	910 (16.4%)	822 (14.7%)	0.02	1176 (10.5%)	1028 (9.3%)	<0.001
CV death	207 (3.2%)	208 (3.2%)	0.96	319 (3.0%)	285 (2.7%)	0.15
MI	698 (10.8%)	621 (9.6%)	0.02	673 (6.1%)	564 (5.2%)	0.001
Ischemic stroke	93 (1.4%)	74 (1.1%)	0.14	294 (2.6%)	250 (2.2%)	0.06
GUSTO moderate or severe bleeding	290 (4.5%)	391 (6.1%)	<0.001	267 (2.5%)	438 (4.2%)	<0.001
TIMI clinically significant bleeding	755 (11.7%)	1065 (16.5%)	<0.001	1241 (11.1%)	1759 (15.8%)	<0.001
Fatal bleeding	8 (0.1%)	15 (0.2%)	0.15	20 (0.2%)	29 (0.3%)	0.19
Intracranial hemorrhage	12 (0.2%)	40 (0.6%)	<0.001	53 (0.5%)	102 (1.0%)	<0.001

CV, cardiovascular.

*TRACER primary efficacy end point.

†TRA 2P-TIMI 50 primary efficacy end point and TRACER key secondary end point.

The TRA 2P-TIMI 50 trial studied vorapaxar in a secondary prevention cohort of 26,449 patients, assessing vorapaxar in patients with established chronic atherothrombotic disease. The trial included three populations: (i) patients with recent spontaneous MI (within 2 weeks to 1 year), (ii) patients with recent ischemic stroke (within 2 weeks to 1 year), and (iii) patients with documented peripheral arterial disease (PAD). Patients were randomly assigned to receive either vorapaxar (2.5 mg daily, without loading dose) or matching placebo in addition to standard of care. The stroke cohort was prematurely discontinued (along with all patients with a history of stroke) following interim DSMB review revealing an excess in intracranial hemorrhages with vorapaxar, while it continued in the remaining cohorts. The main trial results showed a superiority of vorapaxar over placebo with a 13% reduction in the primary end point (composite of CV death, MI, or stroke) with a 9.3% rate in the vorapaxar group and 10.5% rate in the placebo group (HR, 0.87; 95% CI, 0.80–0.94; $P < 0.001$). There was a significant increase in bleeding with vorapaxar. GUSTO moderate or severe bleeding was observed in 4.2% of patients in the vorapaxar group and 2.5% in the placebo group (HR, 1.66; 95% CI, 1.43–1.93). There was a significant increase in the rate of intracranial hemorrhage in the vorapaxar group (1.0% with vorapaxar vs. 0.5% with the placebo group; HR 1.94; 95% CI, 1.39–2.70) [20].

The greatest benefit was observed in the post-MI cohort. Among the 17,779 patients who qualified for the study following an MI, the primary end point was reduced by 20% with vorapaxar (HR 0.80, 95% CI; 0.72–0.89; $p < 0.0001$). The increase in GUSTO moderate or severe was similar to what was observed in the main study (HR 1.61, 95% CI; 1.31–1.97; $p < 0.0001$). Intracranial hemorrhage rates were 0.6% with vorapaxar and 0.4% with placebo ($p = 0.076$). Other serious adverse events were equally distributed between groups. These data suggest that a more favorable efficacy versus bleeding profile with vorapaxar is achieved in secondary prevention of patients with prior MI [19, 20].

Atopaxar

Atopaxar is a selective, potent, and orally active PAR-1 antagonist. Atopaxar is mainly metabolized by CYP3A4, and via feces is its major route of elimination. It has a slower onset of its effects (3.5 h) and is has a faster clearance (half-life 23 h) compared with vorapaxar [21].

Atopaxar has been investigated in phase II trials, in patients with ACS and in patients with stable coronary artery disease in the LANCELOT-ACS and LANCELOT-CAD. The LANCELOT-ACS randomized 603 subjects within 72 h of NSTEMI-ACS to 1 of 3 doses of atopaxar (400 mg loading dose followed by 50, 100, or 200 mg daily) or matching placebo. Major or minor bleeding (CURE) did not differ significantly between the combined atopaxar and placebo groups (3.08% vs. 2.17%, respectively; $P = 0.63$). The incidence of major adverse cardiovascular events (MACE) was similar between the atopaxar and placebo groups (8.03% vs. 7.75%;

$P = 0.93$) and atopaxar reduced ischemia on continuous ECG monitoring (Holter) at 48 h with a relative risk reduction of 34% ($P = 0.02$) [22].

In the LANCELOT-CAD, 720 subjects with confirmed CAD and on aspirin (75–325 mg daily) and/or a thienopyridine (clopidogrel or ticlopidine) were treated for 24 weeks with 4 weeks of posttreatment follow-up, and the primary objective of the study was to assess the safety of atopaxar compared with placebo. Similar results were verified in both bleeding criteria. On the issue of efficacy, there was no significant difference in the combined MACE end point between the combined atopaxar treatment group and placebo (2.6% vs. 4.6%; RR, 0.57; 95% CI, 0.25–1.35; $P = 0.20$). Asymptomatic transient elevation in liver transaminases and dose-dependent QTc prolongation were observed with higher doses of atopaxar in both phase II trials [23].

Future prospective of PAR-1 antagonists

Overall, the TRA 2P-TIMI 50 trial and the TRACER trial provided consistent results (reduction of ischemic events, particularly MI) and have proven the concept that antagonism of thrombin-mediated platelet activation, through the PAR-1 antagonism, translates into a clinical benefit. In terms of bringing PAR-1 antagonism into clinical practice, currently available data support the use of vorapaxar in secondary prevention, mainly in patients with prior MI. In patients with NSTE ACS, the balance between ischemia reduction and bleeding increase, when vorapaxar was largely used as a third agent in most patients, was not favorable. In the presence of a significant bleeding increase, it remains to be seen whether the drug will receive regulatory approval based on available data and in this case what would be the uptake in clinical practice guidelines and in clinical practice. In case of regulatory approval, an appropriate selection of patients, that is, individuals at risk of ischemic event but not excessive risk of bleeding, will be critical.

Finally, with the demonstration of clinical efficacy of PAR-1 antagonism, further research opportunities may arise, including testing vorapaxar with different combinations of antiplatelet agents, in comparison with currently available agents, or in other populations with atherothrombotic disease.

References

1 Fuster, V. and Sweeny, J.M. (2011) Aspirin: a historical and contemporary therapeutic overview. *Circulation*, **123** (**7**), 768–778.
2 Yusuf, S., Zhao, F., Mehta, S.R. *et al.* (2001) Effects of clopidogrel in addition to aspirin in patients with acute coronary syndromes without ST-segment elevation. *The New England Journal of Medicine*, **345** (**7**), 494–502.
3 Wiviott, S.D., Braunwald, E., McCabe, C.H. *et al.* (2007) Prasugrel versus clopidogrel in patients with acute coronary syndromes. *The New England Journal of Medicine*, **357** (**20**), 2001–2015.
4 Wallentin, L., Becker, R.C., Budaj, A. *et al.* (2009) Ticagrelor versus clopidogrel in patients with acute coronary syndromes. *The New England Journal of Medicine*, **361** (**11**), 1045–1057.

5 Eikelboom, J.W., Weitz, J.I., Budaj, A. *et al.* (2002) Clopidogrel does not suppress blood markers of coagulation activation in aspirin-treated patients with non-ST-elevation acute coronary syndromes. *European Heart Journal*, **23 (22)**, 1771–1779.

6 Furie, B. and Furie, B.C. (2008) Mechanisms of thrombus formation. *The New England Journal of Medicine*, **359 (9)**, 938–949.

7 Davì, G. and Patrono, C. (2007) Platelet activation and atherothrombosis. *The New England Journal of Medicine*, **357 (24)**, 2482–2494.

8 Angiolillo, D.J., Capodanno, D. and Goto, S. (2010) Platelet thrombin receptor antagonism and atherothrombosis. *European Heart Journal*, **31 (1)**, 17–28.

9 Coughlin, S.R. (2001) Protease-activated receptors in vascular biology. *Thrombosis and Haemostasis*, **86 (1)**, 298–307.

10 Leonardi, S., Tricoci, P. and Becker, R.C. (2010) Thrombin receptor antagonists for the treatment of atherothrombosis: therapeutic potential of vorapaxar and E-5555. *Drugs*, **70 (14)**, 1771–1783.

11 Kahn, M.L., Nakanishi-Matsui, M., Shapiro, M.J., Ishihara, H. and Coughlin, S.R. (1999) Protease-activated receptors 1 and 4 mediate activation of human platelets by thrombin. *The Journal of Clinical Investigation*, **103 (6)**, 879–887.

12 Molino, M., Bainton, D.F., Hoxie, J.A., Coughlin, S.R. and Brass, L.F. (1997) Thrombin receptors on human platelets. *Initial localization and subsequent redistribution during platelet activation. The Journal of Biological Chemistry*, **272 (9)**, 6011–6017.

13 Coughlin, S.R. (2005) Protease-activated receptors in hemostasis, thrombosis and vascular biology. *Journal of Thrombosis and Haemostasis*, **3 (8)**, 1800–1814.

14 Vandendries, E.R., Hamilton, J.R., Coughlin, S.R., Furie, B. and Furie, B.C. (2007) Par4 is required for platelet thrombus propagation but not fibrin generation in a mouse model of thrombosis. *Proceedings of the National Academy of Sciences of the United States of America*, **104 (1)**, 288–292.

15 Kosoglou, T., Reyderman, L., Tiessen, R.G. *et al.* (2012) Pharmacodynamics and pharmacokinetics of the novel PAR-1 antagonist vorapaxar (formerly SCH 530348) in healthy subjects. *European Journal of Clinical Pharmacology*, **68 (3)**, 249–258.

16 Statkevich, P., Kosoglou, T., Preston, R.A. *et al.* (2012) Pharmacokinetics of the novel PAR-1 antagonist vorapaxar in patients with hepatic impairment. *European Journal of Clinical Pharmacology*, **68 (11)**, 1501–1508.

17 Chintala, M., Strony, J., Yang, B., Kurowski, S. and Li, Q. (2010) SCH 602539, a protease-activated receptor-1 antagonist, inhibits thrombosis alone and in combination with cangrelor in a Folts model of arterial thrombosis in cynomolgus monkeys. *Arteriosclerosis, Thrombosis, and Vascular Biology*, **30 (11)**, 2143–2149.

18 Becker, R.C., Moliterno, D.J., Jennings, L.K. *et al.* (2009) Safety and tolerability of SCH 530348 in patients undergoing non-urgent percutaneous coronary intervention: a randomized, double-blind, placebo-controlled phase II study. *Lancet*, **373 (9667)**, 919–928.

19 Tricoci, P., Huang, Z., Held, C. *et al.* (2012) Thrombin-receptor antagonist vorapaxar in acute coronary syndromes. *The New England Journal of Medicine*, **366 (1)**, 20–33.

20 Morrow, D.A., Braunwald, E., Bonaca, M.P. *et al.* (2012) Vorapaxar in the secondary prevention of atherothrombotic events. *The New England Journal of Medicine*, **366 (15)**, 1404–1413.

21 Kogushi, M., Matsuoka, T., Kawata, T. *et al.* (2011) The novel and orally active thrombin receptor antagonist E5555 (Atopaxar) inhibits arterial thrombosis without affecting bleeding time in guinea pigs. *European Journal of Pharmacology*, **657** (**1–3**), 131–137.

22 O'Donoghue, M.L., Bhatt, D.L., Wiviott, S.D. *et al.* (2011) Safety and tolerability of atopaxar in the treatment of patients with acute coronary syndromes: the lessons from antagonizing the cellular effects of Thrombin–Acute Coronary Syndromes Trial. *Circulation*, **123** (**17**), 1843–1853.

23 Wiviott, S.D., Flather, M.D., O'Donoghue, M.L. *et al.* (2011) Randomized trial of atopaxar in the treatment of patients with coronary artery disease: the lessons from antagonizing the cellular effect of Thrombin–Coronary Artery Disease Trial. *Circulation*, **123** (**17**), 1854–1863.

Section IV

Percutaneous Coronary Intervention and Antiplatelet Therapy

25 Dual Antiplatelet Therapy Prior to Percutaneous Coronary Intervention

Fabio Mangiacapra, Annunziata Nusca, Rosetta Melfi, and Germano di Sciascio

Campus Bio-Medico University of Rome, Rome, Italy

Antiplatelet therapy has been a cornerstone of the pharmacological treatment of patients undergoing percutaneous coronary intervention (PCI) since the beginning of interventional cardiology. Optimal platelet inhibition is crucial to prevent thrombotic procedural complications, as coronary manipulation may induce trauma to the endothelium and deeper layers of the vessel wall, which in turn results in inflammatory cell and platelet activation [1, 2]. This condition may be even more pronounced in patients with acute coronary syndrome (ACS) in whom platelet reactivity is already increased at baseline [3], and enhanced inflammatory status is present especially at the level of coronary circulation [4, 5] (Table 25.1).

Dual antiplatelet therapy (DAPT) for patients undergoing PCI includes acetylsalicylic acid (ASA) and an inhibitor of the P2Y12 platelet ADP receptor. While ASA is consistently recommended in all patients, the choice of the P2Y12 platelet ADP receptor inhibitor depends mainly on the clinical setting. First-generation thienopyridine ticlopidine was the first P2Y12 receptor blocker used in patients treated with PCI. However, due to lower side effects and better tolerability, it has been replaced by second-generation thienopyridine clopidogrel [6]. The latter still represents the cornerstone of DAPT for most patients, although newer, more potent P2Y12 receptor blockers have been recently introduced in clinical practice. Given the availability of various options, a thorough evaluation of ischemic and bleeding risk should be made on an individual basis in order to maximize the net clinical benefit deriving from the balance between protection from ischemic events and prevention of bleeding. Although recent studies have failed to prove any benefit from tailoring antiplatelet therapy on the basis of platelet function test results [7, 8], on-treatment platelet reactivity still represents an important marker of risk for both ischemic and bleeding complications, by which a therapeutic window may be identified [9, 10, 11].

Antiplatelet Therapy in Cardiovascular Disease, First Edition. Edited by Ron Waksman, Paul A. Gurbel, and Michael A. Gaglia, Jr.

Table 25.1 Options for dual antiplatelet therapy (DAPT) prior to percutaneous coronary intervention (PCI)

	Acetylsalicylic acid (ASA)	P2Y12 receptor inhibitors
Stable coronary artery disease (CAD)	81–325 mg for patients on chronic therapy 325 mg for patients not on chronic therapy	Clopidogrel 600 mg at least 2 h before PCI Clopidogrel 300 mg at least 6 h before PCI
Non-ST-segment-elevation acute coronary syndrome (NSTEACS)	81–325 mg for patients on chronic therapy 325 mg for patients not on chronic therapy	Clopidogrel 600 mg as early as possible before or at the time of PCI Prasugrel 60 mg promptly once coronary anatomy is defined (no later than 1 h after PCI) Ticagrelor 180 mg as early as possible before or at the time of PCI
ST-segment-elevation myocardial infarction (STEMI)	81–325 mg for patients on chronic therapy 325 mg for patients not on chronic therapy	All drugs should be administered as soon as possible after diagnosis Prasugrel 60 mg Ticagrelor 180 mg Clopidogrel 600 mg if prasugrel or ticagrelor is either not available or contraindicated

Acetylsalicylic acid

Most of the studies investigating the effects of ASA in patients with coronary artery disease (CAD) were performed before the widespread use of PCI. However, the consistent evidence of clinical benefit from this drug [12] has led to the general recommendation of ASA as standard therapy for CAD patients, irrespective of their management (i.e., invasive vs. conservative). The only placebo-controlled randomized study of ASA alone in patients undergoing PCI was the Multi-Hospital Eastern Atlantic Restenosis Trial (M-HEART) II [13], which showed a significant reduction of adverse clinical events in comparison to placebo (30% vs. 41%). Due to the lack of randomized studies, uncertainty remains regarding the optimal dose of ASA to be administered before PCI. Currently, for patients already on chronic ASA therapy, a further 81–325 mg dose is recommended before PCI, whereas for patients not on ASA, a nonenteric 325 mg dose before PCI is recommended [14]. In patients presenting with ACS, ASA should be administered as soon as possible after hospitalization.

P2Y12 receptor inhibitors

Stable CAD

The beneficial effects of clopidogrel have been extensively demonstrated in patients with stable CAD, and several investigations have been performed to explore different loading doses before stenting in order to minimize thrombotic risk. The Clopidogrel for the Reduction of Events During Observation (CREDO) trial [15] showed a 38% relative risk reduction of death, myocardial infarction (MI), and urgent target vessel revascularization (TVR) at 28 days in patients undergoing elective or urgent PCI and pretreated with 300 mg loading dose of clopidogrel before the procedure versus the assumption of clopidogrel, without loading dose, at the time of intervention ($p = 0.05$). Accordingly, a 300 mg clopidogrel loading dose has represented the conventional therapy for P2Y12 inhibition in patients undergoing elective PCI for several years. Following pharmacodynamic studies demonstrating greater platelet inhibition with higher (600 mg) clopidogrel loading dose, the Antiplatelet therapy for Reduction of Myocardial Damage during Angioplasty (ARMYDA)-2 study [16] assessed in a randomized head-to-head comparison a 600 mg and a 300 mg loading dose of clopidogrel in low- to moderate-risk patients undergoing PCI. The primary end point (30-day occurrence of death, MI, TVR) occurred in 4% of patients in the high versus 12% of patients in the conventional loading dose group ($p = 0.041$), with 600 mg clopidogrel load associated with a 52% risk reduction of periprocedural MI at multivariate analysis (OR, 0.48; 95% CI, 0.15–0.97; $p = 0.044$). Interestingly, no higher inhibition of platelet aggregation or clinical benefit was observed with increasing the loading dose (900 mg) compared with 600 mg in the Assessment of the Best Loading Dose of Clopidogrel to Blunt Platelet Activation, Inflammation and Ongoing Necrosis (ALBION) [17] and the Intracoronary Stenting and Antithrombotic Regimen: Choose Between 3 High Oral Doses for Immediate Clopidogrel Effect (ISAR-CHOICE) [18] studies. On the basis of these findings, the latest updates of both ACCF/AHA/SCAI [14] and ESC/EACTS [19] guidelines for myocardial revascularization recommend that a 600 mg loading dose of clopidogrel be administered at least 2 h before elective PCI. However, according to the ESC/EACTS guidelines [19], a 300 mg loading dose, ideally administered the day before the planned procedure or at least 6 h before, may also be considered as an appropriate antiplatelet strategy.

Other crucial issues regarding clopidogrel loading in patients with stable CAD have been further investigated. The potential benefit of a drug reload in patients already on chronic clopidogrel treatment was tested in the ARMYDA-4 study [20], where a further 600 mg loading dose in patients on chronic therapy with 75 mg/day clopidogrel did not translate into significant clinical benefit in patients with stable CAD undergoing coronary stenting. Furthermore, whether in-laboratory clopidogrel loading (i.e., after coronary angiogram and immediately before PCI) provides similar protection from periprocedural ischemic complications compared with pretreatment several hours before the procedure was investigated in the ARMYDA-5 [21] and PRAGUE-8 [22] trials. The results from both these randomized trials showed no significant difference in 30-day major adverse cardiovascular event (MACE) incidence in "preloaded" patients compared with those receiving a 600 mg clopidogrel load immediately before PCI, suggesting that a selective antiplatelet strategy for patients with previously unknown coronary anatomy is safe and may prevent the potential bleeding risk associated with DAPT when coronary bypass surgery is required instead of percutaneous revascularization.

Of note, both ACCF/AHA/SCAI [14] and ESC/EACTS [19] guidelines do not recommend the use of newer P2Y12 inhibitors (i.e., prasugrel and ticagrelor) as antiplatelet agents for patients with stable CAD, given the absence of specific clinical studies investigating this issue. Nevertheless, given their greater platelet inhibition, emerging evidence suggests a potential role of newer P2Y12 inhibitors especially in high-risk patients with persistent high platelet reactivity despite clopidogrel [23, 24]. However, despite these positive results from pharmacodynamic studies, the net clinical benefit (possible reduction of ischemic events without significant increase in bleeding) of these new antiplatelet drugs in patients with stable CAD is yet to be demonstrated.

Non-ST-segment-elevation acute coronary syndrome (NSTEACS)

Non-ST-segment-elevation acute coronary syndrome (NSTEACS) includes a large range of clinical settings and patient characteristics. DAPT is universally accepted as the optimal treatment to reduce thrombotic risk in NSTEACS patients undergoing PCI. The effects of clopidogrel in addition to aspirin have been well established in patients with NSTEACS. In the Clopidogrel in Unstable angina to prevent Recurrent Events (CURE) trial [25], clopidogrel (300 mg loading dose and then 75 mg/day) was shown to reduce the relative risk of the composite end point of cardiovascular death, nonfatal MI, and stroke by 20% versus aspirin alone in patients with NSTEACS. In the subgroup of patients receiving PCI [26], the benefit of clopidogrel was even higher, with 30% relative risk reduction of death, MI, and repeat revascularization. A higher dose of clopidogrel (600 mg) has been tested in the setting of ACS in the Clopidogrel and Aspirin Optimal Dose Usage to Reduce Recurrent Events – Seventh Organization to Assess Strategies in Ischemic Symptoms (CURRENT-OASIS 7) trial [27]. In this study, no significant difference was observed between a 600 mg and a 300 mg dose of clopidogrel in reducing the primary outcome of death, MI, or stroke at 30 days. However, a higher dose of clopidogrel showed a significant benefit in the subgroup of patients undergoing PCI, especially in reducing the rates of stent thrombosis [28].

Several investigations on the pharmacodynamic properties of clopidogrel have highlighted at least three limitations of this drug: delayed onset of action, large interindividual variability in platelet response, and irreversibility of its inhibitory effect on platelets [29]. These aspects are of particular importance in the setting of patients with ACS, where a more pronounced thrombotic milieu is expected and rapid and effective platelet inhibition is key in preventing thrombotic complications. Newer P2Y12 receptor inhibitors may, at least in part, overcome these limitations of clopidogrel.

Prasugrel is a third-generation thienopyridine that also irreversibly binds to the P2Y12 receptor, with a more rapid onset of action, a stronger inhibitory effect, and a lower variability on platelet response [30, 31]. In the Trial to Assess Improvement in Therapeutic Outcomes by Optimizing Platelet Inhibition with Prasugrel – Thrombolysis in Myocardial Infarction 38 (TRITON-TIMI 38) study, among ACS patients undergoing PCI [32, 33], those pretreated with prasugrel (60 mg followed by 10 mg/day after PCI) showed significantly lower rates of the primary end point (cardiovascular death, MI, or stroke) compared with patients pretreated with clopidogrel (300 mg followed by 75 mg/day after PCI) (9.7% vs. 11.9%, $p < 0.001$; 19% risk reduction). In particular, stent thrombosis was significantly reduced with prasugrel (1.13% vs. 2.35%, $p < 0.0001$; 52% risk reduction), both in patients treated with drug-eluting stents (0.84% vs. 2.31%, $p < 0.0001$; 64% risk reduction) and in those receiving bare-metal stents (1.27% vs. 2.41%, $p = 0.0009$; 48% risk reduction). Interestingly, a higher rate of Thrombolysis in Myocardial Infarction (TIMI) major bleeding not related to coronary artery bypass grafting (CABG) was observed for prasugrel, although this difference did not reach statistical significance (2.4% vs. 1.9%, $p = 0.06$). However, in the TRITON-TIMI 38, prasugrel was only administered after coronary angiography when the decision to proceed to PCI was made, and no data are available on the efficacy and safety of this drug in all-comer patients in whom coronary anatomy is unknown. Due to the proven increase in bleeding events, prasugrel is contraindicated in patients with active pathological bleeding or a history of transient ischemic attack (TIA) or stroke. Furthermore, in patients older than 75 years, prasugrel is generally not recommended, except in those with diabetes or a history of prior MI, in whom its protective effect appears to be greater. Prasugrel should also be used with caution in patients with body weight <60 kg, propensity to bleed, and concomitant use of medications that increase the risk of bleeding (e.g., warfarin, heparin, fibrinolytic therapy, or chronic use of nonsteroidal anti-inflammatory drugs).

Ticagrelor is an oral, reversible, short-acting, nonthienopyridine P2Y12 receptor antagonist. It has a direct antiplatelet action and is less dependent from metabolic activation [34]. The PLATelet Inhibition and Patient Outcomes (PLATO) trial [35] compared ticagrelor (180 mg loading dose, 90 mg twice daily thereafter) and clopidogrel (300–600 mg loading dose, 75 mg daily thereafter) in patients admitted for ACS. At 12 months, the incidence of the composite end point (cardiovascular death, MI, and stroke) was significantly reduced in the ticagrelor group (9.8% vs. 11.7%, $p < 0.001$; risk reduction 16%). The benefit was maintained for the single components of the composite end points, including cardiovascular mortality (4.5% vs. 5.9%, $p < 0.001$) and MI (5.8% vs. 6.9%, $p = 0.005$). No significant difference in the rates of overall major bleeding was observed, but ticagrelor was associated with higher incidence of major bleeding not related to CABG (4.5% vs. 3.8%, $p = 0.03$).

In a study-level meta-analysis [36] including 32,893 patients from DISPERSE-2 [37], PLATO [35], and TRITON-TIMI 38 [32], an indirect comparison between prasugrel and ticagrelor has shown no significant difference in the risk of the composite ischemic end point of death, MI, and stroke between the two drugs. The use of prasugrel was however associated with lower risk of probable/definite stent thrombosis ($p = 0.02$) but increased risk of any TIMI major bleeding ($p = 0.007$).

Given the important prognostic role of both ischemic and hemorrhagic events in patients with NSTEACS, choosing the appropriate antiplatelet strategy according to both risks may represent the optimal practice. Current ACCF/AHA guidelines [38] recommend a loading dose of P2Y12 receptor inhibitor be administered in NSTEACS patients for whom PCI is planned. The availability of three agents for antagonizing platelet ADP receptors makes it possible to individualize antiplatelet therapy. One of the following regimens is recommended: clopidogrel 600 mg as early as possible before or at the time of PCI, prasugrel 60 mg administered promptly once coronary anatomy is defined and a decision is made to proceed with PCI and anyway no later than 1 h after PCI, and ticagrelor 180 mg given as early as possible before or at the time of PCI.

ST-segment-elevation myocardial infarction (STEMI)

In patients with ST-segment-elevation myocardial infarction (STEMI), platelet reactivity plays an important role in determining initial patency of the infarct-related artery and myocardial reperfusion after primary PCI. Both these factors have been shown to significantly impact on immediate- and long-term clinical outcomes. Achieving a profound and timely platelet inhibition is therefore crucial in determining prognosis of STEMI patients.

Clopidogrel has been the cornerstone of DAPT also for STEMI patients for nearly 15 years until newer P2Y12 receptor inhibitors have became available. Limited data are available regarding the choice of the loading dose of clopidogrel in patients with STEMI undergoing primary PCI, mainly coming from an observational study suggesting that a 600 mg loading dose is associated with improvements in procedural angiographic end points and 1-year clinical outcomes compared with a 300 mg dose [39] and the ARMYDA-6 MI study [40]. The latter is the only available randomized study comparing the two loading doses of clopidogrel and has shown that pretreatment with a 600 mg load before primary PCI was associated with a reduction of the infarct size compared with a 300 mg dose, as well as with improvement of angiographic results, residual cardiac function, and 30-day MACE.

For patients undergoing PCI after fibrinolysis, the recommended loading dose of clopidogrel should be 300 mg within 24 h and 600 mg more than 24 h after receiving fibrinolytic therapy [14].

The evidence for the use of prasugrel in patients with STEMI undergoing PCI derives from TRITON-TIMI 38 [41]. In this subset of patients, prasugrel was associated with a significant reduction of the primary end point (composite of cardiovascular death, nonfatal MI, or nonfatal stroke) at 30 days compared with clopidogrel (6.5% vs. 9.5%, $p = 0.0017$). This benefit persisted at 15-month follow-up (10.0% vs. 12.4%, $p = 0.0221$). Interestingly, in STEMI patients, prasugrel was not associated with an excess in TIMI major bleeding unrelated to cardiac surgery at 30 days ($p = 0.3359$) and 15 months ($p = 0.6451$), while only TIMI major bleeding after CABG surgery was significantly increased with prasugrel ($p = 0.0033$). This resulted in a significant net clinical benefit in favor of prasugrel, even when including CABG-related major bleeding in the composite net end point ($p = 0.0412$, number needed to treat = 42).

Ticagrelor has also shown in the PLATO trial [42] clinical benefit compared with clopidogrel in the subset of patients with STEMI undergoing primary PCI. The reduction of the primary end point (MI, stroke, or cardiovascular death) with ticagrelor versus clopidogrel (10.8% vs. 9.4%) was consistent with the overall PLATO results, although not reaching statistical significance ($p = 0.07$). However, when taken as single end points, MI (4.7% vs. 5.8%, $p = 0.03$), total mortality (9.8% vs. 11.3, $p = 0.05$), and definite stent thrombosis (1.6% vs. 2.4%, $p = 0.03$) were significantly reduced with ticagrelor. Of note, among STEMI patients, no increase in TIMI major bleeding was observed in the ticagrelor group ($p = 0.66$).

Based on this evidence, the latest recommendations for STEMI patients undergoing PCI privilege the use of prasugrel (60 mg in clopidogrel-naive patients, if no history of prior stroke/TIA, age <75 years) or ticagrelor (180 mg) as initial agents for P2Y12 receptor inhibition in association with aspirin [14, 43]. Clopidogrel 600 mg still remains an option when prasugrel or ticagrelor is either not available or contraindicated.

References

1 Serrano, C.V.J., Ramires, J.A., Venturinelli, M. *et al.* (1997) Coronary angioplasty results in leukocyte and platelet activation with adhesion molecule expression. Evidence of inflammatory responses in coronary angioplasty. *Journal of the American College of Cardiology*, **29**, 1276–1283.

2 Mangiacapra, F., Bartunek, J., Bijnens, N. *et al.* (2012) Peri-procedural variations of platelet reactivity during elective percutaneous coronary intervention. *Journal of Thrombosis and Haemostasis*, **10 (12)**, 2452–2461.

3 Gurbel, P.A., Bliden, K.P., Hayes, K.M., and Tantry, U. (2004) Platelet activation in myocardial ischemic syndromes. *Expert Review of Cardiovascular Therapy*, **2**, 535–545.

4 Libby, P. (1995) Molecular bases of the acute coronary syndromes. *Circulation*, **91**, 2844–2850.

5 De Servi, S., Mariani, M., Mariani, G., and Mazzone, A. (2005) C-reactive protein increase in unstable coronary disease cause or effect? *Journal of the American College of Cardiology*, **46**, 1496–1502.

6 Bhatt, D.L., Bertrand, M.E., Berger, P.B. *et al.* (2002) Meta-analysis of randomized and registry comparisons of ticlopidine with clopidogrel after stenting. *Journal of the American College of Cardiology*, **39**, 9–14.

7 Price, M.J., Berger, P.B., Teirstein, P.S. *et al.* (2011) Standard- vs. high-dose clopidogrel based on platelet function testing after percutaneous coronary intervention: the GRAVITAS randomized trial. *JAMA*, **305**, 1097–1105.

8 Trenk, D., Stone, G.W., Gawaz, M. *et al.* (2012) A randomized trial of prasugrel versus clopidogrel in patients with high platelet reactivity on clopidogrel after elective percutaneous coronary intervention with implantation of drug-eluting stents: results of the TRIGGER-PCI (Testing Platelet Reactivity In Patients Undergoing Elective Stent Placement on Clopidogrel to Guide Alternative Therapy With Prasugrel) study. *Journal of the American College of Cardiology*, **59**, 2159–2164.

9 Bonello, L., Tantry, U.S., Marcucci, R. *et al.* (2010) Consensus and future directions on the definition of high on-treatment platelet reactivity to adenosine diphosphate. *Journal of the American College of Cardiology*, **56**, 919–933.

10 Mangiacapra, F., Patti, G., Barbato, E. *et al.* (2012) A therapeutic window for platelet reactivity for patients undergoing elective percutaneous coronary intervention: results of the ARMYDA-PROVE (Antiplatelet therapy for Reduction of MYocardial Damage during Angioplasty-Platelet Reactivity for Outcome Validation Effort) study. *JACC. Cardiovascular Interventions*, **5**, 281–289.

11 Tantry, U.S., Jeong, Y.H., Navarese, E.P., and Gurbel, P.A. (2012) Platelet function measurement in elective percutaneous coronary intervention patients: exploring the concept of a P2Y(1)(2) inhibitor therapeutic window. *JACC. Cardiovascular Interventions*, **5**, 290–292.

12 Antithrombotic Trialists' Collaboration (2002) Collaborative meta-analysis of randomised trials of antiplatelet therapy for prevention of death, myocardial infarction, and stroke in high risk patients. *BMJ*, **324**, 71–86.

13 Savage, M.P., Goldberg, S., Bove, A.A. *et al.* (1995) Effect of thromboxane A2 blockade on clinical outcome and restenosis after successful coronary angioplasty. Multi-Hospital Eastern Atlantic Restenosis Trial (M-HEART II). *Circulation*, **92**, 3194–3200.

14 Levine, G.N., Bates, E.R., Blankenship, J.C. *et al.* (2011) 2011 ACCF/AHA/SCAI guideline for percutaneous coronary intervention. A report of the American College of Cardiology Foundation/American Heart Association Task Force on Practice Guidelines and the Society for Cardiovascular Angiography and Interventions. *Journal of the American College of Cardiology*, **58**, e44–e122.

15 Steinhubl, S.R., Berger, P.B., Mann, J.Tr. *et al.* (2002) Early and sustained dual oral antiplatelet therapy following percutaneous coronary intervention: a randomized controlled trial. *JAMA*, **288**, 2411–2420.

16 Patti, G., Colonna, G., Pasceri, V., Pepe, L.L., Montinaro, A. and Di Sciascio, G. (2005) Randomized trial of high loading dose of clopidogrel for reduction of periprocedural myocardial infarction in patients undergoing coronary intervention: results from the ARMYDA-2 (Antiplatelet therapy for Reduction of MYocardial Damage during Angioplasty) study. *Circulation*, **111**, 2099–2106.

17 Montalescot, G., Sideris, G., Meuleman, C. *et al.* (2006) A randomized comparison of high clopidogrel loading doses in patients with non-ST-segment elevation acute coronary syndromes: the ALBION (Assessment of the Best Loading Dose of Clopidogrel to Blunt Platelet Activation, Inflammation and Ongoing Necrosis) trial. *Journal of the American College of Cardiology*, **48**, 931–938.

18 von Beckerath, N., Taubert, D., Pogatsa-Murray, G., Schomig, E., Kastrati, A. and Schomig, A. (2005) Absorption, metabolization, and antiplatelet effects of 300-, 600-, and 900-mg loading doses of clopidogrel: results of the ISAR-CHOICE (Intracoronary Stenting and Antithrombotic Regimen: Choose Between 3 High Oral Doses for Immediate Clopidogrel Effect) Trial. *Circulation*, **112**, 2946–2950.

19 Wijns, W., Kolh, P., Danchin, N. *et al.* (2010) Guidelines on myocardial revascularization. *European Heart Journal*, **31**, 2501–2555.

20 Di Sciascio, G., Patti, G., Pasceri, V., Colonna, G., Mangiacapra, F. and Montinaro, A. (2010) Clopidogrel reloading in patients undergoing percutaneous coronary intervention on chronic clopidogrel therapy: results of the ARMYDA-4 RELOAD (Antiplatelet therapy for Reduction of MYocardial Damage during Angioplasty) randomized trial. *European Heart Journal*, **31**, 1337–1343.

21 Di Sciascio, G., Patti, G., Pasceri, V., Gatto, L., Colonna, G., and Montinaro, A. (2010b) Effectiveness of in-laboratory high-dose clopidogrel loading versus routine pre-load in patients undergoing percutaneous coronary intervention: results of the ARMYDA-5 PRELOAD (Antiplatelet therapy for Reduction of MYocardial Damage during Angioplasty) randomized trial. *Journal of the American College of Cardiology*, **56**, 550–557.

22 Widimsky, P., Motovska, Z., Simek, S. *et al.* (2008) Clopidogrel pre-treatment in stable angina: for all patients >6 h before elective coronary angiography or only for angiographically selected patients a few minutes before PCI? A randomized multicentre trial PRAGUE-8. *European Heart Journal*, **29**, 1495–1503.

23 Angiolillo, D.J., Badimon, J.J., Saucedo, J.F. *et al.* (2011) A pharmacodynamic comparison of prasugrel vs. high-dose clopidogrel in patients with type 2 diabetes mellitus and coronary artery disease: results of the Optimizing anti-Platelet Therapy In diabetes MellitUS (OPTIMUS)-3 Trial. *European Heart Journal*, **32**, 838–846.

24 Gurbel, P.A., Bliden, K.P., Butler, K. *et al.* (2009) Randomized double-blind assessment of the ONSET and OFFSET of the antiplatelet effects of ticagrelor versus clopidogrel in patients with stable coronary artery disease: the ONSET/OFFSET study. *Circulation*, **120**, 2577–2585.

25 Yusuf, S., Zhao, F., Mehta, S.R., Chrolavicius, S., Tognoni, G., and Fox, K.K. (2001) Effects of clopidogrel in addition to aspirin in patients with acute coronary syndromes without ST-segment elevation. *The New England Journal of Medicine*, **345**, 494–502.

26 Mehta, S.R., Yusuf, S., Peters, R.J. *et al.* (2001) Effects of pretreatment with clopidogrel and aspirin followed by long-term therapy in patients undergoing percutaneous coronary intervention: the PCI-CURE study. *Lancet*, **358**, 527–533.

27 Mehta, S.R., Bassand, J.P., Chrolavicius, S. *et al.* (2010a) Dose comparisons of clopidogrel and aspirin in acute coronary syndromes. *The New England Journal of Medicine*, **363**, 930–942.

28 Mehta, S.R., Tanguay, J.F., Eikelboom, J.W. *et al.* (2010b) Double-dose versus standard-dose clopidogrel and high-dose versus low-dose aspirin in

individuals undergoing percutaneous coronary intervention for acute coronary syndromes (CURRENT-OASIS 7): a randomised factorial trial. *Lancet*, **376**, 1233–1243.

29 Angiolillo, D.J., Fernandez-Ortiz, A., Bernardo, E. *et al.* (2007) Variability in individual responsiveness to clopidogrel: clinical implications, management, and future perspectives. *Journal of the American College of Cardiology*, **49**, 1505–1516.

30 Damman, P., Woudstra, P., Kuijt, W.J., de Winter, R.J., and James, S.K. (2012) P2Y12 platelet inhibition in clinical practice. *Journal of Thrombosis and Thrombolysis*, **33**, 143–153.

31 Wallentin, L. (2009) P2Y(12) inhibitors: differences in properties and mechanisms of action and potential consequences for clinical use. *European Heart Journal*, **30**, 1964–1977.

32 Wiviott, S.D., Braunwald, E., McCabe, C.H. *et al.* (2007) Prasugrel versus clopidogrel in patients with acute coronary syndromes. *The New England Journal of Medicine*, **357**, 2001–2015.

33 Wiviott, S.D., Braunwald, E., McCabe, C.H. *et al.* (2008) Intensive oral antiplatelet therapy for reduction of ischaemic events including stent thrombosis in patients with acute coronary syndromes treated with percutaneous coronary intervention and stenting in the TRITON-TIMI 38 trial: a subanalysis of a randomised trial. *Lancet*, **371**, 1353–1363.

34 Husted, S., Emanuelsson, H., Heptinstall, S., Sandset, P.M., Wickens, M., and Peters, G. (2006) Pharmacodynamics, pharmacokinetics, and safety of the oral reversible P2Y12 antagonist AZD6140 with aspirin in patients with atherosclerosis: a double-blind comparison to clopidogrel with aspirin. *European Heart Journal*, **27**, 1038–1047.

35 Wallentin, L., Becker, R.C., Budaj, A. *et al.* (2009) Ticagrelor versus clopidogrel in patients with acute coronary syndromes. *The New England Journal of Medicine*, **361**, 1045–1057.

36 Biondi-Zoccai, G., Lotrionte, M., Agostoni, P. *et al.* (2011) Adjusted indirect comparison meta-analysis of prasugrel versus ticagrelor for patients with acute coronary syndromes. *International Journal of Cardiology*, **150**, 325–331.

37 Cannon, C.P., Husted, S., Harrington, R.A. *et al.* (2007) Safety, tolerability, and initial efficacy of AZD6140, the first reversible oral adenosine diphosphate receptor antagonist, compared with clopidogrel, in patients with non-ST-segment elevation acute coronary syndrome: primary results of the DISPERSE-2 trial. *Journal of the American College of Cardiology*, **50**, 1844–1851.

38 Jneid, H., Anderson, J.L., Wright, R.S. *et al.* (2012) 2012 ACCF/AHA focused update of the guideline for the management of patients with unstable angina/non-ST-elevation myocardial infarction (updating the 2007 guideline and replacing the 2011 focused update): a report of the American College of Cardiology Foundation/American Heart Association Task Force on Practice Guidelines. *Journal of the American College of Cardiology*, **60**, 645–681.

39 Mangiacapra, F., Muller, O., Ntalianis, A. *et al.* (2010) Comparison of 600 versus 300-mg Clopidogrel loading dose in patients with ST-segment elevation myocardial infarction undergoing primary coronary angioplasty. *The American Journal of Cardiology*, **106**, 1208–1211.

40 Patti, G., Barczi, G., Orlic, D. *et al.* (2011) Outcome comparison of 600- and 300-mg loading doses of clopidogrel in patients undergoing primary percutaneous coronary intervention for ST-segment elevation myocardial infarction: results from the ARMYDA-6 MI (Antiplatelet therapy for

Reduction of MYocardial Damage during Angioplasty-Myocardial Infarction) randomized study. *Journal of the American College of Cardiology*, **58**, 1592–1599.

41 Montalescot, G., Wiviott, S.D., Braunwald, E. *et al.* (2009) Prasugrel compared with clopidogrel in patients undergoing percutaneous coronary intervention for ST-elevation myocardial infarction (TRITON-TIMI 38): double-blind, randomised controlled trial. *Lancet*, **373**, 723–731.

42 Steg, P.G., James, S., Harrington, R.A. *et al.* (2010) Ticagrelor versus clopidogrel in patients with ST-elevation acute coronary syndromes intended for reperfusion with primary percutaneous coronary intervention: A Platelet Inhibition and Patient Outcomes (PLATO) trial subgroup analysis. *Circulation*, **122**, 2131–2141.

43 Steg, P.G., James, S.K., Atar, D. *et al.* (2012) ESC Guidelines for the management of acute myocardial infarction in patients presenting with ST-segment elevation: The Task Force on the management of ST-segment elevation acute myocardial infarction of the European Society of Cardiology (ESC). *European Heart Journal*, **33**, 2569–2619.

26 Duration of Dual Antiplatelet Therapy after Drug-Eluting Stent Implantation

Joshua P. Loh and Ron Waksman

MedStar Washington Hospital Center, Washington, DC, USA

Introduction

In the last decade, percutaneous coronary intervention (PCI) with drug-eluting stents (DES) has largely replaced PCI with bare-metal stents (BMS) due to their superior antirestenotic properties. However, the optimal duration of dual antiplatelet therapy (DAPT) with aspirin and a thienopyridine after DES implantation remains unknown. With early-generation DES, it was shown that premature discontinuation of DAPT [<3 months for sirolimus-eluting stents (SES) and <6 months for paclitaxel-eluting stents (PES)] strongly predicts stent thrombosis (ST) [1, 2]. Moreover, additional safety concerns arose from observational reports on increased risks of late (30 days to 1 year) and very late (>1 year) ST compared to BMS [3]. These late thrombotic events were hypothesized to be due to delayed vessel healing [4] and have led many to promote longer durations of DAPT for DES. In fact, current guidelines from American societies recommend DAPT for at least 12 months [5], while the European Society of Cardiology recommends 6–12 months after DES implantation [6]. These recommendations, however, were not based on any strong prospective randomized data, but rather on consensus opinion derived from earlier trials involving thienopyridine dosing strategies [7, 8] and observational studies suggesting lower death and myocardial infarction (MI) rates with prolonged DAPT [9, 10]. Moreover, prolonging DAPT increases bleeding risks [11], and post-PCI bleeding leads to deleterious long-term outcomes [12]. Hence, uncertainty exists regarding DAPT duration in the absence of solid clinical evidence while striking a balance between reducing ST and increment bleeding risk.

Antiplatelet Therapy in Cardiovascular Disease, First Edition. Edited by Ron Waksman, Paul A. Gurbel, and Michael A. Gaglia, Jr.
© 2014 John Wiley & Sons, Ltd. Published 2014 by John Wiley & Sons, Ltd.

Prolonged DAPT duration greater than 12 months

Several observational studies that specifically analyzed DAPT duration and ST risk were unable to demonstrate that prolonged DAPT greater than 12 months neither prevents very late ST [13] nor exerts any benefit in preventing death and MI [13, 14]. In contrast, other studies have reported reductions in death and MI [9, 15], but did not specifically address late ST events. Several current randomized trials seek to address the issue of varying DAPT durations after DES implantation (Table 26.1).

In the Correlation of Clopidogrel Therapy Discontinuation in Real-World Patients Treated with Drug-Eluting Stent Implantation/Evaluation of the Long-Term Safety after Zotarolimus-Eluting Stent, Sirolimus-Eluting Stent, or Paclitaxel-Eluting Stent Implantation for Coronary Lesions-Late Coronary Arterial Thrombotic Events (REAL/ZEST-LATE) [16], 2701 patients who were event-free 12 months after DES implantation were randomized to continue DAPT or just aspirin monotherapy. The study found no significant difference in 2-year cardiac death or MI and a trend toward the increased composite risk of MI, stroke, and death with prolonged DAPT. In the PROlonging Dual antiplatelet treatment after Grading stent-induced Intimal hyperplasia studY (PRODIGY) [18], 1970 patients who were event-free for 30 days after stenting (DES or BMS) were randomized to 6 versus 24 months' DAPT. The study found no difference in death, MI, or stroke at 2 years. In addition, there was no benefit of prolonged DAPT in reducing ST, but there was a significantly increased risk of bleeding. In view of the low ischemic and bleeding events in both trials, these findings are not definitive. A larger, ongoing trial [Dual AntiPlatelet Therapy (DAPT), NCT00977938] will compare greater than 20,000 patients randomized to 12 versus 30 months of DAPT. The trial is powered to assess major bleeding events and is due to be completed in 2014. There are also several other ongoing randomized trials addressing the efficacy and safety of DAPT beyond 12 months (Table 26.1), which, upon completion, should add clarity to its benefits/risks. Based on current evidence, prolonging DAPT beyond 12 months does not appear to mitigate ST risk while at the same time increases bleeding risk and should not be recommended in all patients receiving a DES.

Shortened DAPT duration less than 12 months

Perhaps more provocative are studies addressing whether DAPT is even needed for the full 12 months after stenting. This is a particularly important clinical question in patients who are unable to tolerate the full DAPT duration due to increased bleeding risks and unplanned noncardiac surgery or in patients with low drug adherence. Several observational studies have found that the protective effect of DAPT on ST was only observed within the first 6 months after DES implantation [2, 20]. Moreover, the temporal relationship between DAPT discontinuation

Table 26.1 Randomized studies evaluating different dual antiplatelet therapy (DAPT) durations.

Study	Inclusion group	DAPT duration	Stent type(s)	Primary outcome (follow-up)	Secondary end points	Status/Reference
REAL/ZEST-LATE	2,701 12-month event-free	12 versus 24 months	PES, SES, ZES	No difference in cardiac death or MI (24 months)	No difference in ST, TVR, or major bleed (TIMI)	Completed [16]
EXCELLENT	1,443	6 versus 12 months	EES, SES	No difference in death/MI/ ischemia-driven TVR (12 months)	ST numerically higher in 6 month's DAPT	Completed [17]
PRODIGY	1,970 30-day event-free	6 versus 24 months	PES, EES, E-ZES, BMS	No difference in death/MI/ stroke (2 years)	Higher risk of bleed with prolonged DAPT	Completed [18]
RESET	2,148	3 (E-ZES) versus 12 months (other DES)	E-ZES, R-ZES, EES, SES	No difference in cardiac death/MI/ST/TVR/bleeding (1 year)	No difference in individual component end points	Completed [19]
ISAR-SAFE	6,000 6-month event-free	6 versus 12 months	DES	Death/MI/stroke/major bleed (15 months)	Individual component end points	Ongoing NCT0661206
ITALIC	3,200	6 versus 12 months	EES	Death/MI/TVR/stroke/major bleed (1 year)	Composite outcome (2, 3 years)	Ongoing NCT00780156
OPTIMIZE	3,120	3 versus 12 months	E-ZES	Death/MI/stroke/major bleed (1 year)	ST	Ongoing NCT01113372
SECURITY	4,000 Stable	6 versus 12 months	Second-generation DES	ST (2 year)	Death/MI/TVR	Ongoing NCT00944333

OPTIDUAL	1,966 12-month event-free	12 versus 48 months	DES	Death/MI/stroke/major bleed (4 years)	ST, TVR, minor bleed	Ongoing NCT00822536
ARCTIC-2	2,466 12-month event-free	12 versus 18 months	DES	Time to death/MI/TVR/ST/ stroke	Time to component end points	Completed enrollment NCT00827411
DES-LATE	5,000 12-month event-free	12 versus 24 months	DES	Death/MI/stroke (2 years)	ST, TIMI bleed, TVR	Ongoing NCT01186126
DAPT	20,645 12-month event-free	12 versus 30 months	DES, BMS	Death/MI/stroke and ST (33 months)	Major bleed (GUSTO)	Ongoing NCT00977938

BMS, bare-metal stent; DAPT, dual antiplatelet therapy; DES, drug-eluting stent; E-ZES, Endeavor zotarolimus-eluting stent; EES, everolimus-eluting stent; MI, myocardial infarction; PES, paclitaxel-eluting stent; R-ZES, Resolute zotarolimus-eluting stent; SES, sirolimus-eluting stent; ST, stent thrombosis; TVR, target vessel revascularization; ZES, zotarolimus-eluting stent and ST events was no longer apparent beyond 6 months. A large registry, however, described persistent ST risk beyond 6 months, but this association to DAPT discontinuation is limited because of low ST event rates beyond 6 months [21].

The results of several recent randomized trials comparing standard to shortened DAPT duration suggest that under certain circumstances, a shortened DAPT duration may be feasible. In the Efficacy of Xience/promus versus Cypher to rEduce Late Loss after stENTing) (EXCELLENT) [17], similar target vessel failure rates were demonstrated in 1443 patients randomized at index PCI to 6 versus 12 months' DAPT, suggesting noninferiority of shortened to standard DAPT duration. Bleeding rates were low and were not significantly different although numerically they were twofold higher with 12 months' DAPT. In the REal Safety and Efficacy of 3-month dual antiplatelet Therapy following Endeavor zotarolimus-eluting stent (RESET) trial [19], 2148 patients of low anatomical risk profile were randomized to receive an Endeavor zotarolimus-eluting stent (E-ZES) (Medtronic, Santa Rosa, CA)/3 months' DAPT versus other DES/12 months' DAPT. The results showed no significant differences in 1-year death, MI, ST, revascularization, or bleeding, suggesting noninferiority of E-ZES with shortened DAPT to standard therapy. In these two trials, however, the noninferiority margins were considered wide for the low event rates encountered to prove their hypotheses of the safety of a shortened DAPT duration in low-risk patients. Several ongoing trials with greater than 16,000 patients enrolled and with contemporary DES use (Table 26.1) will hopefully give a clearer direction of the efficacy and safety of 3 or 6 months' DAPT against 12 months' DAPT.

Stent-specific considerations

The current guidelines recommending DAPT duration after DES implantation are based on data from early-generation DES (primarily PES and SES). Meanwhile, newer-generation DES with biocompatible or biodegradable polymers and thin-strut platforms have largely replaced early-generation DES in clinical use. The newer-generation DES have proven to be equal or superior in antirestenotic effect while demonstrating a consistently better safety profile in reducing late or very late ST [22, 23]. Moreover, differential rates of vessel healing were reported across different DES platforms and favored the newer-generation DES [24]. Thus, a potential determinant of DAPT duration may be the type of DES implanted. This was hypothesized in RESET [19], where E-ZES (which has a supposed better safety profile due to early vessel healing) coupled with a short DAPT duration was noninferior to other DES with a longer DAPT duration. However, in two randomized trials [25, 26], SES were associated with an equal or lower risk of ST compared to E-ZES. Based on current clinical data, the everolimus-eluting stent (EES) has recently received the *Conformité Européenne* (CE) mark recommending a minimal DAPT duration of only 3 months. Also, on the basis of encouraging results demonstrating reductions in ST [22], the Randomized Clinical Evaluation of the BioFreedom™ Stent (LEADERS FREE) trial [NCT01623180] [27] will assess 1 month of DAPT for patients at high bleeding risk undergoing PCI with biodegradable polymer DES compared to BMS.

Although the results were in no way definitive, a recent analysis from PRODIGY indicates heterogeneity across stent types in response to different DAPT durations [28], suggesting that optimal DAPT duration may be stent specific. Adverse events were significantly higher for ZES on prolonged DAPT, while more ST events occurred in PES with short DAPT duration. There was no difference in primary outcome in short versus prolonged DAPT for BMS, PES, and EES. Thus, stent-specific optimization with shorter duration of DAPT may be on the horizon as more evidence accumulates regarding the safety profile of newer DES.

Patient-specific considerations

An important consideration is the risk profile of the patient (i.e., clinical presentation) and the complexity of the anatomy, which may warrant longer DAPT. Current guidelines recommend 12 months of DAPT in ACS patients regardless of stent type, which is based on strong evidence. Patients (e.g., renal failure, diabetes) and lesions (e.g., bifurcations, diffuse disease) at higher thrombotic risk [1, 21] should require at least 12 months' DAPT. Moreover, higher-risk patients with established vascular disease and a prior thrombotic event may benefit from prolonged DAPT for the prevention of further thrombotic events irrespective of stent placement [29].

DAPT interruption

Another important issue related to DAPT is interruption/discontinuation. Several studies have established a temporal relationship with regard to ST events after DAPT discontinuation within 6 months of DES implantation, but this relationship becomes indistinct after 6 months [2, 21]. In a study by Ferreira et al. [30], the authors found that DAPT interruption was not infrequent after DES implantation and occurs in approximately 10.6% of patients, most of the interruption was temporary (median 7 days), and brief DAPT interruptions 1 month after DES do not have a major impact on the future ischemic risks. Moreover, if aspirin was maintained, short-term discontinuation of clopidogrel appeared safe [31]. An ongoing registry [Patterns of Non-Adherence to Dual Anti-Platelet Regimen In Stented Patients (PARIS), NCT00998127] will assess the different modes of nonadherence to DAPT and its impact on clinical outcomes.

Summary

Current evidence supporting the duration of DAPT after DES is inadequate. There is increasing evidence that greater than 6 months of DAPT after DES implantation does not appear to lessen risk of late/very late ST, while prolonging DAPT beyond 12 months may increase bleeding events. Newer-generation DES appear safer compared to early-generation DES in reducing ST risk, but more evidence is required before stent-specific recommendations are made regarding varying DAPT duration. Patient-specific considerations are important in deciding DAPT duration and should be a balance between thrombotic risk and bleeding risk. Brief DAPT interruptions after the first month of DES do not appear to have a major impact on clinical outcomes.

References

1 Iakovou, I., Schmidt, T., Bonizzoni, E. *et al.* (2005) Incidence, predictors, and outcome of thrombosis after successful implantation of drug-eluting stents. *JAMA*, **293**, 2126–2130.

2 Airoldi, F., Colombo, A., Morici, N. *et al.* (2007) Incidence and predictors of drug-eluting stent thrombosis during and after discontinuation of thienopyridine treatment. *Circulation*, **116**, 745–754.

3 Lagerqvist, B., James, S.K., Stenestrand, U. *et al.* (2007) Long-term outcomes with drug-eluting stents versus bare-metal stents in Sweden. *The New England Journal of Medicine*, **356**, 1009–1019.

4 Joner, M., Finn, A.V., Farb, A. *et al.* (2006) Pathology of drug-eluting stents in humans: delayed healing and late thrombotic risk. *Journal of the American College of Cardiology*, **48**, 193–202.

5 Levine, G.N., Bates, E.R., Blankenship, J.C. *et al.* (2011) 2011 ACCF/AHA/SCAI guideline for percutaneous coronary intervention. A report of the American College of Cardiology Foundation/American Heart Association Task Force on Practice Guidelines and the Society for Cardiovascular Angiography and Interventions. *Journal of the American College of Cardiology*, **58**, e44–e122.

6 Wijns, W., Kolh, P., Danchin, N. *et al.* (2010) Guidelines on myocardial revascularization. *European Heart Journal*, **31**, 2501–2555.

7 Mehta, S., Yusuf, S., Peters, R. *et al.* (2001) Effects of pretreatment with clopidogrel and aspirin followed by long-term therapy in patients undergoing percutaneous coronary intervention: the PCI-CURE study. *Lancet*, **358**, 527–533.

8 Steinhubl, S.R., Berger, P.B., Mann, J.T. *et al.* (2002) Early and sustained dual oral antiplatelet therapy following percutaneous coronary intervention: a randomized controlled trial. *JAMA*, **288**, 2411–2420.

9 Eisenstein, E.L., Anstrom, K.J., Kong, D.F. *et al.* (2007) Clopidogrel use and long-term clinical outcomes after drug-eluting stent implantation. *JAMA*, **297**, 159–168.

10 Brar, S.S., Kim, J., Brar, S.K. *et al.* (2008) Long-term outcomes by clopidogrel duration and stent type on a diabetic population with de novo coronary artery lesions. *Journal of the American College of Cardiology*, **51**, 2220–2227.

11 Tada, T., Natsuaki, M., Morimoto, T. *et al.* (2012) Duration of dual antiplatelet therapy and long-term clinical outcome after coronary drug-eluting stent implantation: landmark analyses from the CREDO-Kyoto PCI/CABG Registry Cohort-2. *Circulation. Cardiovascular Interventions,* **5**, 381–391.

12 Rao, S.V., Dai, D., Subherwal, S. *et al.* (2012) Association between periprocedural bleeding and long-term outcomes following percutaneous coronary intervention in older patients. *JACC: Cardiovascular Interventions,* **5**, 958–965.

13 Park, D.W., Yun, S.C., Lee, S.W. *et al.* (2008) Stent thrombosis, clinical events, and influence of prolonged clopidogrel use after placement of drug-eluting stent: data from an observational cohort study of drug-eluting versus bare-metal stents. *JACC: Cardiovascular Interventions,* **1**, 494–503.

14 Harjai, K.J., Shenoy, C., Orshaw, P. & Boura, J. (2009) Dual antiplatelet therapy for more than 12 months after percutaneous coronary intervention: insights from the Guthrie PCI Registry. *Heart,* **95**, 1579–1586.

15 Faxon, D.P., Lawler, E., Young, M., Gaziano, M. & Kinlay, S. (2012) Prolonged clopidogrel use after bare metal and drug-eluting stent placement: the Veterans Administration drug-eluting stent study. *Circulation. Cardiovascular Interventions,* **5**, 372–380.

16 Park, S.J., Park, D.W., Kim, Y.H. *et al.* (2010) Duration of dual antiplatelet therapy after implantation of drug-eluting stents. *The New England Journal of Medicine,* **362**, 1374–1382.

17 Gwon, H.C., Hahn, J.Y., Park, K.W. *et al.* (2012) Six-month versus 12-month dual antiplatelet therapy after implantation of drug-eluting stents: the Efficacy of Xience/Promus Versus Cypher to Reduce Late Loss After Stenting (EXCELLENT) randomized, multicenter study. *Circulation,* **125**, 505–513.

18 Valgimigli, M., Campo, G., Monti, M. *et al.* (2012) Short- versus long-term duration of dual-antiplatelet therapy after coronary stenting: a randomized multicenter trial. *Circulation,* **125**, 2015–2026.

19 Kim, B.K., Hong, M.K., Shin, D.H. *et al.* (2012) A new strategy for discontinuation of dual antiplatelet therapy: the RESET Trial (REal Safety and Efficacy of 3-month dual antiplatelet Therapy following Endeavor zotarolimus-eluting stent implantation). *Journal of the American College of Cardiology,* **60**, 1340–1348.

20 Schulz, S., Schuster, T., Mehilli, J. *et al.* (2009) Stent thrombosis after drug-eluting stent implantation: incidence, timing, and relation to discontinuation of clopidogrel therapy over a 4-year period. *European Heart Journal,* **30**, 2714–2721.

21 van Werkum, J.W., Heestermans, A.A., Zomer, A.C. *et al.* (2009) Predictors of coronary stent thrombosis: the Dutch stent thrombosis registry. *Journal of the American College of Cardiology,* **53**, 1399–1409.

22 Palmerini, T., Biondi-Zoccai, G., Della Riva, D. *et al.* (2012) Stent thrombosis with drug-eluting and bare-metal stents: evidence from a comprehensive network meta-analysis. *Lancet,* **379**, 1393–1402.

23 Stefanini, G.G., Byrne, R.A., Serruys, P.W. *et al.* (2012) Biodegradable polymer drug-eluting stents reduce the risk of stent thrombosis at 4 years in patients undergoing percutaneous coronary intervention: a pooled analysis of individual patient data from the ISAR-TEST 3, ISAR-TEST 4, and LEADERS randomized trials. *European Heart Journal,* **33**, 1214–1222.

24 Joner, M., Nakazawa, G., Finn, A.V. *et al.* (2008) Endothelial cell recovery between comparator polymer-based drug-eluting stents. *Journal of the American College of Cardiology,* **52**, 333–342.

25 Camenzind, E., Wijns, W., Mauri, L. *et al.* (2012) Stent thrombosis and major clinical events at 3 years after zotarolimus-eluting or sirolimus-eluting coronary stent implantation: a randomised, multicentre, open-label, controlled trial. *Lancet*, **380**, 1396–1405.

26 Rasmussen, K., Maeng, M., Kaltoft, A. *et al.* (2010) Efficacy and safety of zotarolimus-eluting and sirolimus-eluting coronary stents in routine clinical care (SORT OUT III): a randomised controlled superiority trial. *Lancet*, **375**, 1090–1099.

27 Urban, P., Abizaid, A., Chevalier, B. *et al.* (2013) Rationale and design of the LEADERS FREE trial: a randomized double-blind comparison of the BioFreedom drug-coated stent vs the Gazelle bare metal stent in patients at high bleeding risk using a short (1 month) course of dual antiplatelet therapy. *American Heart Journal*, **16**, 704–709.

28 Valgimigli, M., Borghesi, M., Tebaldi, M. *et al.* (2013) Should duration of dual antiplatelet therapy depend on the type and/or potency of implanted stent? A pre-specified analysis from the PROlonging Dual antiplatelet treatment after Grading stent-induced Intimal hyperplasia studY (PRODIGY). *European Heart Journal*, **34**, 909–919.

29 Bhatt, D.L., Flather, M.D., Hacke, W. *et al.* (2007) Patients with prior myocardial infarction, stroke, or symptomatic peripheral arterial disease in the CHARISMA trial. *Journal of the American College of Cardiology*, **49**, 1982–1988.

30 Ferreira-González, I., Marsal, J.R., Ribera, A. *et al.* (2012) Double antiplatelet therapy after drug-eluting stent implantation: risk associated with discontinuation within the first year. *Journal of the American College of Cardiology*, **60**, 1333–1339.

31 Eisenberg, M.J., Richard, P.R., Libersan, D. *et al.* (2009) Safety of short-term discontinuation of antiplatelet therapy in patients with drug-eluting stents. *Circulation*, **119**, 1634–1642.

27 Antiplatelet Therapy for Patients with Acute Coronary Syndromes

Michael A. Gaglia, Jr. and Ray V. Matthews

University of Southern California Keck School of Medicine, Los Angeles, CA, USA

Acetylsalicylic acid

Aspirin acts by irreversibly inhibiting platelet cyclooxygenase-1, preventing the formation of thromboxane A1 and thus diminishing platelet aggregation. Although a precursor of aspirin was derived from the willow tree and utilized as an analgesic and antipyretic as early as 400 BC, it was not recognized as an effective antiplatelet therapy for acute coronary syndromes (ACS) until the 1970s. This data was summarized by a large meta-analysis conducted by the Antiplatelet Trialists' Collaboration in 1994, showing that among nine randomized trials of aspirin in acute or suspected myocardial infarction (MI), there was a highly significant reduction in vascular death, MI, and stroke (10.6% vs. 14.4% at 1 month, $p < 0.0001$) [1]. This result was largely driven by the ISIS-2 trial, a randomized 2-by-2 study of streptokinase and aspirin in acute MI [2].

Although the recommended maintenance dose of aspirin remains somewhat controversial, another meta-analysis of randomized trials of high-risk patients in 2002 showed a similar reduction in vascular events for doses between 75 and 1500 mg [3]. This is in part because the cyclooxygenase pathway is well inhibited at low doses of aspirin. There is some evidence that bleeding increases with aspirin dose. A retrospective analysis of the CURE trial has shown that patients with non-ST segment elevation myocardial infarction (NSTEMI) undergoing percutaneous coronary intervention (PCI) taking clopidogrel and aspirin less than 100 mg have similar rates of ischemic events, but less major bleeding, than patients taking higher maintenance doses of aspirin [4]. Similarly, analysis of the CURRENT-OASIS 7 trial did not show a benefit of aspirin 325 mg versus 81 mg among patients with NSTEMI in regard to ischemic outcomes, although major bleeding was also similar [5]. In addition, a recent meta-analysis of ACS patients showed higher-dose aspirin was

Antiplatelet Therapy in Cardiovascular Disease, First Edition. Edited by Ron Waksman, Paul A. Gurbel, and Michael A. Gaglia, Jr.
© 2014 John Wiley & Sons, Ltd. Published 2014 by John Wiley & Sons, Ltd.

associated with higher rates of major bleeding at 1 month [6]. Low-dose aspirin (75–162 mg) would therefore appear to provide similar efficacy to higher doses, but with less bleeding, in regard to long-term therapy following an ACS.

Clopidogrel

Clopidogrel irreversibly inhibits platelet ADP (P2Y12) receptors, which increases levels of vasodilator-stimulated phosphoprotein and thereby decreases activation of glycoprotein IIb/IIIa receptors. In the CAPRIE trial, clopidogrel was studied as an alternative to aspirin. Clopidogrel 75 mg was shown to be slightly more effective than aspirin 325 mg among a high-risk population of nearly 20,000 patients, which included patients with recent MI (5.3% vs. 5.8%, $p = 0.04$); rates of bleeding were similar [7]. Clopidogrel was then studied as an adjunct to aspirin therapy in the CURE trial, which included 12,562 patients with NSTEMI or unstable angina (UA). Clopidogrel (300 mg loading dose, 75 mg maintenance dose) and aspirin, as compared to aspirin alone, significantly reduced the rate of cardiovascular death, MI, or stroke (9.3% vs. 11.4%, $p < 0.001$). Major bleeding, however, was more frequent in the clopidogrel group (3.7% vs. 2.7%, $p = 0.001$) [8]. Among the 21% of patients in CURE that were treated with PCI, there appeared to be similar benefit from the addition of clopidogrel to aspirin in regard to cardiovascular death, MI, or urgent target vessel revascularization after 30 days (4.5% vs. 6.4%, $p = 0.03$) [9]. Furthermore, this benefit extended up to 1 year following PCI. Clopidogrel has thus been shown to be effective in NSTEMI and UA patients undergoing either medical or invasive management; although there are no dedicated trials examining the addition of clopidogrel specifically in STEMI, current guidelines nonetheless recommend its routine use for most ACS (including STEMI) [10, 11].

Some uncertainty remains regarding the optimal loading dose of clopidogrel. The CURRENT-OASIS 7 trial compared a 600 mg loading dose, 150 mg maintenance dose for 1 week, and 75 mg thereafter versus a 300 mg loading dose and 75 mg maintenance dose in patients with NSTEMI and UA. Although there was no benefit to the higher dose in the overall trial, there was a reduction in stent thrombosis in the PCI subgroup (1.6% vs. 2.3%, $p = 0.001$); this came at the cost of slightly higher rates of major bleeding (2.5% vs. 2.0%, $p = 0.01$) [5]. Pharmacodynamic studies would also appear to suggest that higher loading doses of clopidogrel have a faster onset and greater magnitude of platelet inhibition [12, 13]. In addition, a meta-analysis of clinical outcomes suggested loading doses greater than 300 mg reduced death and MI without a significant increase in bleeding [14]. Guidelines therefore indicate that a 600 mg loading dose of clopidogrel be given as soon as possible for patients with ACS (300 mg if fibrinolytics have been administered) [15].

Prasugrel

Prasugrel is also a thienopyridine that irreversibly inhibits the P2Y12 receptor, but it achieves more rapid and complete platelet inhibition than clopidogrel. A loading dose of 60 mg and maintenance dose of 10 mg of prasugrel was compared to a loading dose of 300 mg and maintenance dose of 75 mg of clopidogrel in the TRITON-TIMI 38 randomized trial, which included 13,608 patients with both STEMI and moderate- to high-risk NSTEMI or UA undergoing invasive management. The primary end point, which included cardiovascular death, MI, or stroke, was significantly lower with prasugrel at up to 15 months (9.9% vs. 12.1%, $p < 0.001$) [16]. This difference was driven primarily by a reduction in both procedure-related and spontaneous MI (7.4% vs. 9.7%, $p < 0.0001$) [17]. There was no difference in death or stroke, although stent thrombosis and urgent target vessel revascularization were also significantly lower with prasugrel.

The primary safety end point of non-CABG-related TIMI major bleeding, however, was significantly higher with prasugrel (2.4% vs. 1.8%, $p = 0.03$); rates of major bleeding among patients undergoing CABG were even higher (13.4% vs. 3.2%, $p < 0.0001$). *Post hoc* subanalysis revealed three groups in whom bleeding risk outweighed ischemic benefit: age greater than 75 years, weight less than 60 kg, and history of transient ischemic attack (TIA) or stroke. Current guidelines thus state that prasugrel is contraindicated in patients with a history of TIA or stroke and caution against its use in patients greater than 75 years or less than 60 kg [11]. Labeling information suggests a 5 mg dose for patients less than 60 kg, but there is little prospective data regarding the lower dose [18]. The practicality of a loading dose of prasugrel before PCI is also limited because of concerns regarding potential bleeding in patients ultimately requiring CABG.

Unlike clopidogrel, prasugrel is not currently indicated for noninvasive management of ACS. Prasugrel was again compared to clopidogrel in TRILOGY ACS, among 7243 patients less than 75 years with medically managed ACS. In regard to death, MI, or stroke, there was no difference between prasugrel and clopidogrel at up to 30 months (13.9% vs. 16.0%, $p = 0.21$). There did not appear to be a difference in non-CABG-related GUSTO severe or life-threatening bleeding [19].

Ticagrelor

Ticagrelor is a novel and potent P2Y12 antagonist, also with more rapid and complete platelet inhibition than clopidogrel; but unlike the thienopyridines, it binds reversibly to platelet receptors. It was first studied in the PLATO randomized trial, which compared a loading dose of 180 mg and maintenance dose of 90 mg twice a day of ticagrelor to a loading dose of 300–600 mg and maintenance dose of 75 mg once daily of clopidogrel among 18,624 patients with STEMI and high-risk NSTEMI/UA [20].

Unlike TRITON-TIMI 38, ticagrelor was administered upstream before coronary anatomy was known. Furthermore, both invasively and medically managed patients were included, as were patients already on clopidogrel at baseline. The primary end point of vascular death, MI, and stroke at 12 months occurred less frequently with ticagrelor versus clopidogrel (9.8% vs. 11.7%, $p < 0.001$). Importantly, this difference was driven by less vascular death (4.0% vs. 5.1%, $p = 0.001$) and less MI (5.8% vs. 6.9%, $p = 0.005$). All-cause death and stent thrombosis were also less common with prasugrel, although there was no difference in stroke. There was a higher rate of PLATO-defined non-CABG major bleeding with ticagrelor (4.5% vs. 3.8%, $p = 0.03$).

Post hoc analysis, however, showed that there did not appear to be a benefit of ticagrelor over clopidogrel among patients in North America. Furthermore, it appeared that the great majority of patients in North America were on a higher aspirin maintenance dose of 325 mg. Although an FDA advisory panel was skeptical of the biological plausibility of such an interaction between ticagrelor and high-dose aspirin [21], the drug carries a black box warning in the USA to avoid maintenance doses of aspirin greater than 100 mg [22].

Glycoprotein IIb/IIIa inhibitors

Glycoprotein IIb/IIIa inhibitors (GPIs) act by inhibiting the final step in platelet aggregation, the cross-linking of platelets by fibrinogen binding to glycoprotein IIb/IIIa receptors. There are three GPIs utilized clinically: abciximab, a monoclonal antibody; tirofiban, a nonpeptide inhibitor; and eptifibatide, a peptide inhibitor. Contemporary use of the GPIs, however, is complicated by the fact that they were initially studied before the routine use of dual antiplatelet therapy and early invasive management. Much of this data is summarized by a 2002 meta-analysis of 31,402 non-ST-elevation ACS patients receiving a GPI or placebo who did not undergo early revascularization or receive routine thienopyridines; this study showed a benefit in regard to death or MI at 30 days in higher-risk patients [23]. Similarly, a meta-analysis of 27,115 STEMI patients receiving abciximab or placebo showed a benefit in regard to mortality for patients undergoing primary PCI (but not fibrinolysis); again, patients were not pretreated with a P2Y12 inhibitor [24].

More contemporary trials, however, have been conducted upon a background of routine P2Y12 inhibition; furthermore, bivalirudin, an antithrombin parenteral anticoagulant, has emerged as an alternative to heparin. The ACUITY trial examined, in part, the role of bivalirudin alone, heparin plus GPI, and bivalirudin plus GPI in 13,819 non-ST-elevation ACS patients undergoing early invasive management. Bivalirudin versus heparin plus GPI demonstrated similar rates of ischemia, but major bleeding was markedly reduced (3.0% vs. 5.7%, $p < 0.001$) [25].

9207 patients in the GPI arms of ACUITY were also randomized to immediate upstream versus provisional (i.e., given only if PCI pursued) GPI.

There was no difference in ischemic end points between immediate and provisional GPI, although the margin for noninferiority of provisional therapy was not met (7.1% vs. 7.9%, $p = 0.044$ for noninferiority); there was less major bleeding in the provisional group (4.9% vs. 6.1%, $p = 0.009$ for superiority) [26]. Similarly, the EARLY ACS trial examined early versus provisional eptifibatide in 9492 patients with non-ST-elevation ACS receiving primarily heparin. This study also showed no ischemic benefit to upstream versus provisional GPI therapy, and increased bleeding and need for transfusion with the former [27]. It would therefore appear that there is a questionable benefit to routine upstream GPI administration in NSTEMI or UA patients receiving a P2Y12 inhibitor. Current guidelines emphasize their use only in high-risk NSTEMI or UA patients without undue risk of bleeding [28].

Bivalirudin was also studied in 3602 STEMI patients undergoing primary PCI, compared to heparin plus GPI in the HORIZONS-AMI trial. At 30 days, bivalirudin resulted in a lower rate of net adverse clinical events, a combination of bleeding and cardiovascular events (9.2% vs. 12.1%, $p = 0.005$). This end point was primarily driven by less major bleeding (4.9% vs. 8.3%, $p > 0.001$). There did appear to be a significant increase in stent thrombosis after 24 h with bivalirudin (1.3% vs. 0.3%, $p < 0.001$); at 30 days, however, this difference was not significant (2.5% vs. 1.9%, $p = 0.30$) [29]. This increase in very early stent thrombosis could have been due to inadequate P2Y12 and thrombin inhibition, as two-thirds of patients receiving bivalirudin also received preprocedural heparin and only 60% overall received a 600 mg loading dose of clopidogrel. There was no evidence, however, of an interaction between treatment group and either preprocedural heparin or clopidogrel loading dose.

The timing of GPI administration in STEMI has also been recently studied. In the FINESSE trial, 2452 patients received either abciximab at the time of PCI, abciximab before PCI, or abciximab plus half-dose reteplase before PCI, with a background of heparin and clopidogrel therapy. Prehospital abciximab did not show a benefit in regard to cardiovascular events, but there was an increase in TIMI major and minor bleeding with or without reteplase [30]. There does not appear to be a benefit to routine prehospital GPI in either STEMI or NSTEMI patients. In the setting of adequate P2Y12 inhibition, the benefit of routine GPI with heparin anticoagulation remains obscure; recent studies suggest that routine GPI with bivalirudin anticoagulation is unnecessary.

Conclusion

Current US guidelines do not endorse one P2Y12 inhibitor over another, despite more potent platelet inhibition and improved clinical outcomes with the newer agents. In addition, they do not endorse bivalirudin over heparin plus a GPI, despite less bleeding and potentially less overall mortality with the former. This acknowledges concerns regarding bleeding risk, cost, patient compliance, and the relative paucity of data for newer

P2Y12 inhibitors and concerns regarding cost and increased risk of thrombosis with bivalirudin. Available clinical data, however, suggest that more potent P2Y12 blockade in concert with more targeted anticoagulant therapy may bring us closer to the elusive therapeutic window that balances bleeding and thrombotic risk.

References

1 Antiplatelet Trialists Collaboration (1994) Collaborative overview of randomised trials of antiplatelet therapy—I: Prevention of death, myocardial infarction, and stroke by prolonged antiplatelet therapy in various categories of patients. *BMJ*, **308 (6921)**, 81–106.

2 Second International Study of Infarct Survival Collaborative Group (1988) Randomised trial of intravenous streptokinase, oral aspirin, both, or neither among 17,187 cases of suspected acute myocardial infarction: ISIS-2. *Lancet*, **2 (8607)**, 349–360.

3 Antithrombotic Trialists C (2002) Collaborative meta-analysis of randomised trials of antiplatelet therapy for prevention of death, myocardial infarction, and stroke in high risk patients. *BMJ*, **324 (7329)**, 71–86.

4 Jolly, S.S., Pogue, J., Haladyn, K. *et al.* (2009) Effects of aspirin dose on ischaemic events and bleeding after percutaneous coronary intervention: insights from the PCI-CURE study. *European Heart Journal*, **30 (8)**, 900–907.

5 Investigators C-O, Mehta, S.R., Bassand, J.P. *et al.* (2010) Dose comparisons of clopidogrel and aspirin in acute coronary syndromes. *The New England Journal of Medicine*, **363 (10)**, 930–942.

6 Berger, J.S., Sallum, R.H., Katona, B. *et al.* (2012) Is there an association between aspirin dosing and cardiac and bleeding events after treatment of acute coronary syndrome? A systematic review of the literature. *American Heart Journal*, **164 (2)**, 153.e5–162.e5.

7 Committee CS (1996) A randomised, blinded, trial of clopidogrel versus aspirin in patients at risk of ischaemic events (CAPRIE) CAPRIE Steering Committee. *Lancet*, **348 (9038)**, 1329–1339.

8 Yusuf, S., Zhao, F., Mehta, S.R., Chrolavicius, S., Tognoni, G., and Fox, K.K. (2001) Effects of clopidogrel in addition to aspirin in patients with acute coronary syndromes without ST-segment elevation. *The New England Journal of Medicine*, **345 (7)**, 494–502.

9 Mehta, S.R., Yusuf, S., Peters, R.J. *et al.* (2001) Effects of pretreatment with clopidogrel and aspirin followed by long-term therapy in patients undergoing percutaneous coronary intervention: the PCI-CURE study. *Lancet*, **358 (9281)**, 527–533.

10 Anderson, J.L., Adams, C.D., Antman, E.M. *et al.* (2007) ACC/AHA 2007 guidelines for the management of patients with unstable angina/non ST-elevation myocardial infarction executive summary: a report of the American College of Cardiology/American Heart Association Task Force on Practice Guidelines (Writing Committee to Revise the 2002 Guidelines for the Management of Patients With Unstable Angina/Non ST-Elevation Myocardial Infarction) Developed in Collaboration with the American College of Emergency Physicians, the Society for Cardiovascular Angiography and Interventions, and the Society of Thoracic Surgeons Endorsed by the American Association of Cardiovascular and Pulmonary Rehabilitation and the Society for Academic Emergency Medicine. *Journal of the American College of Cardiology*, **50 (7)**, 652–726.

11 Kushner, F.G., Hand, M., Smith, S.C., Jr *et al.* (2009) focused updates: ACC/AHA guidelines for the management of patients with ST-elevation myocardial infarction (Updating the 2004 Guideline and 2007 Focused Update) and ACC/AHA/SCAI guidelines on percutaneous coronary intervention (Updating the 2005 Guideline and 2007 Focused Update): a report of the American College of Cardiology Foundation/American Heart Association Task Force on Practice Guidelines. *Journal of the American College of Cardiology*, **54 (23)**, 2205–2241.

12 Montalescot, G., Sideris, G., Meuleman, C. *et al.* (2006) A randomized comparison of high clopidogrel loading doses in patients with non-ST-segment elevation acute coronary syndromes: the ALBION (Assessment of the Best Loading Dose of Clopidogrel to Blunt Platelet Activation, Inflammation and Ongoing Necrosis) trial. *Journal of the American College of Cardiology*, **48 (5)**, 931–938.

13 von Beckerath, N., Taubert, D., Pogatsa-Murray, G., Schomig, E., Kastrati, A., and Schomig, A. (2005) Absorption, metabolization, and antiplatelet effects of 300-, 600-, and 900-mg loading doses of clopidogrel: results of the ISAR-CHOICE (Intracoronary Stenting and Antithrombotic Regimen: Choose Between 3 High Oral Doses for Immediate Clopidogrel Effect) Trial. *Circulation*, **112 (19)**, 2946–2950.

14 Lotrionte, M., Biondi-Zoccai, G.G., Agostoni, P. *et al.* (2007) Meta-analysis appraising high clopidogrel loading in patients undergoing percutaneous coronary intervention. *The American Journal of Cardiology*, **100 (8)**, 1199–1206.

15 Levine, G.N., Bates, E.R., Blankenship, J.C. *et al.* (2011) ACCF/AHA/SCAI guideline for percutaneous coronary intervention. A report of the American College of Cardiology Foundation/American Heart Association Task Force on Practice Guidelines and the Society for Cardiovascular Angiography and Interventions. *Journal of the American College of Cardiology*, **58 (24)**, e44–e122.

16 Wiviott, S.D., Braunwald, E., McCabe, C.H. *et al.* (2007) Prasugrel versus clopidogrel in patients with acute coronary syndromes. *The New England Journal of Medicine*, **357 (20)**, 2001–2015.

17 Morrow, D.A., Wiviott, S.D., White, H.D. *et al.* (2009) Effect of the novel thienopyridine prasugrel compared with clopidogrel on spontaneous and procedural myocardial infarction in the Trial to Assess Improvement in Therapeutic Outcomes by Optimizing Platelet Inhibition with Prasugrel-Thrombolysis in Myocardial Infarction 38: an application of the classification system from the universal definition of myocardial infarction. *Circulation*, **119 (21)**, 2758–2764.

18 Prasugrel: drug information. 2012. Lexi-Comp Online, Hudson, OH.

19 Roe, M.T., Armstrong, P.W., Fox, K.A. *et al.* (2012) Prasugrel versus clopidogrel for acute coronary syndromes without revascularization. *The New England Journal of Medicine*, **367 (14)**, 1297–1309.

20 Wallentin, L., Becker, R.C., Budaj, A. *et al.* (2009) Ticagrelor versus clopidogrel in patients with acute coronary syndromes. *The New England Journal of Medicine*, **361 (11)**, 1045–1057.

21 Gaglia, M.A., Jr and Waksman, R. (2011) Overview of the 2010 Food and Drug Administration Cardiovascular and Renal Drugs Advisory Committee meeting regarding ticagrelor. *Circulation*, **123 (4)**, 451–456.

22 Ticagrelor: drug information. 2012. Lexi-Comp Online, Hudson, OH.

23 Boersma, E., Harrington, R.A., Moliterno, D.J. *et al.* (2002) Platelet glycoprotein IIb/IIIa inhibitors in acute coronary syndromes: a meta-analysis of all major randomised clinical trials. *Lancet*, **359 (9302)**, 189–198.

24 De Luca, G., Suryapranata, H., Stone, G.W. *et al.* (2005) Abciximab as adjunctive therapy to reperfusion in acute ST-segment elevation myocardial infarction: a meta-analysis of randomized trials. *JAMA*, **293 (14)**, 1759–1765.

25 Stone, G.W., McLaurin, B.T., Cox, D.A. *et al.* (2006) Bivalirudin for patients with acute coronary syndromes. *The New England Journal of Medicine*, **355 (21)**, 2203–2216.

26 Stone, G.W., Bertrand, M.E., Moses, J.W. *et al.* (2007) Routine upstream initiation vs deferred selective use of glycoprotein IIb/IIIa inhibitors in acute coronary syndromes: the ACUITY Timing trial. *JAMA*, **297 (6)**, 591–602.

27 Giugliano, R.P., White, J.A., Bode, C. *et al.* (2009) Early versus delayed, provisional eptifibatide in acute coronary syndromes. *The New England Journal of Medicine*, **360 (21)**, 2176–2190.

28 Jneid, H., Anderson, J.L., Wright, R.S. *et al.* (2012) ACCF/AHA focused update of the guideline for the management of patients with unstable angina/non-ST-elevation myocardial infarction (updating the 2007 guideline and replacing the 2011 focused update): a report of the American College of Cardiology Foundation/American Heart Association Task Force on Practice Guidelines. *Journal of the American College of Cardiology*, **60 (7)**, 645–681.

29 Stone, G.W., Witzenbichler, B., Guagliumi, G. *et al.* (2008) Bivalirudin during primary PCI in acute myocardial infarction. *The New England Journal of Medicine*, **358 (21)**, 2218–2230.

30 Ellis, S.G., Tendera, M., de Belder, M.A. *et al.* (2008) Facilitated PCI in patients with ST-elevation myocardial infarction. *The New England Journal of Medicine*, **358 (21)**, 2205–2217.

28 Antiplatelet Therapy in Stable Coronary Artery Disease

Ana Laynez and Ron Waksman

MedStar Washington Hospital Center, Washington, DC, USA

Introduction

Chronic stable angina (CSA) is the most common manifestation of ischemic heart disease in the developed world and is associated with impaired quality of life and increased mortality. It is a clinical syndrome, sometimes disabling, characterized by chest, jaw, shoulder, back, or arm discomfort related to stress or exercise that terminates with rest or nitroglycerin administration, generally the expression of an imbalance between myocardial oxygen demand and supply. When the angina appears with effort and with no changes in its onset in the last month, the angina is classified as stable, and it implies no complications or unfavorable evolution in an immediate future.

The effective management of this highly prevalent condition is largely dependent on the identification of the prevailing pathogenic mechanism, the implementation of lifestyle changes, and the appropriate use of pharmacological agents and revascularization techniques. Medical treatment must be focused on symptoms release and, basically, on the improvement of patient prognosis by reducing the incidence of thrombotic complications, such as acute myocardial infarction (MI) and death.

Aspirin

The first meta-analysis that analyzed the efficacy of aspirin in coronary artery disease, including patients with CSA, included 145 trials and 29 treatment comparisons. It was published by the Antithrombotic Trialists' Collaboration and studied patients with different vascular entity. It concluded that the use of 75–325 mg/day of aspirin during a long period of time was efficient against MI, death, and stroke [1]. Later, in 2002, a

---

Antiplatelet Therapy in Cardiovascular Disease, First Edition. Edited by Ron Waksman, Paul A. Gurbel, and Michael A. Gaglia, Jr.
© 2014 John Wiley & Sons, Ltd. Published 2014 by John Wiley & Sons, Ltd.

Table 28.1 Aspirin in CSA studies.

Study	N	Patient population	Aspirin mg/day	Follow-up
Cardiff-I [3], 1974	1239	Men with a prior MI	300	13 months
Danish Low Dose [4], 1988	301	Prior carotid endarterectomy	50–100	23 months
UK-TIA [5], 1991	1620	Prior TIA or minor stroke	300	50 months
SALT [6], 1991	1360	Prior TIA or stroke	75	32 months
ESPS-2 [7], 1996	3298	Prior TIA or stroke	50	24 months
SAPAT [8], 1992	2035	CSA	75	50 months

new meta-analysis with 287 studies issued up to 1997, was published. 212,000 patients were analyzed, including patients with CSA. It concluded again that aspirin, as an antiplatelet agent, protects most of the population at high risk of ischemic vascular events [2]. Seven studies with patients with CSA stand out in this meta-analysis (Table 28.1). The most important one, the Swedish angina pectoris aspirin trial, with 2035 patients with CSA treated with sotalol for symptoms control, studied the effect of 75 mg aspirin compared to placebo [8]. This was the first prospective study to show the beneficial effect of aspirin in the reduction of MI and death in CSA. Those patients under aspirin showed a 34% reduction in primary events (MI and sudden death; 95% CI, 24–49%; $p = 0.003$) compared to patients under placebo and a reduction in secondary events (vascular events, vascular death, death by any reason, stroke) from 22% in the group with placebo compared to 32% in the group having aspirin.

Previously, 22,071 male medical doctors with no previous history of acute MI, stroke, or TIA were studied in a double-blind randomized study, where the effect of 325 mg of aspirin in primary prevention was analyzed [9]. From the whole studied population, 333 patients with CSA were analyzed in a posterior substudy. They were randomized into two groups whether they received aspirin 325 mg or placebo, and the effect of the aspirin in secondary prevention was analyzed. Those patients treated with aspirin presented a total reduction of primary event (first MI) of 12.9% compared to 3.9% in the placebo's group (relative risk (RR), 0. 30; 95% CI, 0.14–0.63; $P = 0.003$) [10].

Doses

ACT trial [2] also provided a valuable information related to the effect of different doses of aspirin in patients at high risk of cardiovascular (CV) events. Different groups depending on the dose used were compared (<75 mg, 75–150 mg, 160–325 mg and 500–1500 mg). A similar risk reduction in CV events was observed when the different groups were compared against each other, not seeing significant differences between low and high doses of aspirin in terms of effectiveness. That led to conclude that with similar results, a lower dose is preferable in terms of avoiding bleeding complications. Few studies from the meta-analysis used doses of less than 75 mg of aspirin, so no final conclusions on this dose could be made.

Side effects and aspirin resistance

A minority of patients develops hypersensitivity to aspirin, manifested clinically in different situations, such as respiratory tract disease or urticaria and angioedema [11, 12].

The main adverse effect of aspirin is an increased risk of bleeding mainly from the gastrointestinal (GI) tract but also very rarely intracranial bleeding. It is important to recognize patients with higher risk of bleeding and to consider an alternative antiplatelet agent for them. In the US Preventive Services Task Force report on the use of aspirin for the primary prevention of CV disease, the magnitude of increase in risk was approximately two to three times higher in patients with a history of GI ulcer and twice as high for men as women [13].

It is assumed that between 5.5% and 60% of patients treated with aspirin may develop a degree of aspirin resistance, depending on the definition used and parameters measured [14]. Aspirin resistance could clinically refer to patients with maintained ischemic events despite appropriate use of aspirin. Patients who are not compliant with aspirin therapy or those who are not prescribed with aspirin when clinically indicated could be also considered as aspirin resistant. The effect of the interaction with other medical agents could be also interpreted as resistance. In the laboratory, aspirin resistance suggests the inability of the drug to achieve a specific level of platelet inhibition in *ex vivo* studies [15]. Clinical resistance or treatment failure with aspirin therapy is known to be present in nearly 50% of patients; however, true pharmacological resistance is much less common. Different trials have analyzed the effect of real pharmacological resistance in patients with high risk of ischemic events and have concluded that aspirin resistance was associated with a higher risk of adverse events compared with those responsive to aspirin [16].

Clopidogrel

Large multicenter, randomized controlled trials have provided clinical evidence supporting the benefit of clopidogrel as antiplatelet therapy in patients with acute coronary syndrome (unstable angina, non-ST-elevation MI) and in patients undergoing percutaneous coronary intervention (PCI) [17, 18, 19, 20].

The first multicenter, randomized controlled trial that provided clinical evidence supporting the use of clopidogrel as antiplatelet agent in patients

Table 28.2 Clopidogrel in CSA studies

Study	Patient population	Follow-up	Primary end point	RRR (%)
CAPRIE [21]	19,185 with MI/ stroke/peripheral artery disease	1–3 years (mean 1.91 years)	CV death, MI, or stroke	8.7
CHARISMA [22]	15,603 with CV disease or multiple risk factors for CV disease	Median of 28 days	CV death, MI, or stroke	7

at high risk of ischemic events was the CAPRIE trial [21] (Table 28.2). 19,185 patients with recent MI, stroke, or symptomatic peripheral disease were randomized to clopidogrel 75 mg or aspirin 325 mg and followed up during a mean time of 1.91 years. It was reported in the trial that 44% of the population studied had a history of stable coronary artery disease, but were not classified as patients with CSA. Primary efficacy outcomes were a composite of stroke, MI, or vascular death; the safety of the treatment was also assessed. No difference in mortality between the two groups was seen, with 3.11% in the aspirin group versus 3.05% in the clopidogrel group (RR 2.2%, 95% CI: −9.9 to 12.9). There was no reduction in vascular death either (2.06% in aspirin group vs. 1.90% in clopidogrel group, RR 7.6%, 95% CI: −6.9 to 20.1). However, an 8.7% relative risk reduction for the composite outcome of vascular death, MI, or stroke associated with the use of clopidogrel was observed, from 5.83% in patients treated with aspirin to 5.32% in clopidogrel group (95% CI: 0.3–16.5). When each group was analyzed separately, the weakest difference between both drugs was seen in the group of patients with recent MI (RRR −3.7%, 95% CI: −22.1 to 12). Regarding the safety of the drugs, there was a similar incidence of abnormal liver function, GI disturbances, and intracranial bleeding. The appearance of rash was more likely in the clopidogrel group (6.02% vs. 4.61%) than in the aspirin group. On the other hand, patients on clopidogrel were less likely to have a severe GI bleeding than those on aspirin (0.49% vs. 0.71%). In conclusion, the total benefit of clopidogrel compared to aspirin was very small, with an absolute reduction in the composite end point of only 0.51%. No separate analysis in patients with CSA was performed and the weakest difference was observed in the group of patients of recent MI group (who are known to be at higher risk of thrombotic events than patients with CSA).

The CHARISMA trial [22] (Table 28.2) showed, in patients with stable coronary disease or asymptomatic patients with multiple CV risk factors, that the combination of clopidogrel plus aspirin versus aspirin alone was not significantly more effective in the reduction of the rate of

MI, stroke, or death from CV causes (6.8% with clopidogrel plus aspirin and 7.3% with placebo plus aspirin, RR, 0.93; 95% CI: 0.83–1.05). With regard to the safety, a slight increase in the risk of moderate to severe bleeding in the combination therapy group was also seen (2.1% in clopidogrel plus aspirin group vs. 1.3% in the aspirin group; RR 1.62; 95% CI: 1.27–2.08).

Lately, in a retrospective analysis of the CHARISMA trial [23], dual antiplatelet therapy was compared to aspirin alone as a primary prevention strategy showing an increase in CV death in the clopidogrel plus aspirin group (3% vs. 1.8%, $p = 0.07$). The cause of this dual antiplatelet therapy damage was not found. However, it has been suggested that dual antiplatelet therapy with aspirin and clopidogrel for primary prevention of atherothrombotic events not only brings no benefits but also increases the risk of bleeding.

Clopidogrel side effects

Purpura, diarrhea, rash, and pruritus are the most frequent side effects of clopidogrel (≤5% of cases). Routine hematological monitoring is not required, since clopidogrel is not associated with an increased risk of neutropenia [21]. In comparison to ticlopidine, the overall incidence of thrombotic thrombocytopenic purpura (TTP) is lower. Although being metabolized by the liver, clopidogrel has no great impact on hepatic enzyme induction. It is recommended to be cautious when using clopidogrel in combination with nonsteroidal anti-inflammatory drugs or warfarin due to an increased risk of bleeding.

GPS IIB/IIIA

IV glycoprotein IIb/IIIa inhibitors have demonstrated a reduction of fatal CV complications after PCI. That has led to develop trials to prove their effectiveness as oral medication in coronary disease (acute coronary syndrome and patients with coronary disease undergoing PCI). A meta-analysis that analyzed three trials comparing oral glycoprotein IIb/IIIa inhibitor with or without background aspirin versus aspirin concluded that oral glycoprotein IIb/IIIa inhibitor therapy was associated with 31% increased mortality (OR = 1.31; 95% CI: 1.12–1.53; $P = 0.0001$) and ischemic events or sudden death (OR = 1.22; 95% CI: 0.91–1.63). An explanation for these findings could not be found, and the final conclusion was that the problem was likely to be multifactorial [24].

The only trial published that studied the effect of oral glycoprotein IIb/IIIa inhibitor in patients with CSA was designed to compare the dose–response effect on the inhibition of platelet aggregation of roxifiban (DMP754) and its safety and tolerability compared to placebo [25]. Ninety-eight patients were randomized to receive either placebo or 1 of 8 oral dosages of roxifiban, and 22 patients were enrolled in a multiple-dose regimen and followed up during 30 days. The final results showed that the induction of platelet inhibition by roxifiban was dose dependent with higher levels of platelet inhibition with higher dose, as well as higher incidence of minor bleeding events. That made roxifiban a possible alternative as an antiplatelet agent in patients with CSA, but not better as aspirin or clopidogrel. Further studies should be run to confirm the results.

Conclusions

In conclusion, aspirin should be recommended to patients diagnosed with coronary artery disease, with no contraindications to its use. It reduces the probability of ischemic events in patients with CSA, being effective at doses from 75 to 325 mg/day, with no evidence that lower or higher doses improve the results.

Clopidogrel has also shown similar beneficial effects in stable angina. That makes this agent a good alternative in patients with aspirin allergy or intolerance.

No major benefits have been shown in the use of oral glycoprotein IIb/IIIa inhibitors in patients with CSA yet.

References

1 Antiplatelet Trialists' Collaboration (1994) Collaborative overview of randomised trials of antiplatelet therapy. I. Prevention of death, myocardial infarction, and stroke by prolonged antiplatelet therapy in various categories of patients. *BMJ*, **308 (6921)**, 81–106.

2 Collaboration AT (2002) Collaborative meta-analysis of randomised trials of antiplatelet therapy for prevention of death, myocardial infarction, and stroke in high risk patients. *BMJ*, **324 (7329)**, 71–86.

3 Elwood, P.C., Cochrane, A.L., Burr, M.L. *et al.* (1974) A randomized controlled trial of acetyl salicylic acid in the secondary prevention of mortality from myocardial infarction. *British Medical Journal*, **1 (5905)**, 436–440.

4 Boysen, G., Sorensen, P.S., Juhler, M. *et al.* (1988) Danish very-low-dose aspirin after carotid endarterectomy trial. *Stroke*, **19 (10)**, 1211–1215.

5 Farrell, B., Godwin, J., Richards, S. & Warlow, C. (1991) The United Kingdom transient ischaemic attack (UK-TIA) aspirin trial: final results. *Journal of Neurology, Neurosurgery and Psychiatry*, **54 (12)**, 1044–1054.

6 SALT Collaborative Group (1991) Swedish Aspirin Low-Dose Trial (SALT) of 75 mg aspirin as secondary prophylaxis after cerebrovascular ischaemic events. *Lancet*, **338 (8779)**, 1345–1349.

7 Diener, H., Forbes, C., Riekkinen, P., Sivenius, J., Smets, P. & Lowenthal, A. (1997) European Stroke Prevention Study 2. *Efficacy and safety data. Journal of the Neurological Sciences*, **151** (Suppl), S1–S77.

8 Juul-Moller, S., Edvardsson, N., Jahnmatz, B., Rosen, A., Sorensen, S. & Omblus, R. (1992) Double-blind trial of aspirin in primary prevention

of myocardial infarction in patients with stable chronic angina pectoris. The Swedish Angina Pectoris Aspirin Trial (SAPAT) Group. *Lancet*, **340 (8833)**, 1421–1425.

9 Manson, J.E., Grobbee, D.E., Stampfer, M.J. *et al.* (1990) Aspirin in the primary prevention of angina pectoris in a randomized trial of United States physicians. *The American Journal of Medicine*, **89 (6)**, 772–776.

10 Ridker, P.M., Manson, J.E., Gaziano, J.M., Buring, J.E. & Hennekens, C.H. (1991) Low-dose aspirin therapy for chronic stable angina. A randomized, placebo-controlled clinical trial. *Annals of Internal Medicine*, **114 (10)**, 835–839.

11 Jenkins, C., Costello, J. & Hodge, L. (2004) Systematic review of prevalence of aspirin induced asthma and its implications for clinical practice. *BMJ*, **328 (7437)**, 434.

12 Grattan, C.E. (2003) Aspirin sensitivity and urticaria. *Clinical and Experimental Dermatology*, **28 (2)**, 123–127.

13 US Preventive Services Task Force (2009) Aspirin for the prevention of cardiovascular disease: U.S. Preventive Services Task Force recommendation statement. *Annals of Internal Medicine*, **150 (6)**, 396–404.

14 Muir, A.R., McMullin, M.F., Patterson, C. & McKeown, P.P. (2009) Assessment of aspirin resistance varies on a temporal basis in patients with ischaemic heart disease. *Heart*, **95 (15)**, 1225–1229.

15 Grosser, T., Fries, S., Lawson, J.A., Kapoor, S.C., Grant, G.R. & FitzGerald, G.A. (2013) Drug resistance and pseudoresistance: an unintended consequence of enteric coating aspirin. *Circulation*, **127 (3)**, 377–385.

16 Eikelboom, J.W., Hirsh, J., Weitz, J.I., Johnston, M., Yi, Q. & Yusuf, S. (2002) Aspirin-resistant thromboxane biosynthesis and the risk of myocardial infarction, stroke, or cardiovascular death in patients at high risk for cardiovascular events. *Circulation*, **105 (14)**, 1650–1655.

17 Sabatine, M.S., Cannon, C.P., Gibson, C.M. *et al.* (2005) Addition of clopidogrel to aspirin and fibrinolytic therapy for myocardial infarction with ST-segment elevation. *New England Journal of Medicine*, **352 (12)**, 1179–1189.

18 Chen, Z.M., Jiang, L.X., Chen, Y.P. *et al.* (2005) Addition of clopidogrel to aspirin in 45,852 patients with acute myocardial infarction: randomised placebo-controlled trial. *Lancet*, **366 (9497)**, 1607–1621.

19 Yusuf, S., Zhao, F., Mehta, S.R., Chrolavicius, S., Tognoni, G. & Fox, K.K. (2001) Effects of clopidogrel in addition to aspirin in patients with acute coronary syndromes without ST-segment elevation. *New England Journal of Medicine*, **345 (7)**, 494–502.

20 Mehta, S.R., Bassand, J.P., Chrolavicius, S. *et al.* (2010) Dose comparisons of clopidogrel and aspirin in acute coronary syndromes. *New England Journal of Medicine*, **363 (10)**, 930–942.

21 CAPRIE Steering Committee (1996) A randomised, blinded, trial of clopidogrel versus aspirin in patients at risk of ischaemic events (CAPRIE). CAPRIE Steering Committee. *Lancet*, **348** (9038), 1329–1339.

22 Bhatt, D.L., Fox, K.A., Hacke, W. *et al.* (2006) Clopidogrel and aspirin versus aspirin alone for the prevention of atherothrombotic events. *New England Journal of Medicine*, **354 (16)**, 1706–1717.

23 Wang, T.H., Bhatt, D.L., Fox, K.A. *et al.* (2007) An analysis of mortality rates with dual-antiplatelet therapy in the primary prevention

population of the CHARISMA trial. *European Heart Journal*, **28 (18)**, 2200–2207.

24 Newby, L.K., Califf, R.M., White, H.D. *et al.* (2002) The failure of orally administered glycoprotein IIb/IIIa inhibitors to prevent recurrent cardiac events. *The American Journal of Medicine*, **112 (8)**, 647–658.

25 Murphy, J., Wright, R.S., Gussak, I. *et al.* (2003) The use of roxifiban (DMP754), a novel oral platelet glycoprotein IIb/IIIa receptor inhibitor, in patients with stable coronary artery disease. *American Journal of Cardiovascular Drugs*, **3 (2)**, 101–112.

29 Antiplatelet Therapy for Patients with Peripheral Arterial Disease

Aung Myat,[1] Yousif Ahmad,[2,3] and Simon R. Redwood[1]

[1]King's College London BHF Centre of Research Excellence, The Rayne Institute, St Thomas' Hospital, London, UK

[2]National Heart and Lung Institute, Imperial College London, London, UK

[3]University of Birmingham Centre for Cardiovascular Sciences, City Hospital, Birmingham, UK

Introduction

Peripheral arterial disease (PAD) is a broad term that encompasses all vascular sites including carotid, vertebral, upper extremity, mesenteric, renal, and lower extremity vessels. To that end, much of the focus of this chapter has been restricted to the antiplatelet management of lower extremity artery disease (LEAD). On the whole, PAD is a common clinical problem, its prevalence rising steeply after the age of 50 years along with the presence of other cardiovascular risk factors [1]. Cigarette smoking, diabetes mellitus, dyslipidemia, and hypertension all significantly increase the risk of PAD [2]. Atherosclerosis is the most common cause of PAD, and since this is a systemic disorder, physicians must be aware of its propensity to affect other vascular beds and lead to critical organ damage. Patients with PAD have markedly increased rates of coronary artery disease (CAD) and cerebrovascular disease [3, 4]. This increased risk of myocardial infarction (MI) and stroke [5] informs the prognosis of PAD, with cardiovascular events being the leading cause of mortality in these patients [6]. The recognition of this cohort of patients as being at high cardiovascular risk has prompted a paradigm shift in their management over recent years: rather than predomination of vascular surgical procedures, it is now appreciated that these patients require comprehensive multidisciplinary medical management with a focus on modification of cardiovascular risk factors and protection against potentially catastrophic coronary and cerebrovascular events. Antiplatelet therapy forms a cornerstone of this management strategy, alongside exercise programs and aggressive risk-factor modification (smoking cessation, blood pressure control, lipid-lowering drugs, and strict glycemic control for patients with diabetes).

Antiplatelet Therapy in Cardiovascular Disease, First Edition. Edited by Ron Waksman, Paul A. Gurbel, and Michael A. Gaglia, Jr.
© 2014 John Wiley & Sons, Ltd. Published 2014 by John Wiley & Sons, Ltd.

Antiplatelet therapy

Having established that patients with PAD are a high cardiovascular risk group, it stands to reason that antiplatelet therapy would be of prognostic benefit. This benefit was most clearly established by a meta-analysis (MA) conducted by the Antithrombotic Trialists' Collaboration, comparing antiplatelet therapy with control in 135,000 high-risk vascular patients in 287 studies [7]. This included an analysis of 9716 patients with PAD, studied in 42 trials. For these patients, treatment with antiplatelet therapy conferred a 23% reduction in adverse cardiovascular events (vascular death, MI, and stroke). The benefit of antiplatelet therapy was consistent regardless of whether patients had peripheral bypass procedures, peripheral angioplasty, or suffered intermittent claudication. The majority of the trials included in this analysis used aspirin as the antiplatelet agent, and different doses of aspirin were also studied. There was a significantly smaller (13%) reduction in cardiovascular events in patients treated with less than 75 mg daily, but higher doses of aspirin were not beneficial compared to 75–150 mg. Moreover higher doses have been associated with increased gastrointestinal disturbance, including hemorrhage [8]. As well as preventing adverse coronary and cerebrovascular events, MA data has also suggested that antiplatelet therapy leads to a reduction in arterial occlusion and revascularization procedures when used in patients with intermittent claudication [9, 10].

Clopidogrel has been compared to aspirin for the secondary prevention of cardiovascular events in the CAPRIE trial [11]. This study included a subgroup of 6452 patients with PAD and demonstrated that clopidogrel was associated with a statistically significant 23.8% ($p = 0.0028$) reduction in the composite of ischemic stroke, MI, and vascular death. The effect on overall mortality was minimal, and clopidogrel was at least as well tolerated as aspirin.

The CHARISMA trial [12] is the only large randomized trial to compare a strategy of dual antiplatelet therapy (DAPT) with aspirin and clopidogrel to aspirin alone for the prevention of atherothrombotic events in patients at high risk. The overall study was negative, with no clear benefit of DAPT being proven over and above aspirin alone for the prevention of MI, stroke, or cardiovascular death. A *post hoc* analysis focusing on PAD patients ($n = 3096$) was subsequently performed [13]. Here, the composite primary efficacy (cardiovascular death, MI, and stroke) and safety end points occurred with similar frequency in patients treated with either antiplatelet strategy. The combination of clopidogrel with aspirin therapy reduced the rate of MI (2.3% vs. 3.7%; hazard ratio [HR], 0.63; 95% confidence interval [CI], 0.42–0.96; $P = 0.029$) and the rate of hospitalization for ischemic events (16.5% vs. 20.1%; HR, 0.81; 95% CI, 0.68–0.95; $P = 0.011$) but caused an increased rate of minor bleeding (34.4% vs. 20.8%; odds ratio [OR], 1.99; 95% CI, 1.69–2.34; $P < 0.001$). The trial investigators suggest therefore that patients perceived to be at a low bleeding but high atherothrombotic risk may gain some added benefit from DAPT.

Oral anticoagulation (OAC) has been shown to reduce major cardiovascular events in patients with CAD [14], and it has therefore been hypothesized that the addition of an anticoagulant to aspirin may also be benefit for PAD patients. MA data has proved inconclusive in establishing the efficacy and safety of OAC with or without aspirin in the context of PAD [15]. The WAVE trial compared a strategy of warfarin (INR 2.0–3.0) in addition to aspirin with aspirin alone in 2161 patients with PAD [16]. Combination therapy was no more effective than aspirin alone for the prevention of MI, stroke, or cardiovascular death. Life-threatening bleeding, however, was significantly increased in the combination therapy group (**relative risk, 3.41; 95% CI, 1.84 to 6.35; P<0.001**), including fatal bleeds and hemorrhagic stroke.

Percutaneous therapy

Percutaneous transluminal angioplasty (PTA) can be used to achieve successful revascularization with small procedural risk in symptomatic patients with PAD [17]. The main drawback of this technique has historically been treatment failure, with restenosis observed in half of treatment segments within one year [18]. Despite initially promising results, a string of randomized trials failed to demonstrate a sustained benefit of bare-metal stents (BMS) over balloon angioplasty [19, 20, 21]. A trial comparing self-expanding nitinol stents to stand-alone balloon angioplasty demonstrated improved anatomical and clinical results at 6 and 12 months with the stent group [22]. All patients in this trial received aspirin and clopidogrel DAPT for three months and continued on aspirin indefinitely thereafter. Despite the improved outcomes in the stent group, late restenosis remained a significant clinical concern, occurring in 37% of stent-treated patients after one year. In an attempt to overcome this significant limitation, work has been undertaken to examine the use of drug-eluting stents (DES) for patients with symptomatic PAD.

The Zilver PTX study [23] evaluated the efficacy and safety of paclitaxel-coated DES ($n = 236$) versus PTA ($n = 238$) for femoropopliteal disease. Of the PTA group, 120 suffered acute PTA failure and proceeded to a secondary randomization to provisional DES ($n = 61$) or BMS ($n = 59$). Patency was achieved in 83.1% of the DES group compared to 32.8% of the control group ($p < 0.001$). This translated in to superior 12-month event-free survival in the DES cohort (90.4% vs. 82.6%, $p = 0.004$). All patients in the trial were treated with a minimum of 60 days DAPT (aspirin and clopidogrel), and aspirin was continued indefinitely. Of note, 60% of patients remained on DAPT 24 months after the procedure – the majority of these patients had an additional indication for DAPT, which is plausible owing to the high rates of CAD among patients with PAD. Following reassuring longer-term data, the FDA has now approved the use of the Zilver PTX stent [24].

Furthermore, a recent randomized study evaluated the long-term effects of sirolimus-eluting stents compared to BMS for the treatment of infrapopliteal disease [25]. All patients were treated with indefinite aspirin and clopidogrel for 6 months, and mean follow-up was over 1000 days. The DES group demonstrated improved event-free survival (65.8% vs. 44.6%, log rank $p = 0.02$) and lower rates of amputation ($p = 0.03$) and target vessel revascularization ($p = 0.06$). Symptomatic status of patients assessed by using the Rutherford-Becker metric was also significantly improved with the use of DES ($p = 0.006$).

Treatment after peripheral artery bypass graft surgery

In the main, the recommendations for antiplatelet therapy after peripheral artery bypass surgery are similar to those made in general for patients with PAD. An MA of sixteen studies demonstrated benefit of antiplatelet therapy (with aspirin alone or aspirin and dipyridamole) for patients receiving infrainguinal bypasses [26]. Graft patency at twelve months was improved with antiplatelet therapy, with the benefits more pronounced in patients receiving prosthetic grafts compared to venous grafts. The CASPAR study [27] compared aspirin and clopidogrel DAPT versus placebo plus aspirin after below-knee bypass grafting. After twelve months, there was no overall difference between the two groups (HR, 0.98; 95% CI, 0.78–1.23), although patients receiving a prosthetic graft fared better with combination therapy (HR, 0.65; 95% CI, 0.45–0.95; $p = 0.025$). The addition of OAC with warfarin to antiplatelet drugs has not been associated with improved graft patency and leads to significant increases in hemorrhage [28, 29].

Conclusions

Antiplatelet therapy is an essential component of PAD management in general and LEAD in particular. Current US guidelines have assigned a class IA recommendation for antiplatelet therapy to "reduce the risk of MI, stroke and vascular death in individuals with symptomatic atherosclerotic lower extremity PAD, including those with intermittent claudication or critical limb ischemia, prior lower extremity revascularization (endovascular or surgical), or prior amputation for lower extremity ischemia" [30]. More specifically, a class IB recommendation has been assigned individually to aspirin in daily doses of 75–325 mg and clopidogrel at 75 mg [30]. Conversely, a class IIIB recommendation of potential harm has been attached to the addition of warfarin (in the absence of a proven indication for OAC therapy) to antiplatelet treatment to reduce the risk of adverse cardiovascular ischemic events in lower extremity PAD [30]. Current European guidelines prefer a class IC recommendation for antiplatelet therapy in patients with symptomatic PAD [31].

Patients with PAD are at high cardiovascular risk and have a worse prognosis than those with coronary and cerebrovascular disease. The use

Table 29.1 Landmark trials of antiplatelet therapy for peripheral arterial disease (PAD).

Study	Type	Year	N	Type of disease	Antithrombotic agent	Primary end point	Result
ATTC [7]	MA	2002	9214	All PAD	ASA, ticlopidineversus placebo	Vascular death, MI, stroke	23% reduction with antiplatelet therapy
CAPRIE [11]	RCT	1996	6452	All PAD	Clopidogrel versus ASA	Vascular death, MI, stroke	24% reduction with clopidogrel
CHARISMA [12, 13]	RCT	2009	3096	All PAD	Clopidogrel + ASA versus ASA alone	Vascular death, MI, stroke	No reduction with DAPT compared to ASA alone except for MI and hospitalization
WAVE [15]	RCT	2007	2161	All PAD	Warfarin + ASA versus ASA alone	Vascular death, MI, stroke	No reduction with addition of OAC
Cochrane Review [26]	MA	2008	966	Infrainguinal bypass surgery	ASA or ASA + dipyridamole versus placebo	Graft patency	41% reduction with antiplatelet therapy
CASPAR [27]	RCT	2010	851	Below-knee bypass grafting	Clopidogrel + ASA versus ASA alone	Graft patency, amputation, death	No benefit with DAPT except for those receiving prosthetic grafts
DBOAA [28]	RCT	2000	2690	Infrainguinal bypass surgery	Warfarin + ASA versus ASA alone	Graft patency	No reduction with addition of OAC

DAPT, dual antiplatelet therapy; MA, meta-analysis; MI, myocardial infarction; OAC, oral anticoagulation; PAD, peripheral arterial disease; RCT, randomized controlled trial of antiplatelet agents has been shown to significantly attenuate the risk of vascular death, nonfatal MI, and nonfatal stroke (Table 29.1). Along with reducing adverse cardiovascular events, antiplatelet therapy also has a significant role in maintaining vessel patency following revascularization procedures. The advent of DES should translate into more patients undergoing percutaneous procedures with favorable outcomes. Further research is needed to define the optimal antiplatelet strategy for these patients. For those undergoing peripheral bypass grafting, antiplatelet treatment is associated with improved graft patency and confers a favorable bleeding profile when compared to OAC. The evidence accumulated thus far has suggested that some groups of patients may benefit from DAPT; these findings have thus far only been hypothesis generating, and continued work must be targeted at identifying which cohort of patients may benefit. Current guidelines predate the emergence of the more potent novel antiplatelet drugs such as prasugrel and ticagrelor. Their role in the management of symptomatic PAD remains undefined and also requires further investigation.

References

1 Selvin, E. & Erlinger, T.P. (2004) Prevalence of and risk factors for peripheral arterial disease in the United States: results from the National Health and Nutrition Examination Survey, 1999–2000. *Circulation*, **110**, 738–743.
2 Pasternak, R.C., Criqui, M.H., Criqui, M.H. *et al.* (2004) Atherosclerotic vascular disease conference: writing group I: epidemiology. *Circulation*, **109**, 2605–2612.
3 Aronow, W.S. & Ahn, C. (1994) Prevalence of coexistence of coronary artery disease, peripheral arterial disease, and atherothrombotic brain infarction in men and women > or =62 years of age. *The American Journal of Cardiology*, **74**, 64–65.
4 Ness, J. & Aronow, W.S. (1999) Prevalence of coexistence of coronary artery disease, ischemic stroke, and peripheral arterial disease in older persons, mean age 80 years, in an academic hospital-based geriatrics practice. *Journal of the American Geriatrics Society*, **47**, 1255–1256.
5 Leng, G.C., Lee, A.J., Fowkes, F.G. *et al.* (1996) Incidence, natural history and cardiovascular events in symptomatic and asymptomatic peripheral arterial disease in the general population. *International Journal of Epidemiology*, **25**, 1172–1181.
6 Criqui, M.H., Langer, R.D., Fronek, A. *et al.* (1992) Mortality over a period of 10 years in patients with peripheral arterial disease. *The New England Journal of Medicine*, **326**, 381–386.
7 Antithrombotic Trialists' Collaboration (2002) Collaborative meta-analysis of randomised trials of antiplatelet therapy for prevention of death, myocardial infarction, and stroke in high risk patients. *BMJ*, **324**, 71–86.
8 Roderick, P.J., Wilkes, H.C. & Meade, T.W. (1993) The gastrointestinal toxicity of aspirin: an overview of randomised controlled trials. *British Journal of Clinical Pharmacology*, **35**, 219–226.
9 No Authors Listed (1994) Collaborative overview of randomised trials of antiplatelet therapy – I: prevention of death, myocardial infarction, and stroke by prolonged antiplatelet therapy in various categories of patients. Antiplatelet Trialists' Collaboration. *BMJ*, **308**, 81–106.

10 Girolami, B., Bernardi, E., Prins, M.H. *et al.* (1999) Antithrombotic drugs in the primary medical management of intermittent claudication: a meta-analysis. *Thrombosis and Haemostasis*, **81**, 715–722.

11 CAPRIE Steering Committee (1996) A randomised, blinded, trial of clopidogrel versus aspirin in patients at risk of ischaemic events (CAPRIE). CAPRIE Steering Committee. *Lancet*, **348**, 1329–1339.

12 Bhatt, D.L., Fox, K.A., Hacke, W. *et al.* (2006) Clopidogrel and aspirin versus aspirin alone for the prevention of atherothrombotic events. *The New England Journal of Medicine*, **354**, 1706–1717.

13 Cacoub, P.P., Bhatt, D.L., Steg, P.G., Topol, E.J., Creager, M.A. & CHARISMA Investigators (2009) Patients with peripheral arterial disease in the CHARISMA trial. *European Heart Journal*, **30**, 192–201.

14 Anand, S.S. & Yusuf, S. (1999) Oral anticoagulant therapy in patients with coronary artery disease: a meta-analysis. *JAMA*, **282**, 2058–2067.

15 The Warfarin Antiplatelet Vascular Evaluation Trial Investigators (2007) Oral anticoagulant and antiplatelet therapy and peripheral arterial disease. *The New England Journal of Medicine*, **357**, 217–227.

16 Warfarin Antiplatelet Vascular Evaluation Trial Investigators, Anand, S., Yusuf, S. *et al.* (2007) Oral anticoagulant and antiplatelet therapy and peripheral arterial disease. *The New England Journal of Medicine*, **357**, 217–227.

17 Dormandy, J.A. & Rutherford, R.B. (2000) Management of peripheral arterial disease (PAD). TASC Working Group. TransAtlantic Inter-Society Consensus (TASC). *Journal of Vascular Surgery*, **31**, S1–S296.

18 Johnston, K.W. (1992) Femoral and popliteal arteries: reanalysis of results of balloon angioplasty. *Radiology*, **183**, 767–771.

19 Cejna, M., Thurnher, S., Illiasch, H. *et al.* (2001) PTA versus Palmaz stent placement in femoropopliteal artery obstructions: a multicenter prospective randomized study. *Journal of Vascular and Interventional Radiology*, **12**, 23–31.

20 Grimm, J., Müller-Hülsbeck, S., Jahnke, T., Hilbert, C., Brossmann, J. & Heller, M. (2001) Randomized study to compare PTA alone versus PTA with Palmaz stent placement for femoropopliteal lesions. *Journal of Vascular and Interventional Radiology*, **12**, 935–942.

21 Becquemin, J.P., Favre, J.P., Marzelle, J., Nemoz, C., Corsin, C. & Leizorovicz, A. (2003) Systematic versus selective stent placement after superficial femoral artery balloon angioplasty: a multicenter prospective randomized study. *Journal of Vascular Surgery*, **37**, 487–494.

22 Schillinger, M., Sabeti, S., Loewe, C. *et al.* (2006) Balloon angioplasty versus implantation of nitinol stents in the superficial femoral artery. *The New England Journal of Medicine*, **354**, 1879–1888.

23 Dake, M.D., Ansel, G.M., Jaff, M.R. *et al.* (2011) Paclitaxel-eluting stents show superiority to balloon angioplasty and bare metal stents in femoropopliteal disease: twelve-month Zilver PTX randomized study results. *Circulation. Cardiovascular Interventions*, **4**, 495–504.

24 Dvir, D., Torguson, R. & Waksman, R. (2012) Overview of the 2011 food and drug administration's circulatory system devices panel of the medical devices advisory committee meeting on the Zilver® PTX® drug-eluting peripheral stent. *Cardiovascular Revascularization Medicine*, **13**, 281–285.

25 Rastan, A., Brechtel, K., Krankenberg, H. *et al.* (2012) Sirolimus-eluting stents for treatment of infrapopliteal arteries reduce clinical event rate compared to

bare-metal stents: long-term results from a randomized trial. *Journal of the American College of Cardiology*, **60**, 587–591.

26 Brown, J., Lethaby, A., Maxwell, H., Wawrzyniak, A.J. & Prins, M.H. (2008) Antiplatelet agents for preventing thrombosis after peripheral arterial bypass surgery. *Cochrane Database of Systematic Reviews*, **4** CD00053.

27 Belch, J.J., Dormandy, J., CASPAR Writing Committee *et al.* (2010) Results of the randomized, placebo-controlled clopidogrel and acetylsalicylic acid in bypass surgery for peripheral arterial disease (CASPAR) trial. *Journal of Vascular Surgery*, **52**, 825–833 833.e1–2.

28 No Authors Listed (2000) Efficacy of oral anticoagulants compared with aspirin after infrainguinal bypass surgery (The Dutch Bypass Oral Anticoagulants or Aspirin Study): a randomised trial. *Lancet*, **355**, 346–351.

29 Johnson, W.C., Williford, W.O. & Department of Veterans Affairs Cooperative Study #362 (2002) Benefits, morbidity, and mortality associated with long-term administration of oral anticoagulant therapy to patients with peripheral arterial bypass procedures: a prospective randomized study. *Journal of Vascular Surgery*, **35**, 413–421.

30 Rooke, T.W., Hirsch, A.T., Misra, S. *et al.* (2011) 2011 ACCF/AHA focused update of the guideline for the management of patients with peripheral artery disease (updating the 2005 guideline): a report of the American College of Cardiology Foundation/American Heart Association Task Force on Practice Guidelines: developed in collaboration with the Society for Cardiovascular Angiography and Interventions, Society of Interventional Radiology, Society for Vascular Medicine, and Society for Vascular Surgery. *Circulation*, **124**, 2020–2045.

31 Tendera, M., Aboyans, V., Bartelink, M.L. *et al.* (2011) ESC guidelines on the diagnosis and treatment of peripheral artery diseases: document covering atherosclerotic disease of extracranial carotid and vertebral, mesenteric, renal, upper and lower extremity arteries: the Task Force on the Diagnosis and Treatment of Peripheral Artery Diseases of the European Society of Cardiology (ESC). *European Heart Journal*, **32**, 2851–2906.

30 Bleeding Risk and Outcomes of Patients Undergoing Percutaneous Coronary Intervention Treated with Antiplatelets

Sa'ar Minha and Ron Waksman

MedStar Washington Hospital Center, Washington, DC, USA

Introduction

The merits of antiplatelet therapy for patients undergoing percutaneous coronary intervention (PCI) are well established. The outcome benefits outweigh the inherent, increased bleeding risk, which is the most common, noncardiac adverse event of PCI. Although this increased risk usually manifests as easily bruising, when severe, it is associated with an increased propensity for morbidity and mortality. This chapter will focus on the bleeding risk that accompanies the antiplatelet therapy associated with PCI.

Scope of problem

The exact rate of bleeding associated with each antiplatelet agent is not completely clear. Reported bleeding rates vary greatly mainly due to heterogeneity in bleeding definitions and patient populations included. When different definitions were applied to evaluate the rates of "major bleeding" in a population of patients undergoing PCI in the context of non-ST-elevation myocardial infarction, the rate ranged from 1.2% to 8.2% [1]. Further, the ability to properly assess the bleeding rate of a specific agent, even when uniform definition is being used, is hampered by adjunctive therapies, such as other antithrombotic agents and concomitant anticoagulant usage.

A thorough discussion regarding the different bleeding definitions will follow this chapter. In brief, bleeding definitions commonly utilize both clinical events and laboratory parameters to define "major" and

Antiplatelet Therapy in Cardiovascular Disease, First Edition. Edited by Ron Waksman, Paul A. Gurbel, and Michael A. Gaglia, Jr.
© 2014 John Wiley & Sons, Ltd. Published 2014 by John Wiley & Sons, Ltd.

"minor" bleeding. Thrombolysis in Myocardial Infarction (TIMI) [2] and Global Utilization of Strategies To Open Occluded Arteries (GUSTO) [3] are two of the most commonly used definitions, although originated in the thrombolysis era. More recently, a professional consortium has suggested a standardized set of definitions to be used in clinical trials [4]. When these and other definitions were used in pivotal clinical trials [5, 6, 7, 8], the major bleeding rate ranged from 1.5% to 3.7%. Data from "real-life" registries have reported higher incidences of major bleeding (9.2–12.0%), which demonstrate the aforementioned heterogeneity [9, 10]. Increased bleeding risk translates into increased mortality risk [11, 12].

Bleeding predictors

Percutaneous coronary intervention-related major bleeding stems are the result of both patient and procedural parameters. Old age, female gender, impaired renal function, anemia, and cardiogenic shock at presentation are patient characteristics associated with major bleeding, while the use of intra-aortic balloon pump counterpulsation and concomitant use of antithrombotic and glycoprotein IIb/IIIa inhibitors (GPI) are two important procedural aspects associated with major bleeding [13, 14, 15]. Contemporary data from Thrombolysis in Myocardial Infarction 38 (TRITON-TIMI 38), which compared the risk and benefits of two dual antiplatelet therapies in acute coronary syndrome (ACS) patients, demonstrated that within the entire patient cohort, history of stroke or transient ischemic event, age greater than 75 years, and body weight less than 60 kg were all associated with a higher risk for serious bleeding irrespective of the antiplatelet regimen used (HR 1.58, 95% CI 1.10–2.29, $p = 0.01$; HR 2.58, 95% CI 2.13–3.13, $p < 0.001$; and HR 2.30, 95% CI 1.74–3.05, $p < 0.001$, respectively). More specifically, within the subgroups of elderly patients and those with low body weight, prasugrel was associated with a significantly higher risk for bleeding compared with clopidogrel [16].

Femoral access bleeding is reported to be the most common bleeding site associated with PCI, accounting for greater than 50% of all major bleeding events with an incidence of approximately 2–8% [13, 14, 16, 17, 18, 19], although contemporary evidence has demonstrated a decline in the rates of femoral artery-related major bleeding in the last decade [19, 20]. Femoral access bleeding is followed by gastrointestinal, retroperitoneal, and other major organ bleeding. Femoral sheath size is one of major determinates of access site complications [19, 21]. For example, the odds ratio for major vascular bleeding when using a 7–8Fr sheath size compared with 6Fr is 1.53 (1.28–1.83, 95% CI) and is 1.91 (1.29–2.82, 95% CI) when a 9Fr sheath is compared with 6Fr [19]. Other factors associated with femoral access-related bleeding are procedure length and the intensity and duration of anticoagulation used. Gastrointestinal bleeding (GIB) complicates approximately 1.0% of PCI and is significantly associated with mortality at 30 days and at 1 year (HR 4.87 [2.61–9.08], $p < 0.001$, and HR 3.97 [2.64–5.99], $p < 0.001$, respectively) [22, 23]. Although the incidence of GIB has decreased throughout the years, GIB-related mortality rates have remained constant and are mostly associated with gastrointestinal malignancy [22].

Bleeding and outcome

The association between bleeding events and both short- and long-term mortality was established in numerous clinical trials and registries [11, 14, 16, 19, 24]. These and other studies have demonstrated a 3- to 10-fold increase in mortality risk in patients who bled versus those who did not. Bleeding severity was correlated with this risk [12, 24]. The ability to properly assess the effect of PCI-related bleeding on outcome is limited by the population selected to participate in the clinical trial and the overlap between bleeding risk and mortality risk.

Chhatriwalla *et al.* have collected data from greater than 3.3 million patients who underwent PCI between 2004 to 2011 and sought to evaluate the population's adjusted mortality risk associated with bleeding after PCI. The population-adjusted risk for inhospital mortality was 12% (11.4–12.7%, 95% CI). By utilizing a propensity-matched cohort of patients, it was evident that the number needed to harm was 29 (28–31, 95% CI), with this being consistent across the spectrum of preprocedural patient risk profiles [11]. Beyond the intuitive association between bleeding and short-term mortality, the association of bleeding with long-term mortality was also broadly reported.

In a dataset of greater than 34,000 patients with ACS without ST elevation collected from the Organization to Assess Ischemic Syndromes (OASIS) Registry and the Clopidogrel in Unstable Angina to Prevent Recurrent Events (CURE) trial, Eikelboom *et al.* have reported that the incidence for mortality among patients who bled was 5-fold higher than in patients without bleeding in the first 30 days. On the other hand, "only" a 1.5-fold increased incidence was recorded from 30 days to 6 months [24]. TRITON investigators have reported similar results regarding the impact of bleeding on mortality risk. In their analysis, the mortality risk related to severe bleeding was greatest within the first few days after PCI, while within 40 days, this risk was abolished [16]. When the bleeding events were stratified, it was evident that the association between preprocedural/traumatic bleeding and mortality was of short duration (<1 week), while spontaneous bleeding (GIB) had a longer effect on morality (with a significant hazard ratio for a period of 1 month) [16]. Beyond the high risk for mortality, bleeding was associated with a 5-fold increase in the risk for myocardial infarction, an 8.6-fold increase in the risk for stroke at 30 days, and a 6-fold increase in the risk for stent thrombosis when compared to patients who did not bleed [24, 25].

Avoiding bleeding complications

Avoiding bleeding complications mandates careful consideration and decision-making by consolidating patient characteristics, procedural and pharmacological aspects. PCI mandates concomitant use of anticoagulation and antiplatelets. This combination is needed for prevention of thrombotic events but translates into increased risk for bleeding. Evidence for decreased bleeding indicates that bivalirudin is preferred over unfractionated heparin plus GPI, and similarly, fondaparinux should be considered over enoxaparin [26, 27, 28]. If unfractionated heparin is used, the lowest possible dose should be given. Procedural aspects associated with decreased bleeding rates include using a smaller sheath size [29], fluoroscopic-/ultrasound-guided access site puncture [30], and utilization of transradial access [31]. Although controversial, evidence suggests that vascular closure device usage has decreased the bleeding rate in PCI [28]. Finally, these aforementioned strategies should be tailored as closely as possible to the individual patient. Patients in a high-risk clinical setting (ACS) and with high-risk baseline characteristics should be managed with special care aimed at applying the available evidence-based data to decrease bleeding risk.

Summary

Contemporary antiplatelet therapy has demonstrated improved outcomes in various PCI settings; and such benefits outweigh the inherent bleeding risks. Bleeding rates have decreased throughout the years but are still a significant cause for morbidity and mortality. By applying evidence-based strategies to specific patient subsets, bleeding risk may be minimized.

References

1 Rao, S.V., O'Grady, K., Pieper, K.S. *et al.* (2006) A comparison of the clinical impact of bleeding measured by two different classifications among patients with acute coronary syndromes. *Journal of the American College of Cardiology*, **47 (4)**, 809–816.

2 Rao, A.K., Pratt, C., Berke, A. *et al.* (1988) Thrombolysis in Myocardial Infarction (TIMI) Trial – phase I: hemorrhagic manifestations and changes in plasma fibrinogen and the fibrinolytic system in patients treated with recombinant tissue plasminogen activator and streptokinase. *Journal of the American College of Cardiology*, **11 (1)**, 1–11.

3 The GUSTO investigators (1993) An international randomized trial comparing four thrombolytic strategies for acute myocardial infarction. *The New England Journal of Medicine*, **329 (10)**, 673–682.

4 Mehran, R., Rao, S.V., Bhatt, D.L. *et al.* (2011) Standardized bleeding definitions for cardiovascular clinical trials: a consensus report from the Bleeding Academic Research Consortium. *Circulation*, **123 (23)**, 2736–2747.

5 The PURSUIT Trial Investigators (1998) Inhibition of platelet glycoprotein IIb/IIIa with eptifibatide in patients with acute coronary syndromes. Platelet Glycoprotein IIb/IIIa in Unstable Angina: Receptor Suppression Using Integrilin Therapy. *The New England Journal of Medicine*, **339 (7)**, 436–443.

6 Yusuf, S., Zhao, F., Mehta, S.R., Chrolavicius, S., Tognoni, G., and Fox, K.K. (2001) Clopidogrel in Unstable Angina to Prevent Recurrent Events Trial I. Effects of clopidogrel in addition to aspirin in patients with acute coronary

syndromes without ST-segment elevation. *The New England Journal of Medicine*, **345 (7)**, 494–502.

7 Wiviott, S.D., Braunwald, E., McCabe, C.H. *et al.* (2007) Prasugrel versus clopidogrel in patients with acute coronary syndromes. *The New England Journal of Medicine*, **357 (20)**, 2001–2015.

8 Wallentin, L., Becker, R.C., Budaj, A. *et al.* (2009) Ticagrelor versus clopidogrel in patients with acute coronary syndromes. *The New England Journal of Medicine*, **361 (11)**, 1045–1057.

9 Mortensen, J., Thygesen, S.S., Johnsen, S.P., Vinther, P.M., Kristensen, S.D., and Refsgaard, J. (2008) Incidence of bleeding in 'real-life' acute coronary syndrome patients treated with antithrombotic therapy. *Cardiology*, **111 (1)**, 41–46.

10 Sorensen, R., Hansen, M.L., Abildstrom, S.Z. *et al.* (2009) Risk of bleeding in patients with acute myocardial infarction treated with different combinations of aspirin, clopidogrel, and vitamin K antagonists in Denmark: a retrospective analysis of nationwide registry data. *Lancet*, **374 (9706)**, 1967–1974.

11 Chhatriwalla, A.K., Amin, A.P., Kennedy, K.F. *et al.* (2013) Association between bleeding events and in-hospital mortality after percutaneous coronary intervention. *JAMA*, **309 (10)**, 1022–1029.

12 Rao, S.V., O'Grady, K., Pieper, K.S. *et al.* (2005) Impact of bleeding severity on clinical outcomes among patients with acute coronary syndromes. *The American Journal of Cardiology*, **96 (9)**, 1200–1206.

13 Feit, F., Voeltz, M.D., Attubato, M.J. *et al.* (2007) Predictors and impact of major hemorrhage on mortality following percutaneous coronary intervention from the REPLACE-2 Trial. *The American Journal of Cardiology*, **100 (9)**, 1364–1369.

14 Kinnaird, T.D., Stabile, E., Mintz, G.S. *et al.* (2003) Incidence, predictors, and prognostic implications of bleeding and blood transfusion following percutaneous coronary interventions. *The American Journal of Cardiology*, **92 (8)**, 930–935.

15 Fuchs, S., Kornowski, R., Teplitsky, I. *et al.* (2009) Major bleeding complicating contemporary primary percutaneous coronary interventions-incidence, predictors, and prognostic implications. *Cardiovascular Revascularization Medicine*, **10 (2)**, 88–93.

16 Hochholzer, W., Wiviott, S.D., Antman, E.M. *et al.* (2011) Predictors of bleeding and time dependence of association of bleeding with mortality: insights from the Trial to Assess Improvement in Therapeutic Outcomes by Optimizing Platelet Inhibition With Prasugrel–Thrombolysis in Myocardial Infarction 38 (TRITON-TIMI 38. *Circulation*, **123 (23)**, 2681–2689.

17 Stone, G.W., Witzenbichler, B., Guagliumi, G. *et al.* (2008) Bivalirudin during primary PCI in acute myocardial infarction. *The New England Journal of Medicine*, **358 (21)**, 2218–2230.

18 Stone, G.W., McLaurin, B.T., Cox, D.A. *et al.* (2006) Bivalirudin for patients with acute coronary syndromes. *The New England Journal of Medicine*, **355 (21)**, 2203–2216.

19 Doyle, B.J., Ting, H.H., Bell, M.R. *et al.* (2008) Major femoral bleeding complications after percutaneous coronary intervention: incidence, predictors, and impact on long-term survival among 17,901 patients treated at the Mayo Clinic from 1994 to 2005. *JACC: Cardiovascular Interventions*, **1 (2)**, 202–209.

20 Applegate, R.J., Sacrinty, M.T., Kutcher, M.A. *et al.* (2008) Trends in vascular complications after diagnostic cardiac catheterization and percutaneous

coronary intervention via the femoral artery, 1998 to 2007. *JACC: Cardiovascular Interventions*, **1 (3)**, 317–326.

21 Smilowitz, N.R., Kirtane, A.J., Guiry, M. *et al.* (2012) Practices and complications of vascular closure devices and manual compression in patients undergoing elective transfemoral coronary procedures. *The American Journal of Cardiology*, **110 (2)**, 177–182.

22 Shivaraju, A., Patel, V., Fonarow, G.C., Xie, H., Shroff, A.R. and Vidovich, M.I. (2011) Temporal trends in gastrointestinal bleeding associated with percutaneous coronary intervention: analysis of the 1998–2006 Nationwide Inpatient Sample (NIS) database. *American Heart Journal*, **162 (6)**, 1062. e5–1068.e5.

23 Nikolsky, E., Stone, G.W., Kirtane, A.J. *et al.* (2009) Gastrointestinal bleeding in patients with acute coronary syndromes: incidence, predictors, and clinical implications: analysis from the ACUITY (Acute Catheterization and Urgent Intervention Triage Strategy) trial. *Journal of the American College of Cardiology*, **54 (14)**, 1293–1302.

24 Eikelboom, J.W., Mehta, S.R., Anand, S.S., Xie, C., Fox, K.A. and Yusuf, S. (2006) Adverse impact of bleeding on prognosis in patients with acute coronary syndromes. *Circulation*, **114 (8)**, 774–782.

25 Manoukian, S.V., Feit, F., Mehran, R. *et al.* (2007) Impact of major bleeding on 30-day mortality and clinical outcomes in patients with acute coronary syndromes: an analysis from the ACUITY Trial. *Journal of the American College of Cardiology*, **49 (12)**, 1362–1368.

26 Stone, G.W., White, H.D., Ohman, E.M. *et al.* (2007) Bivalirudin in patients with acute coronary syndromes undergoing percutaneous coronary intervention: a subgroup analysis from the Acute Catheterization and Urgent Intervention Triage strategy (ACUITY) trial. *Lancet*, **369 (9565)**, 907–919.

27 Jolly, S.S., Faxon, D.P., Fox, K.A. *et al.* (2009) Efficacy and safety of fondaparinux versus enoxaparin in patients with acute coronary syndromes treated with glycoprotein IIb/IIIa inhibitors or thienopyridines: results from the OASIS 5 (Fifth Organization to Assess Strategies in Ischemic Syndromes) trial. *Journal of the American College of Cardiology*, **54 (5)**, 468–476.

28 Marso, S.P., Amin, A.P., House, J.A. *et al.* (2010) Association between use of bleeding avoidance strategies and risk of periprocedural bleeding among patients undergoing percutaneous coronary intervention. *JAMA*, **303 (21)**, 2156–2164.

29 Buchler, J.R., Ribeiro, E.E., Falcao, J.L. *et al.* (2008) A randomized trial of 5 versus 7 French guiding catheters for transfemoral percutaneous coronary stent implantation. *Journal of Interventional Cardiology*, **21 (1)**, 50–55.

30 Seto, A.H., Abu-Fadel, M.S., Sparling, J.M. *et al.* (2010) Real-time ultrasound guidance facilitates femoral arterial access and reduces vascular complications: FAUST (Femoral Arterial Access With Ultrasound Trial). *JACC: Cardiovascular Interventions*, **3 (7)**, 751–758.

31 Rao, S.V., Ou, F.S., Wang, T.Y. *et al.* (2008) Trends in the prevalence and outcomes of radial and femoral approaches to percutaneous coronary intervention: a report from the National Cardiovascular Data Registry. *JACC: Cardiovascular Interventions*, **1 (4)**, 379–386.

31 Bleeding Definitions

Sameer Bansilal[1], Deborah E. Aronson[1], and Roxana Mehran[1,2]

[1]The Icahn School of Medicine at Mount Sinai, New York, NY, USA
[2]Cardiovascular Research Foundation, New York, NY, USA

Introduction

Over the last two decades, several potent antithrombotics have been developed with a focus on reduction of ischemic outcomes, with less attention to the inevitable increase in bleeding risk. As regimens continue to emerge and evolve, it has become increasingly complex to balance the ischemic and bleeding risks in acute coronary syndrome (ACS) patients. Agents include intravenous antithrombotics such as fondaparinux, bivalirudin, and cangrelor; oral antiplatelet agents such as clopidogrel, prasugrel, and ticagrelor; oral anticoagulants such as rivaroxaban, dabigatran, and apixaban; and several novel and derivative agents that are in various phases of testing. While these more potent agents have significantly reduced ischemic outcomes, using them in combination as is frequently necessary post percutaneous coronary intervention (PCI), is associated with an increased risk of bleeding.

It has been shown that major bleeding post PCI is associated with significant increases in both short- and long-term morbidity and mortality [1, 2]. In a pooled analysis of 34,146 ACS patients from registries and clinical trials, Eikelboom *et al.* found that major bleeding was associated with a 5-fold increase in the 30-day mortality and the risk increased incrementally with bleeding event severity [3]. In the Acute Catheterization and Urgent Intervention Triage Strategy (ACUITY) trial, major bleeding was associated with a 7-fold increased risk of mortality and higher rates of composite ischemia (23.1% vs. 6.8%) and stent thrombosis (3.4% vs. 0.6%) [2]. In an ACUITY substudy, the risk of myocardial infarction (MI) and mortality (up to 1 year post procedure) both increased linearly with bleeding severity [4].

Antiplatelet Therapy in Cardiovascular Disease, First Edition. Edited by Ron Waksman, Paul A. Gurbel, and Michael A. Gaglia, Jr.
© 2014 John Wiley & Sons, Ltd. Published 2014 by John Wiley & Sons, Ltd.

Heterogeneous bleeding definitions

To understand the safety profile of a therapy, it is essential to accurately characterize bleeding events. Multiple bleeding definitions were derived from several seminal clinical studies, in their attempt to best characterize such events (Table 31.1).

The Thrombolysis in Myocardial Infarction (TIMI) [5] and Global Use of Strategies to Open Occluded Arteries (GUSTO) [6] trials were based on combinations of three major principal components, namely, clinical events including overt bleeding, access site hematoma, and cardiac tamponade; laboratory parameters including changes in hemoglobin (Hg) and hematocrit (Hct) levels; and outcomes including death, hemodynamic compromise, and transfusion (Figure 31.1) [7]. In both cases, bleeding was classified by severity using the subjective terms minimal, mild, and major for TIMI and mild, moderate, and severe in GUSTO. The TIMI definition neglects precise Hg measurement timing and relies overly on laboratory measurements without the clinical context, while GUSTO is largely a clinical events based definition and does not take Hg drops or blood transfusion quantification into account, which alters interpretation considerably. For example, a patient undergoing PCI with a Hg drop of 2 g/L, with no obvious bleeding site, and who received a transfusion is classified by TIMI as major, but has no appropriate classification according to GUSTO. In the randomized, controlled trial, Superior Yield of the New Strategy of Enoxaparin, Revascularization and Glycoprotein IIb/IIIa Inhibitors (SYNERGY) [8], the safety and efficacy of enoxaparin, a low-molecular-weight heparin, was compared with unfractionated heparin in 10,027 patients. The authors found enoxaparin had a higher rate of TIMI major bleeding but GUSTO severe bleeding was not statistically significant.

Subsequently, several more definitions were derived including Acute Catheterization and Urgent Intervention Triage Strategy (ACUITY), Harmonizing Outcomes With Revascularization and Stents in Acute Myocardial Infarction (HORIZONS-AMI) [9], Randomized Evaluation in Percutaneous Coronary Intervention Linking Angiomax to Reduced Clinical Events (REPLACE-2) [10], Global Registry of Acute Coronary Events (GRACE) [11], Intracoronary Stenting and Antithrombotic Regimen (ISAR) [12], Ticagrelor and Clopidogrel in Patients With Acute Coronary Syndrome (PLATO), and Clopidogrel in Unstable Angina to Prevent Recurrent Events (CURE) that combined, modified, or added criteria. However, many of these definitions are also limited by intracategory variability. For example, bleeding with a Hg drop of greater than 5 g/dL is considered major bleeding in TIMI but not in ACUITY and HORIZONS, while retroperitoneal bleeding is classified as major for GUSTO, ACUITY, and HORIZONS but minor on the TIMI scale [13, 14].

Table 31.1 Definitions of Major or Severe Bleeding in Randomized Controlled Clinical Trials

Type of bleeding	GUSTO	TIMI phase I	TIMI phase II	REPLACE-2	OASIS-5 ESSENCE	CURE	STEEPLE	ACUITY HORIZONS	PLATO
Intracranial/intracerebral	+	+	+	+	+	+	+	+	+
Intraocular	−	−	−	+	+	+	+	+	+
Retroperitoneal	−	−	−	+	+	+	+	+	−
Bleeding causing hemodynamic compromise	+	−	−	−	−	−	−	−	+
Cardiac tamponade	−	+	+	−	−	−	−	−	+
Bleeding requiring surgical intervention	−	−	−	−	−	+	+	+	+
Hematoma >5cm at the puncture site	−	−	−	−	−	−	−	+	−
Transfusion, units	≥1	≥1	≥1	≥2	≥2	≥2	≥1	≥1	≥4
Decrease in Hgb with overt bleeding, g/dL	−	≥5.0*	≥3.0	≥3.0	≥3.0	−	≥3.0	≥3.0	≥5.0
Decrease in Hgb without overt bleeding, g/dL	−	−	−	≥4.0	−	≥5.0	−	≥4.0	−

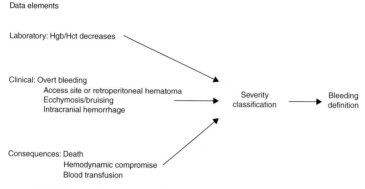

Data elements

Laboratory: Hgb/Hct decreases

Clinical: Overt bleeding
  Access site or retroperitoneal hematoma
  Ecchymosis/bruising
  Intracranial hemorrhage

Severity classification

Bleeding definition

Consequences: Death
  Hemodynamic compromise
  Blood transfusion

Figure 31.1 Constructing a bleeding definition from three principal components. (Source: Adapted from Rao S and Mehran R 2012 [7]. Reproduced with permission of Wolters Kluwer Health.)

The need for standardization

The high degree of variability regarding the patient population and study parameters translated into stark contrasts in the definitions, leading to estimates of major bleeding ranging from 1.5% for eptifibatide in the PURSUIT study to 9.1% for enoxaparin in the SYNERGY trial. This not only made clinical event committee adjudication difficult, but on a more practical level, did not allow for practitioners to make any cross-trial bleeding event comparisons to guide their decision making [15]. It became apparent that discrepancy among definitions could vastly alter the interpretation of the safety, in that, a more restrictive bleeding definition causes fewer events to meet the criteria resulting in a reduced bleeding rate and vice versa. Depending on the definition, an agent with significant bleeding risk could look 'safe'; conversely an agent with a reasonably safe profile could appear 'harmful'.

In an analysis of 119,020 patients with ACS from 6 contemporary antithrombotic trials, Quinlan *et al.* [16] found the bleeding definition to be a significant contributor to variability in major bleeding rates (0.6% in COMMIT to 11.2% in PLATO). They found that bleeding event classification variability was attenuated when a standardized definition (TIMI criteria) was applied across trials. With this new insight in hand, investigators across the research spectrum collaborated to identify and best employ the most relevant clinical elements to create a quantitative and universal standardized bleeding definition to better facilitate the accurate evaluation of new drugs and regimens [8, 17].

The Standardized BARC definition

The Bleeding Academic Research Consortium (BARC) bleeding definitions were created as part of a large scale research collaboration to improve upon and employ the most salient and standardized components.

Table 31.2 The Bleeding Academic Research Consortium (BARC) bleeding definition.

Type 0:	No bleeding
Type 1:	Bleeding that is not actionable (and does not cause patient to seek treatment)
Type 2:	Any overt, actionable sign of hemorrhage requiring diagnostics, nonsurgical intervention leading to hospitalization or treatment
Type 3a:	Overt bleeding plus hemoglobin (Hg) drop of 3 to <5 g/dL
	Transfusion with overt bleeding
Type 3b:	Overt bleeding plus Hg drop ≥5 g/dL
	Cardiac tamponade
	Bleeding requiring surgical intervention or intravenous vasoactive agents
Type 3c:	Intracranial hemorrhage (via autopsy, imaging, or lumbar puncture confirmation)
	Intraocular bleeding compromising vision
Type 4:	CABG-related bleeding within 48 h
Type 5:	Definite fatal bleeding (overt, autopsy, or via imaging confirmation)

CABG, coronary artery bypass graf. (Source: Adapted from Mehran R et al. 2011 [8]. Reproduced with permission of Wolters Kluwer Health.)

This attempt at standardizing bleeding events is more robustly universalized in that it eliminates the use of subjective nomenclature (major, minor, mild, severe) in favor of a hierarchal, quantitative, alphanumerical 0–5 scale (Table 31.2). In a significant step forward from all previous definitions, the BARC definitions specifically address bleeding associated with CABG and related to patient adherence. BARC type 4 CABG-related bleeding is a crucial delineation in that CABG-related bleeding is almost inevitable as it is performed in a fully anticoagulated state. The importance of this is best highlighted in the PLATO trial, where both TIMI- and protocol-defined bleeding indicated an increase in non-CABG-related bleeding; however, when CABG-related bleeding was combined with the primary end point, differences were abolished [18]. The BARC definition takes patient cessation of antithrombotic therapy into account, assigned as type 1 bleeding, which incorporates patient perspective and provides insight into antithrombotic therapy adherence (Table 31.1) [8]. Similar bleeding definitions are now being utilized in the field of trancatheter valve implanatation (VARC definition) [19].

Ndrepepa et al., performed a BARC validation study in 12,459 patients with coronary artery disease (CAD) undergoing PCI from 6 ISAR trials BARC-defined bleeding was independently associated with 1-year mortality in these patients. There was also a progressive increase in mortality after 1-year follow-up in accordance with increasing severity of BARC-defined hierarchical bleeding. The predictive accuracy of BARC was found to be comparable to both the TIMI (minor + major) and REPLACE-2 definitions, though BARC's greater sensitivity seems to have been achieved at the cost of a slightly lower specificity for 1-year mortality [20]. Recently, Vranckx et al. presented data on 12,944 patients with NSTEACS from the TRACER trial [21].

Once again, there was a clear relation between higher grades of BARC bleeding and increased mortality.

Valuable insight could be gained from additional BARC validation studies that extend prospectively to patients across the CAD spectrum including those with ST-elevation MI and patients undergoing surgical and endovascular procedures. The BARC consensus bleeding definition has enhanced and will continue to promote better understanding of clinical data within and across trials worldwide.

References

1 Rao, S.V., Eikelboom, J.A., Granger, C.B., Harrington, R.A., Califf, R.M., and Bassand, J.P. (2007 May) Bleeding and blood transfusion issues in patients with non-ST-segment elevation acute coronary syndromes. *European Heart Journal*, **28 (10)**, 1193–1204.

2 Manoukian, S.V., Feit, F., Mehran, R. *et al.* (2007) Impact of major bleeding on 30-day mortality and clinical outcomes in patients with acute coronary syndromes: an analysis from the ACUITY Trial. *Journal of the American College of Cardiology*, **49 (12)**, 1362–1368.

3 Eikelboom, J.W., Mehta, S.R., Anand, S.S., Xie, C., Fox, K.A., and Yusuf, S. (2006) Adverse impact of bleeding on prognosis in patients with acute coronary syndromes. *Circulation*, **114 (8)**, 774–782.

4 Mehran, R., Pocock, S.J., Stone, G.W. *et al.* (2009) Associations of major bleeding and myocardial infarction with the incidence and timing of mortality in patients presenting with non-ST-elevation acute coronary syndromes: a risk model from the ACUITY trial. *European Heart Journal*, **30 (12)**, 1457–1466.

5 Chesebro, J.H., Knatterud, G., Roberts, R. *et al.* (1987) Thrombolysis in Myocardial Infarction (TIMI) Trial Phase I: a comparison between intravenous tissue plasminogen activator and intravenous streptokinase. Clinical findings through hospital discharge. *Circulation*, **76 (1)**, 142–154.

6 Anonymous (1993) An international randomized trial comparing four thrombolytic strategies for acute myocardial infarction. The GUSTO investigators. *The New England Journal of Medicine*, **329 (10)**, 673–682.

7 Rao, S.V. and Mehran, R. (2012) Evaluating the bite of the BARC. *Circulation*, **125 (11)**, 1344–1346.

8 Mehran, R., Rao, S.V., Bhatt, D.L. *et al.* (2011) Standardized bleeding definitions for cardiovascular clinical trials: a consensus report from the Bleeding Academic Research Consortium. *Circulation*, **123 (23)**, 2736–2747.

9 Mehran, R., Lansky, A.J., Witzenbichler, B. *et al.* (2009) Bivalirudin in patients undergoing primary angioplasty for acute myocardial infarction (HORIZONS-AMI): 1-year results of a randomised controlled trial. *Lancet*, **374 (9696)**, 1149–1159.

10 Lincoff, A.M., Bittl, J.A., Harrington, R.A. *et al.* (2003) Bivalirudin and provisional glycoprotein IIb/IIIa blockade compared with heparin and planned glycoprotein IIb/IIIa blockade during percutaneous coronary intervention: REPLACE-2 randomized trial. *JAMA*, **289 (7)**, 853–863.

11 Moscucci, M., Fox, K.A., Cannon, C.P. *et al.* (2003) Predictors of major bleeding in acute coronary syndromes: the Global Registry of Acute Coronary Events (GRACE). *European Heart Journal*, **24 (20)**, 1815–1823.

12 Schomig, A., Neumann, F.J., Kastrati, A. *et al.* (1996) A randomized comparison of antiplatelet and anticoagulant therapy after the placement

of coronary-artery stents. *The New England Journal of Medicine*, **334 (17)**, 1084–1089.

13 Stone, G.W., McLaurin, B.T., Cox, D.A. *et al.* (2006) Bivalirudin for patients with acute coronary syndromes. *The New England Journal of Medicine*, **355 (21)**, 2203–2216.

14 Rao, A.K., Pratt, C., Berke, A. *et al.* (1988) Thrombolysis in Myocardial Infarction (TIMI) Trial-phase I: hemorrhagic manifestations and changes in plasma fibrinogen and the fibrinolytic system in patients treated with recombinant tissue plasminogen activator and streptokinase. *Journal of the American College of Cardiology*, **11 (1)**, 1–11.

15 Rao, S.V., O'Grady, K., Pieper, K.S. *et al.* (2006) A comparison of the clinical impact of bleeding measured by two different classifications among patients with acute coronary syndromes. *Journal of the American College of Cardiology*, **47 (4)**, 809–816.

16 Quinlan, D.J., Eikelboom, J.W., Goodman, S.G. *et al.* (2011) Implications of variability in definition and reporting of major bleeding in randomized trials of oral P2Y12 inhibitors for acute coronary syndromes. *European Heart Journal*, **32 (18)**, 2256–2265.

17 Rao, S.V., O'Grady, K., Pieper, K.S. *et al.* (2005) Impact of bleeding severity on clinical outcomes among patients with acute coronary syndromes. *The American Journal of Cardiology*, **96 (9)**, 1200–1206.

18 Wallentin, L., Becker, R.C., Budaj, A. *et al.* (2009) Ticagrelor versus clopidogrel in patients with acute coronary syndromes. *The New England Journal of Medicine*, **361 (11)**, 1045–1057.

19 Leon, M.B., Piazza, N., Nikolsky, E. *et al.* (2011) Standardized endpoint definitions for transcatheter aortic valve implantation clinical trials: a consensus report from the Valve Academic Research Consortium. *European Heart Journal*, **32 (2)**, 205–217.

20 Ndrepepa, G., Schuster, T., Hadamitzky, M. *et al.* (2012) Validation of the Bleeding Academic Research Consortium definition of bleeding in patients with coronary artery disease undergoing percutaneous coronary intervention. *Circulation*, **125 (11)**, 1424–1431.

21 Vranckx, P., Tricoci, P., Huang, Van De Werf, F. *et al.* (2013) Clinical validation of BARC definitions of bleeding after an ACS in the TRACER trial. *European Heart Journal*, **34 (1)**, 23–24.

Section V

Antiplatelet Responsiveness

32 Personalizing Antiplatelet Therapy

Paul A. Gurbel[1,2,4], Young-Hoon Jeong[3], and Udaya S. Tantry[1]

[1] Sinai Hospital of Baltimore, Baltimore, MD, USA
[2] Johns Hopkins University School of Medicine, Baltimore, MD, USA
[3] Gyeongsang National University Hospital, Jinju-si, South Korea
[4] Duke University School of Medicine, Durham, NC, USA

Dual antiplatelet therapy (DAPT) with aspirin and a $P2Y_{12}$ receptor blocker is the most important pharmacological therapy administered to the high-risk percutaneous coronary intervention (PCI)/acute coronary syndromes (ACS) patient to block platelet reactivity and recurrent ischemic event occurrence. Although the clinical efficacy of DAPT has been demonstrated in a wide range of high-risk coronary artery disease (CAD) patients, clopidogrel therapy is also associated with an unpredictable pharmacodynamic response where approximately one in three clopidogrel-treated patients will have high platelet reactivity (HPR). HPR assessed by multiple laboratory tests has been linked to post-PCI ischemic event occurrence in observational studies of thousands of patients. Despite the fundamental importance of unblocked $P2Y_{12}$ receptors in the genesis of thrombosis, the clear demonstration of clopidogrel nonresponsiveness, and even the identification of genes associated with resistance – *CYP2C19*2 and *3* – cardiologists largely don't determine platelet function or identify genetic polymorphisms in their high-risk patients treated with clopidogrel to ensure that an antiplatelet effect is actually present. Indeed, this "nonselective" or "one-size-fits-all" approach to clopidogrel, the most widely used $P2Y_{12}$ inhibitor to prevent a catastrophic thrombotic event occurrence, is paradoxical in comparison to the objective assessments and adjustments frequently made during treatment with most other cardiovascular drugs [1].

There has been a long-term reluctance to assess platelet function due to potential introduction of artifacts by laboratory methods, incomplete reflection of the actual *in vivo* thrombotic process, and failure to unequivocally establish a causal relation between the results of the test and thrombotic event occurrence. In the last decade, understanding of platelet receptor physiology has markedly improved; more potent $P2Y_{12}$ receptor blockers that can overcome some of the limitations of clopidogrel have

Antiplatelet Therapy in Cardiovascular Disease, First Edition. Edited by Ron Waksman, Paul A. Gurbel, and Michael A. Gaglia, Jr.
© 2014 John Wiley & Sons, Ltd. Published 2014 by John Wiley & Sons, Ltd.

been developed. The introduction of more user-friendly platelet function assays that can reliably determine the antiplatelet effect of clopidogrel has somewhat changed the latter reluctant mind-set and spurred great interest in antiplatelet therapy monitoring [2].

Small early translational research studies suggested that ischemic risk was not linearly related to on-treatment platelet reactivity to adenosine diphosphate (ADP) but rather occurred above a moderate level of platelet reactivity and provided evidence for a potential threshold of platelet reactivity to ADP or associated with ischemic event occurrence [3, 4]. The goal of $P2Y_{12}$ inhibitor therapy would be to achieve platelet reactivity below this therapeutic target. A recent white paper proposed cutoff values for HPR based on receiver operating characteristic curve (ROC) analyses for different platelet function assays. HPR is now accepted as a risk predictor in the PCI patient; a single periprocedural measurement has predicted both short-term and long-term (up to 2 years) clinical outcomes. Prospective, albeit small, studies provided evidence that HPR may be a modifiable risk factor where tailored incremental loading doses of clopidogrel, prasugrel, and selective glycoprotein (GP)IIb/IIIa receptor blocker administration overcame HPR and were effective in reducing subsequent post-PCI ischemic event occurrence [3, 4].

Box 32.1

2012 ACC/AHA focused update for the management of patients with UA/non-ST-segment-elevation MI (NSTEMI) [5]
Class IIb
1. Platelet function testing to determine platelet inhibitory response in patients with UA/NSTEMI (or after acute coronary syndromes [ACS] and percutaneous coronary intervention [PCI]) on $P2Y_{12}$ receptor inhibitor therapy may be considered if results of testing may alter management (*level of evidence: B*).

2011 ESC Guidelines for the management of ACS in patients presenting without persistent ST-segment elevation [6]
Class IIb
Genotyping and/or platelet function testing may be considered in selected cases when clopidogrel is used (*level of evidence: B*).

2011 ACCF/AHA/SCAI Guideline for Percutaneous Coronary Intervention [7]
Class IIb
1. Platelet function testing may be considered in patients at high risk for poor clinical outcomes (*level of evidence: C*).
2. In patients treated with clopidogrel with high platelet reactivity (HPR), alternative agents, such as prasugrel or ticagrelor, might be considered (*level of evidence: C*).

Class III: No benefit
1. The routine clinical use of platelet function testing to screen patients treated with clopidogrel who are undergoing PCI is not recommended (*level of evidence:* C)

2012 update to the Society of Thoracic Surgeons guideline on use of antiplatelet drugs in patients having cardiac and noncardiac operations [18]
Treatment options for patients on antiplatelet drugs who require urgent operations

Class IIa
For patients on dual antiplatelet therapy (DAPT), it is reasonable to make decisions about surgical delay based on tests of platelet inhibition rather than arbitrary use of a specified period of surgical delay (level B).

Monitoring platelet function
Class IIb
Because of their high negative predictive value, preoperative point-of-care testing to assess bleeding risk may be useful in identifying patients with high residual platelet reactivity after usual doses of antiplatelet drugs and who can undergo operation without elevated bleeding risk (level B). Point-of-care testing to assess perioperative platelet function may be useful in limiting blood transfusion (level B).

Antiplatelet drugs after cardiac operations
Class IIb
Once postoperative bleeding risk is decreased, testing of response to antiplatelet drugs, either with genetic testing or with point-of-care platelet function testing, early after cardiac procedures might be considered to optimize antiplatelet drug effect and minimize thrombotic risk to vein grafts (level B).

   For patients with HPR after usual doses of clopidogrel, it may be helpful to switch to another $P2Y_{12}$ inhibitor (e.g., prasugrel or ticagrelor).

Based on the vast amount of accrued observational data, the recent 2011 American and European guidelines have given a class IIb recommendation in the high-risk patient for platelet function testing or genotyping if the results of testing may alter management [5, 6, 7] (Box 32.1).

Randomized trials of personalized antiplatelet therapy guided by platelet function testing

The GRAVITAS trial was the first large-scale investigation of personalized antiplatelet therapy in the elective PCI patient. In this 6-month study, patients with HPR were randomized to two groups: (A) treatment with a 600 mg extra loading dose of clopidogrel given the day after stenting followed by 150 mg daily therapy or (b) 75 mg clopidogrel therapy. High-dose clopidogrel treatment was ineffective in reducing 6-month composite ischemic event occurrence, and there was an unexpectedly low event rate (2.3%) in both groups [8]. Potential explanations for this neutral observation include (A) suboptimal effectiveness of high-dose clopidogrel to overcome HPR. High-dose clopidogrel reduced the prevalence of HPR at 30 days in only 60% of patients. In support of this hypothesis, in the ELEVATE-TIMI 51 trial, up to 225 mg/day clopidogrel dose was required to overcome the HPR [9]. (B) The cutoff for HPR may have been too high. In a time-dependent covariate Cox regression analysis of on-treatment platelet reactivity in GRAVITAS, PRU >208 was an independent predictor of event-free survival at 60 days (hazard ratio = 0.23; 95% confidence interval [CI] = 0.05– 0.98; P = 0.047) and strongly trended to be an independent predictor at 6 months (hazard ratio = 0.54; 95% CI = 0.28 –1.04; P = 0.06) [10]. (C) The majority of patients enrolled in GRAVITAS were low-risk patients with stable CAD. Only treatment with a highly effective remedy to overcome HPR would have had a chance to produce positive results given the very low event rate.

In the TRIGGER-PCI study conducted in stable elective PCI patients (non-ST-segment-elevation MI (NSTEMI) and ST-segment-elevation MI excluded), >208 PRU was used as the HPR cut point. Instead of a 150 mg daily dose of clopidogrel, a 10 mg daily dose of prasugrel was used in the active arm and was highly effective in reducing the prevalence of HPR; only ~6% of patients had HPR after 90 days of prasugrel therapy. However, the study was terminated early because of futility. There was only 1 occurrence of the primary end point among 236 patients who completed 6 months of follow-up. In addition, ~30% of the enrolled patients declined randomization after being identified as having HPR [11].

Finally in the ARCTIC study, 2440 patients scheduled for planned coronary stenting were randomly assigned to a strategy of platelet function monitoring and drug adjustment or to a conventional strategy without monitoring. In the monitoring arm, one-third of patients had HPR (>235 PRU) before stent implantation, and 80% of these patients immediately received additional clopidogrel, and 2.3% received a prasugrel loading dose. Also, 30% of patients in the monitoring group received GPIIb/IIa therapy compared to 6% in the conventional arm. Platelet function was again checked after 2–4 weeks in the monitoring arm, and therapy was adjusted for patients with HPR. Finally, at the end of the study (at one year), 86% of patients in the conventional arm and 80% in the monitoring arm were on clopidogrel therapy, and only 6% in the conventional arm and 12% in the monitoring arm were on prasugrel therapy. The 1-year primary composite end point of death, myocardial infarction (MI), stent thrombosis, stroke, or urgent revascularization was not different in the monitoring compared to the conventional arm (34.6% vs. 31.1%, hazard ratio, 1.13; 95% CI, 0.98–1.29; P = 0.10). The main secondary end point, stent thrombosis or any urgent revascularization, and also the rate of major bleeding events did not differ significantly between groups. In this trial, the prevalence of ACS patients was low (27% NST-ACS vs. 73% patients with stable CAD); patients at very high risk for early atherothrombotic events, for example, STEMI patients, were excluded from the study; and prasugrel, a superior alternative to overcome HPR as compared to double-dose clopidogrel, was administered only in ~10% of patients [12].

At this time, it appears less certain that we will witness the "proof" from an adequately powered randomized trial of personalized antiplatelet therapy demonstrating the superiority of personalized antiplatelet therapy versus the "unselected" or "one-size-fits-all" approach that is currently most widely employed. Although a major determinant of post-PCI thrombotic event occurrence, HPR is not the sole factor responsible for these events. In contrast, the absence of HPR is the best reassurance thus far for a low likelihood of future ischemic events. The HPR cutoff values reported in many studies are associated with high negative predictive values and low positive predictive values. However, given the overall low prevalence of thrombotic events in these studies, the low positive predictive values and high negative predictive values are understandable. Other factors, including demographic, clinical, and angiographic factors, must be taken into consideration to optimally identify the patients at greatest risk. Along this line, recent studies have suggested that adding clinical variables and genotype to platelet reactivity measurements (a combined risk factor) may improve risk prediction [13, 14].

Finally, a future study demonstrating noninferiority from the selective use of generic clopidogrel and the new $P2Y_{12}$ inhibitors may be more likely. However, low event rates in current practice would require enrollment of a very large number of patients, and the prospect of finding funding for this type of endeavor is not promising. Thus, we must rely on the guidelines and the existing observational data while keeping fully in mind the role that platelet physiology plays in catastrophic event occurrence in the PCI patient.

In addition to the upper threshold for ischemic risk (i.e., HPR), small translational research studies have demonstrated the relation of low platelet reactivity with bleeding. The concept of a "therapeutic window" of $P2Y_{12}$ receptor reactivity associated with both ischemic event occurrence (upper threshold) and bleeding risk (lower threshold) has been proposed. This approach is more meaningful while titrating the dose of more potent $P2Y_{12}$ receptor blockers that are known to be associated with increased incidences of bleeding [3] (Figure 32.1).

Personalized antiplatelet therapy in the surgical patient

The major rationale for 5–7 days' discontinuation of $P2Y_{12}$ receptor inhibitor treatment recommended by the guidelines in patients undergoing CABG was to allow platelet function recovery thereby avoiding excessive perioperative bleeding [15, 16, 17]. A recent study demonstrated that clopidogrel-treated patients undergoing first-time on-pump CABG had the same perioperative bleeding as clopidogrel-naïve

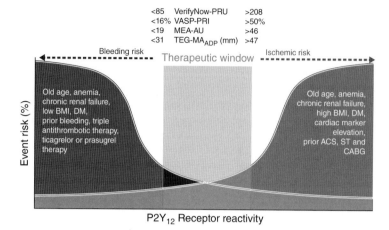

<85	VerifyNow-PRU	>208
<16%	VASP-PRI	>50%
<19	MEA-AU	>46
<31	TEG-MA$_{ADP}$ (mm)	>47

Bleeding risk ◀-------------------- Therapeutic window --------------------▶ Ischemic risk

Event risk (%)

Old age, anemia, chronic renal failure, low BMI, DM, prior bleeding, triple antithrombotic therapy, ticagrelor or prasugrel therapy

Old age, anemia, chronic renal failure, high BMI, DM, cardiac marker elevation, prior ACS, ST and CABG

P2Y$_{12}$ Receptor reactivity

Figure 32.1 The sigmoid cumulative frequency curve in patients with post-percutaneous coronary intervention (PCI) ischemic/thrombotic clinical events relative to platelet reactivity to adenosine diphosphate (ADP). These data support the concept of a therapeutic window for P2Y$_{12}$ blockade. (Source: Adapted from Tantry US et al., 2013 [1]. Reproduced with permission of Elsevier.)

patients when their surgery was timed on the basis of a preoperative assessment of platelet reactivity [16]. Preoperative platelet reactivity was measured by thrombelastography (TEG with platelet mapping). Surgery in patients treated with clopidogrel was scheduled within 24 h of the last dose of clopidogrel in those with a maximum amplitude (MA$_{ADP}$) >50 mm, within 3–5 days of the last dose in those with an MA$_{ADP}$ 35–50 mm, and 5 days after the last dose in those with an MA$_{ADP}$ <35 mm (49). In the 2012 ATS guidelines, there is a class IIa recommendation for platelet function testing in clopidogrel-treated patients to shorten the wait time [18].

Conclusions

Currently, the evidence indicates that HPR and *CYP2C19 LoF* carriage are associated with poorer clinical outcomes in high-risk clopidogrel-treated patients who have undergone PCI. Data from TRITON-TIMI 38 and PLATO trials strongly suggest that prasugrel and ticagrelor are effective alternatives to clopidogrel that overcome the influence of the *LoF* allele carrier status [19, 20]. Pharmacodynamic studies demonstrate that prasugrel and ticagrelor are effective in overcoming HPR during clopidogrel therapy [21]. Therefore, a reasonable strategy is to assess platelet function in high-risk clopidogrel-treated patients (e.g., patients with current or prior ACS, history of stent thrombosis and target vessel revascularization, poor left ventricular function, multivessel stenting, complex anatomy [e.g., bifurcation, long, small stents], high body mass index, and diabetes mellitus and patients cotreated with proton pump inhibitors) and use more potent P2Y$_{12}$ receptor therapy selectively in the patient with HPR. Furthermore, unselected therapy with the new $P2Y_{12}$ receptor blockers is associated with increased bleeding. By personalizing therapy, clinicians find the antiplatelet agent that achieves the optimal level of platelet reactivity for the patient, regardless of the cost. If generic clopidogrel is indeed pharmacodynamically effective in the patient, offering them this less expensive option seems favorable from both cost and efficacy standpoints. The introduction of generic clopidogrel will change practice rapidly and likely increase the role of selective genetic and platelet function testing in patients treated with a coronary stent.

References

1 Tantry, U.S., Bonello, L., Aradi, D., *et al.* (2013) Working Group on On-Treatment Platelet Reactivity. Consensus and update on the definition of on-treatment platelet reactivity to adenosine diphosphate associated with ischemia and bleeding. *Journal of the American College of Cardiology*, **62**, 2261–2273.

2 Hirsh, J. (1987) Hyperactive platelets and complications of coronary artery disease. *The New England Journal of Medicine*, **316**, 1543–1544.

3 Gurbel, P.A., Becker, R.C., Mann, K.G., Steinhubl, S.R. and Michelson, A.D. (2007) Platelet function monitoring in patients with coronary artery disease. *Journal of the American College of Cardiology*, **50**, 1822–1834.

4 Gurbel, P.A. and Tantry, U.S. (2012) Do platelet function testing and genotyping improve outcome in patients treated with antithrombotic agents? Platelet function testing and genotyping improve outcome in patients treated with antithrombotic agents. *Circulation*, **125**, 1276–1287 discussion 1287.

5 Jneid, H., Anderson, J.L., Wright, R.S. *et al.* (2012) 2012 ACCF/AHA focused update of the guideline for the management of patients with unstable angina/ non-ST-elevation myocardial infarction (updating the 2007 guideline and replacing the 2011 focused update): a report of the American College of Cardiology Foundation/American Heart Association Task Force on Practice Guidelines. *Journal of the American College of Cardiology*, **60**, 645–681.

6 Hamm, C.W., Bassand, J.P., Agewall, S. *et al.* (2011) ESC Guidelines for the management of acute coronary syndromes in patients presenting without persistent ST-segment elevation: the Task Force for the management of acute coronary syndromes (ACS) in patients presenting without persistent ST-segment elevation of the European Society of Cardiology (ESC). *European Heart Journal*, **32**, 2999–3054.

7 Levine, G.N., Bates, E.R., Blankenship, J.C. *et al.* (2011) 2011 ACCF/AHA/ SCAI guideline for percutaneous coronary intervention. A report of the American College of Cardiology Foundation/American Heart Association Task Force on practice guidelines and the society for cardiovascular angiography and interventions. *Journal of the American College of Cardiology*, **58**, e44–e122.

8 Price, M.J., Berger, P.B., Teirstein, P.S. *et al.* (2011) Standard- vs high-dose clopidogrel based on platelet function testing after percutaneous coronary intervention: the GRAVITAS randomized trial. *JAMA*, **305**, 1097–1105.

9 Mega, J.L., Hochholzer, W., Frelinger, A.L., 3rd *et al.* (2011) Dosing clopidogrel based on CYP2C19 genotype and the effect on platelet reactivity in patients with stable cardiovascular disease. *JAMA*, **306**, 2221–2228.

10 Price, M.J., Angiolillo, D.J., Teirstein, P.S. *et al.* (2011) Platelet reactivity and cardiovascular outcomes after percutaneous coronary intervention:

a time-dependent analysis of the Gauging Responsiveness with a VerifyNow P2Y12 assay: Impact on Thrombosis and Safety (GRAVITAS) trial. *Circulation*, **124**, 1132–1137.

11 Trenk, D., Stone, G.W., Gawaz, M. *et al.* (2012) A randomized trial of prasugrel versus clopidogrel in patients with high platelet reactivity on clopidogrel after elective percutaneous coronary intervention with implantation of drug-eluting stents: results of the TRIGGER-PCI (Testing Platelet Reactivity in Patients Undergoing Elective Stent Placement on Clopidogrel to Guide Alternative Therapy with Prasugrel) study. *Journal of the American College of Cardiology*, **59**, 2159–2164.

12 Collet, J.P., Cuisset, T., Rangé, G. *et al.* (2012) Bedside monitoring to adjust antiplatelet therapy for coronary stenting. *The New England Journal of Medicine*, **367**, 2100–2109.

13 Geisler, T., Grass, D., Bigalke, B. *et al.* (2008) The residual platelet aggregation after deployment of intracoronary stent (predict) score. *Journal of Thrombosis and Haemostasis*, **6**, 54–61.

14 Fontana, P., Berdagué, P., Castelli, C. *et al.* (2010) Clinical predictors of dual aspirin and clopidogrel poor responsiveness in stable cardiovascular patients from the adrie study. *Journal of Thrombosis and Haemostasis*, **8**, 2614–2623.

15 Chen, L., Bracey, A.W., Radovancevic, R. *et al.* (2004) Clopidogrel and bleeding in patients undergoing elective coronary artery bypass grafting. *The Journal of Thoracic and Cardiovascular Surgery*, **128**, 425–431.

16 Mahla, E., Suarez, T.A., Bliden, K.P. *et al.* (2012) Platelet function measurement-based strategy to reduce bleeding and waiting time in clopidogrel-treated patients undergoing coronary artery bypass graft surgery: the timing based on platelet function strategy to reduce clopidogrel-associated bleeding related to CABG (TARGET-CABG) study. *Circulation. Cardiovascular Interventions*, **5**, 261–269.

17 Kwak, Y.L., Kim, J.C., Choi, Y.S. *et al.* (2010) Clopidogrel responsiveness regardless of the discontinuation date predicts increased blood loss and transfusion requirement after off-pump coronary artery bypass graft surgery. *Journal of the American College of Cardiology*, **56**, 1994–2002.

18 Ferraris, V.A., Saha, S.P., Oestreich, J.H. *et al.* (2012) Society of Thoracic Surgeons. 2012 update to the Society of Thoracic Surgeons guideline on use of antiplatelet drugs in patients having cardiac and noncardiac operations. *Annals of Thoracic Surgery*, **94**, 1761–1781.

19 Mega, J.L., Close, S.L., Wiviott, S.D. *et al.* (2009) Cytochrome P450 genetic polymorphisms and the response to prasugrel: relationship to pharmacokinetic, pharmacodynamic, and clinical outcomes. *Circulation*, **119**, 2553–2560.

20 Wallentin, L., James, S., Storey, R.F. *et al.* (2010) Effect of CYP2C19 and ABCB1 single nucleotide polymorphisms on outcomes of treatment with ticagrelor versus clopidogrel for acute coronary syndromes: a genetic substudy of the PLATO trial. *Lancet*, **376**, 1320–1328.

21 Tantry, U.S., Jeong, Y.H., Navarese, E.P. *et al.* (2013) Influence of genetic polymorphisms on platelet function, response to antiplatelet drugs and clinical outcomes in patients with coronary artery disease. *Expert Review of Cardiovascular Therapy*, **11**, 447–462.

33 Aspirin Resistance

Muthiah Vaduganathan[1] and Eli I. Lev[2,3]

[1] Massachusetts General Hospital, Harvard Medical School, Boston, MA, USA
[2] Rabin Medical Center, Petah-Tikva, Israel
[3] Tel-Aviv University, Tel-Aviv, Israel

Introduction

Approximately a fifth of all persons in the USA currently take aspirin on a routine basis, irrespective of age or indication. This proportion increases to almost 50% in patients over the age of 65 [1]. Despite ongoing debate regarding the utility of chronic aspirin use for primary prophylaxis in patients at high risk for developing cardiovascular disease [2], its central cardioprotective role in patients with coronary artery disease (CAD), peripheral vascular disease, and/or cerebrovascular disease has been well established. A landmark meta-analysis conducted by the Antiplatelet Trialists' Collaboration [3] in the early 1990s including 145 randomized controlled clinical trials and 70,000 high-risk patients showed a robust risk reduction of approximately 25% in serious vascular events (defined as nonfatal myocardial infarction (MI), nonfatal stroke, or vascular death). This risk reduction was consistently demonstrated in patient subgroups, regardless of age, sex, and comorbid illnesses [3]. Indeed, the most recent American Heart Association (AHA)/American College of Cardiology (ACC) guidelines strongly favor the use of aspirin (75–162 mg daily) indefinitely for secondary prevention against atherosclerotic disease (class I, level of evidence A) [4]. In addition, aspirin (with the addition of a thienopyridine) has become the standard therapeutic regimen for patients with acute coronary syndromes (ACS) and for those undergoing percutaneous coronary intervention (PCI) [5].

Over the last decade, however, a preponderance of data has accrued that suggest that the antiplatelet effects of aspirin are nonuniform. In fact, a small, but substantial, proportion of patients may experience suboptimal platelet inhibition despite guideline-recommended dosing of this antiplatelet agent. In recent years, this phenomenon of "aspirin resistance" has transformed from a transient laboratory finding into a potentially clinically relevant entity. Reduced responsiveness to aspirin therapy may place patients at higher risk for adverse ischemic events, highlighting the importance of investigating the mechanisms underlying this phenomenon. The biological response to aspirin therapy is influenced by a number

Antiplatelet Therapy in Cardiovascular Disease, First Edition. Edited by Ron Waksman, Paul A. Gurbel, and Michael A. Gaglia, Jr.

of factors including alterations in drug metabolism and distribution, genetic polymorphisms of molecular pathways, platelet hyperreactivity, and pharmacological interactions. This chapter will focus on the (i) definition and relative prevalence of aspirin resistance, (ii) clinical implications of this phenomenon, (iii) mechanisms of variability and suboptimal response, and (iv) potential methods to overcome aspirin resistance.

Definition, prevalence, and clinical implications of aspirin resistance

The overall definition of "aspirin resistance" is highly dependent on the specific assay, cutoffs (for abnormal values), and patient population. Although consensus working group has established a set of criteria for defining high on-treatment platelet reactivity (HTPR) for clopidogrel [6], to our knowledge, no such standardized definitions exist for aspirin. Most definitions rely on strict laboratory criteria based on various *in vitro* and *ex vivo* platelet assays. It should be noted that a number of studies have defined suboptimal response to aspirin as the upper fraction (e.g., quartile or quintile) of posttreatment residual platelet function in order to avoid issues with arbitrary, nonstandardized definitions. Furthermore, determination of aspirin responsiveness has largely been examined at a single-time point, generally before or after PCI. Platelet function may dynamically change in the periprocedural time period, and thus, platelet response to aspirin may vary with time. Definitive data are lacking regarding the stability of the aspirin resistance phenomenon over time. This emphasizes the dependence of test results on the particular patient setting, clinical status, and population.

Due to these factors, a wide range of prevalence rates have been reported in the literature ranging from less than 1% in certain population to over 60% of patients studied [7, 8, 9]. A well-conducted cross-sectional study by Lordkipanidzé *et al.* [10] compared the prevalence of aspirin resistance in 201 patients with stable CAD using six commonly utilized platelet assays (including light transmission aggregometry (LTA), whole blood aggregometry, Platelet Function Analyzer (PFA)-100, VerifyNow Aspirin assay, urine 11-dehydro-TXB$_2$ concentrations). Approximately 4% of patients were found to be aspirin resistant based on the gold standard LTA stimulated by arachidonic acid (AA). The relative frequency of aspirin resistance for other assays ranged from 6.7% (with VerifyNow Aspirin assay) to 59.5% (with PFA-100). Only few patients were identified by multiple assays to be resistant, and the agreeability between assays was poor [10]. There is especially poor correlation between direct measures of thromboxane metabolites and indirect assays of platelet function [11].

Mounting evidences over the last decade suggest that aspirin resistance is associated with a significantly increased risk of adverse cardiovascular events. In fact, three recent meta-analyses [12, 13, 14] consistently showed that patients with aspirin resistance, measured by a number of laboratory assays, had significantly worse prognosis compared to patients who were aspirin sensitive. Each meta-analysis included over 2000 patients and over 10 independent studies [12, 13, 14]. The pooled odds ratios for combined cardiovascular end points in each meta-analysis were 3.85 (3.08–4.80) [12], 3.8 (2.3–6.1) [13], and 3.11 (1.88–5.15) [14].

Potential mechanisms and targeted approaches to aspirin resistance

Compliance

Mechanism: Poor compliance is likely a major cause of aspirin resistance, or more appropriately of treatment failure [15]. Nonadherence to prescribed therapy in patients with established CAD has consistently been associated with adverse cardiac events [16]. However, assessment of the true magnitude of the contribution of nonadherence to the entire scope of aspirin resistance has been difficult to date. In an interesting study attempting to quantify this effect of noncompliance, Schwartz and colleagues directly observed aspirin ingestion in the approximately 10% of patients originally found to be aspirin resistant by LTA (agonized by AA). The investigators found that all but one patient had substantial platelet responses 2 h after aspirin ingestion, suggesting that noncompliance played a large role in this sample [17].

Targeted approach: The influence of counseling on platelet function parameters in patients prescribed with aspirin therapy after MI was recently examined [18]. The study sample included all patients found to be aspirin resistant based on PFA-100 at baseline. Counseling and dosing escalation significantly lowered rates of aspirin resistance at 1- and 4-week follow-up. At the end of the study, only 1.4% of patients exhibited laboratory evidence of aspirin resistance [18].

Genetic contribution

Mechanism: Rare COX-1 genetic polymorphisms (including A842G and C5OT) and platelet glycoprotein receptors (including Leu33Pro, P1A1/A2) have been reported that may influence aspirin sensitivity [19]. Heritable loci that may influence platelet response to aspirin have been identified in high-risk black and white persons with a strong family history of CAD [20]. Emerging data from genome-wide linkage studies and association data suggest that discrete loci may control platelet phenotypes before and after aspirin therapy [21].

Targeted approach: Currently, there are no available clinically tested rapid tools to assess genetic risk for aspirin resistance.

Drug–drug interactions

Mechanism: The antiplatelet effects of aspirin are widely influenced by a number of pharmacological agents. Nonetheless, relevant clinical implications of these interactions have yet to be substantiated by well-conducted, prospective investigations. Pharmacodynamic reports on specific agents that either potentiate, such as ranitidine, fish oil, and

Ginkgo biloba, or diminish, such as naproxen and gallic acid, aspirin responsiveness are mostly small or inconclusive. One of the few medications that have been shown to clearly alter aspirin efficacy and therefore potentially pose a risk to patients on antiplatelet therapy is ibuprofen. Competitive inhibition is attained by attaching to the Arg120 position, resulting in steric competition with aspirin's ability to acetylate the Ser529 [22, 23]. Furthermore, reduced gastric absorption of aspirin via inactivation by gut-specific esterases may be increased by concomitant intake of proton pump inhibitors, especially in elderly patients [24].

Targeted approach: The clinical relevance of these findings was recently highlighted by a communication from the Food and Drug Administration, which recommended that individuals taking immediate-release (nonenteric-coated) low-dose aspirin should do so at least 30 min before or 8 h after taking ibuprofen to avoid any possible interaction [25]. It is important that clinicians take into consideration potential interactions of aspirin and a variety of medications, paying special attention to side effects such as increased risk of bleeding or failure in antiplatelet therapy.

Increased platelet turnover

Mechanism: There may be transient or dynamic clinical situations that may contribute to increased resistance to antiplatelet therapy in the time period surrounding the event, mediated by increased basal platelet activity or increased platelet turnover. Patients with increased platelet turnover may be at higher risk of being poorly responsive to aspirin therapy. Young, newly produced reticulated platelets are naïve of aspirin exposure as early as 4 h after dosing [26] and thus maintain high platelet function and contribute to persistent thromboxane production. The percentage of reticulated platelets in the peripheral blood has been correlated with rates of aspirin resistance in healthy subjects [27] and in patients with stable CAD [28].

Targeted approach: A significant number of patients that are aspirin resistant based on laboratory data may be dosed at inadequate doses or frequencies. It is noteworthy that the majority of studies investigating this issue have poorly characterized the exact dosing regimen and duration of therapy in each study sample. Patients with CAD taking standard once daily aspirin were vulnerable to increased platelet aggregation by the end of the 24-h treatment window [29]. This phenomenon is known as time-dependent resistance [29]. In a recent study by Rocca *et al.* [30], aspirin 100 mg administered twice daily corrected the observed variability in recovery of platelet COX activity. Another small, but elegant, study showed that twice daily dosing significantly reduced platelet function parameters (LTA, VerifyNow Aspirin, and serum thromboxane levels) compared to once daily dosing in patients with type 2 diabetes (a condition known to have higher rates of platelet turnover [30, 31]) and stable CAD [32].

Heightened basal platelet reactivity

Mechanism: Baseline platelet hyperactivity appears to be a strong indicator of posttreatment residual platelet activity [33]. Platelets play a critical role in the pathogenesis and the evolution of ACS, and heightened platelet reactivity contributes directly to thrombus formation in this setting. Indeed, patients experiencing acute MI have increased rates of aspirin resistance [34]. Other systemic or cardiac perturbations including major cardiovascular surgery may place patients at heightened risk of aspirin resistance in the perioperative period [35].

General management considerations

In select patients, dose escalation may be a viable option in order to overcome resistance that is occurring in a particular setting (ACS, cardiovascular surgery). Aspirin dose escalation has been investigated in the Aspirin-Induced Platelet Effect (ASPECT) study, a double-blind, double-crossover randomized controlled trial of 125 patients with stable CAD, testing different doses (81, 162, and 325 mg daily) and incremental platelet inhibition [36]. Resistance rates using AA-induced LTA in this study were markedly low (ranging from 0% to 6%) across all doses evaluated. Dose-dependent effects were however noted in platelet function parameters that did not rely on AA stimulation [36]. Other approaches have also recently been proposed. We recently reported the effects of omega-3 fatty acid supplementation in overcoming resistance in patients with stable CAD [37]. All baseline aspirin-resistant patients (on low-dose therapy) were randomized to low-dose aspirin plus omega-3 fatty acids versus dose escalation (with aspirin 325 mg daily). Both strategies appeared to equally improve platelet sensitivity to aspirin and reduce platelet reactivity after 30 days [37]. Augmentation of aspirin with other antiplatelet agents may be another potential avenue of therapy. In a prospective study of aspirin-resistant patients with stable CAD, identified by PFA-100, continuation of clopidogrel therapy for an additional 12 months significantly reduced the rates of major adverse cardiovascular events [38]. Finally, in low-risk patients undergoing elective PCI, the addition of tirofiban in aspirin-resistant patients at presentation lowered the risk of postprocedural MI [39]. Despite these hypothesis-generating studies, the definitive role of augmentation with clopidogrel or other novel P2Y12 inhibitors to aspirin is yet to be determined and requires further investigation.

Conclusions

Aspirin is a time-honored agent that has an important role in secondary prevention of cardiovascular disease. Despite this widely recognized benefit, a substantial percentage of patients have suboptimal responses to aspirin therapy. This laboratory finding, known as "aspirin resistance," has emerged as an entity with clinical significance in recent years. No consensus definition exists to help characterize and delimit this patient subset. Due to this poor definition, the estimated prevalence of aspirin resistance ranges from less than 1% to over 60%. Aspirin resistance is associated with a three- to fourfold increased risk of major adverse cardiovascular events in patients with stable CAD. The specific mechanisms that may contribute to aspirin resistance are likely multifactorial but may include poor compliance, improper dosing, gut malabsorption, genetic polymorphisms, drug–drug interactions, increased platelet turnover, and heightened basal platelet activity. Targeted approaches to the management of aspirin-resistant patients are currently being tested in the clinical and research settings. In general, the use of various strategies should continue to address the balance between further reduction in ischemic events and bleeding risks. Strategies should be targeted and tailored based on the patient's likely cause of resistance. Matching the patient's clinical scenario with an appropriate intervention will be essential for therapeutic success.

References

1 Roger, V.L., Go, A.S., Lloyd-Jones, D.M. *et al.* (2012) Heart disease and stroke statistics—2012 update: a report from the American Heart Association. *Circulation*, **125**, e2–e220.

2 Seshasai, S.R., Wijesuriya, S., Sivakumaran, R. *et al.* (2012) Effect of aspirin on vascular and nonvascular outcomes: meta-analysis of randomized controlled trials. *Archives of Internal Medicine*, **172**, 209–216.

3 Antiplatelet Trialists' Collaboration (1994) Collaborative overview of randomised trials of antiplatelet therapy—I: prevention of death, myocardial infarction, and stroke by prolonged antiplatelet therapy in various categories of patients. *BMJ*, **308**, 81–106.

4 Smith, S.C., Jr, Allen, J., Blair, S.N. *et al.* (2006) AHA/ACC guidelines for secondary prevention for patients with coronary and other atherosclerotic vascular disease: 2006 update: endorsed by the National Heart, Lung, and Blood Institute. *Circulation*, **113**, 2363–2372.

5 Kushner, F.G., Hand, M., Smith, S.C., Jr *et al.* (2009) 2009 focused updates: ACC/AHA guidelines for the management of patients with ST-elevation myocardial infarction (updating the 2004 guideline and 2007 focused update) and ACC/AHA/SCAI guidelines on percutaneous coronary intervention (updating the 2005 guideline and 2007 focused update) a report of the American College of Cardiology Foundation/American Heart Association Task Force on Practice Guidelines. *Journal of the American College of Cardiology*, **54**, 2205–2241.

6 Bonello, L., Tantry, U.S., Marcucci, R. *et al.* (2010) Consensus and future directions on the definition of high on-treatment platelet reactivity to adenosine diphosphate. *Journal of the American College of Cardiology*, **56**, 919–933.

7 Cattaneo, M. (2011) Resistance to anti-platelet agents. *Thrombosis Research*, **127** (Suppl 3), S61–S63.

8 Gasparyan, A.Y., Watson, T., and Lip, G.Y. (2008) The role of aspirin in cardiovascular prevention: implications of aspirin resistance. *Journal of the American College of Cardiology*, **51**, 1829–1843.

9 Maree, A.O. and Fitzgerald, D.J. (2007) Variable platelet response to aspirin and clopidogrel in atherothrombotic disease. *Circulation*, **115**, 2196–2207.

10 Lordkipanidze, M., Pharand, C., Schampaert, E. *et al.* (2007) A comparison of six major platelet function tests to determine the prevalence of aspirin resistance in patients with stable coronary artery disease. *European Heart Journal*, **28**, 1702–1708.

11 Gremmel, T., Steiner, S., Seidinger, D., Koppensteiner, R., Panzer, S., and Kopp, C.W. (2011) Comparison of methods to evaluate aspirin-mediated platelet inhibition after percutaneous intervention with stent implantation. *Platelets*, **22**, 188–195.

12 Krasopoulos, G., Brister, S.J., Beattie, W.S., and Buchanan, M.R. (2008) Aspirin "resistance" and risk of cardiovascular morbidity: systematic review and meta-analysis. *BMJ*, **336**, 195–198.

13 Snoep, J.D., Hovens, M.M., Eikenboom, J.C., van der Bom, J.G., and Huisman, M.V. (2007) Association of laboratory-defined aspirin resistance with a higher risk of recurrent cardiovascular events: a systematic review and meta-analysis. *Archives of Internal Medicine*, **167**, 1593–1599.

14 Sofi, F., Marcucci, R., Gori, A.M., Abbate, R., and Gensini, G.F. (2008) Residual platelet reactivity on aspirin therapy and recurrent cardiovascular events—a meta-analysis. *International Journal of Cardiology*, **128**, 166–171.

15 Schwartz, K.A., Schwartz, D.E., Barber, K., Reeves, M., and De Franco, A.C. (2008) Non-compliance is the predominant cause of aspirin resistance in chronic coronary arterial disease patients. *Journal of Translational Medicine*, **6**, 46.

16 Biondi-Zoccai, G.G., Lotrionte, M., Agostoni, P. *et al.* (2006) A systematic review and meta-analysis on the hazards of discontinuing or not adhering to aspirin among 50,279 patients at risk for coronary artery disease. *European Heart Journal*, **27**, 2667–2674.

17 Schwartz, K.A., Schwartz, D.E., Ghosheh, K., Reeves, M.J., Barber, K., and DeFranco, A. (2005) Compliance as a critical consideration in patients who appear to be resistant to aspirin after healing of myocardial infarction. *The American Journal of Cardiology*, **95**, 973–975.

18 von Pape, K.W., Strupp, G., Bonzel, T., and Bohner, J. (2005) Effect of compliance and dosage adaptation of long term aspirin on platelet function with PFA-100 in patients after myocardial infarction. *Thrombosis and Haemostasis*, **94**, 889–891.

19 Lepantalo, A., Mikkelsson, J., Resendiz, J.C. *et al.* (2006) Polymorphisms of COX-1 and GPVI associate with the antiplatelet effect of aspirin in coronary artery disease patients. *Thrombosis and Haemostasis*, **95**, 253–259.

20 Faraday, N., Yanek, L.R., Mathias, R. *et al.* (2007) Heritability of platelet responsiveness to aspirin in activation pathways directly and indirectly related to cyclooxygenase-1. *Circulation*, **115**, 2490–2496.

21 Mathias, R.A., Kim, Y., Sung, H. *et al.* (2010) A combined genome-wide linkage and association approach to find susceptibility loci for platelet function phenotypes in European American and African American families with coronary artery disease. *BMC Medical Genomics*, **3**, 22.

22 Rao, G.H., Johnson, G.G., Reddy, K.R., and White, J.G. (1983) Ibuprofen protects platelet cyclooxygenase from irreversible inhibition by aspirin. *Arteriosclerosis*, **3**, 383–388.

23 Picot, D., Loll, P.J. and Garavito, R.M. (1994) The x-ray crystal structure of the membrane protein prostaglandin H2 synthase-1. *Nature*, **367**, 243–249.

24 Dunn S.P., Macaulay TE. (2011) Drug-drug interactions associated with antiplatelet therapy. *Cardiovascular & Hematological Agents in Medicinal Chemistry*, **9**, 231–240.

25 Ellison, J. and Dager, W. (2007) Recent FDA warning of the concomitant use of aspirin and ibuprofen and the effects on platelet aggregation. *Preventive Cardiology*, **10**, 61–63.

26 Di Minno, G., Silver, M.J., and Murphy, S. (1983) Monitoring the entry of new platelets into the circulation after ingestion of aspirin. *Blood*, **61**, 1081–1085.

27 Guthikonda, S., Lev, E.I., Patel, R. *et al.* (2007) Reticulated platelets and uninhibited COX-1 and COX-2 decrease the antiplatelet effects of aspirin. *Journal of Thrombosis and Haemostasis*, **5**, 490–496.

28 Guthikonda, S., Alviar, C.L., Vaduganathan, M. *et al.* (2008) Role of reticulated platelets and platelet size heterogeneity on platelet activity after dual antiplatelet therapy with aspirin and clopidogrel in patients with stable coronary artery disease. *Journal of the American College of Cardiology*, **52**, 743–749.

29 Henry, P., Vermillet, A., Boval, B. *et al.* (2011) 24-hour time-dependent aspirin efficacy in patients with stable coronary artery disease. *Thrombosis and Haemostasis*, **105**, 336–344.

30 Rocca, B., Santilli, F., Pitocco, D. *et al.* (2012) The recovery of platelet cyclooxygenase activity explains interindividual variability in responsiveness to low-dose aspirin in patients with and without diabetes. *Journal of Thrombosis and Haemostasis*, **10**, 1220–1230.

31 Lordkipanidze, M. and Harrison, P. (2012) Aspirin twice a day keeps new COX-1 at bay. *Journal of Thrombosis and Haemostasis*, **10**, 1217–1219.

32 Capodanno, D., Patel, A., Dharmashankar, K. *et al.* (2011) Pharmacodynamic effects of different aspirin dosing regimens in type 2 diabetes mellitus patients with coronary artery disease. *Circulation. Cardiovascular Interventions*, **4**, 180–187.

33 Frelinger, A.L., 3rd, Furman, M.I., Linden, M.D. *et al.* (2006) Residual arachidonic acid-induced platelet activation via an adenosine diphosphate-dependent but cyclooxygenase-1- and cyclooxygenase-2-independent pathway: a 700-patient study of aspirin resistance. *Circulation*, **113**, 2888–2896.

34 Poulsen, T.S., Jorgensen, B., Korsholm, L., Licht, P.B., Haghfelt, T. and Mickley, H. (2007) Prevalence of aspirin resistance in patients with an evolving acute myocardial infarction. *Thrombosis Research*, **119**, 555–562.

35 Lev, E.I., Ramchandani, M., Garg, R. *et al.* (2007) Response to aspirin and clopidogrel in patients scheduled to undergo cardiovascular surgery. *Journal of Thrombosis and Thrombolysis*, **24**, 15–21.

36 Gurbel, P.A., Bliden, K.P., DiChiara, J. *et al.* (2007) Evaluation of dose-related effects of aspirin on platelet function: results from the Aspirin-Induced Platelet Effect (ASPECT) study. *Circulation*, **115**, 3156–3164.

37 Lev, E.I., Solodky, A., Harel, N. *et al.* (2010) Treatment of aspirin-resistant patients with omega-3 fatty acids versus aspirin dose escalation. *Journal of the American College of Cardiology*, **55**, 114–121.

38 Pamukcu, B., Oflaz, H., Onur, I. *et al.* (2007) Clinical relevance of aspirin resistance in patients with stable coronary artery disease: a prospective follow-up study (PROSPECTAR). *Blood Coagulation and Fibrinolysis*, **18**, 187–192.

39 Campo, G., Fileti, L., de Cesare, N. *et al.* (2010) Long-term clinical outcome based on aspirin and clopidogrel responsiveness status after elective percutaneous coronary intervention: a 3T/2R (tailoring treatment with tirofiban in patients showing resistance to aspirin and/or resistance to clopidogrel) trial substudy. *Journal of the American College of Cardiology*, **56**, 1447–1455.

34 Clopidogrel Resistance

Udaya S. Tantry[1], Kevin P. Bliden[1], Talha Meeran[1,2], and Paul A. Gurbel[1,2]

[1]Sinai Hospital of Baltimore, Baltimore, MD, USA
[2]Johns Hopkins University School of Medicine, Baltimore, MD, USA

Overwhelming evidence exists that the adenosine diphosphate (ADP) $P2Y_{12}$ receptor interaction plays a pivotal role in platelet-rich thrombus generation at the sites of plaque rupture and subsequent ischemic event occurrence in patients with coronary artery disease (CAD). Based on the demonstration of superior efficacy associated with dual antiplatelet therapy of clopidogrel and aspirin in various large-scale clinical trials conducted in high-risk CAD patients, a nonselective or "one-size-fits-all" treatment approach is used by most physicians. Since its first approval in 1997, clopidogrel has revolutionized interventional cardiology and transformed therapy for acute coronary syndrome (ACS)- and percutaneous coronary intervention (PCI)-treated patients [1]. However, a large body of data from observational studies indicates that clopidogrel therapy is associated with major pharmacodynamic (PD) limitations including unpredictable and overall modest effects that have been linked to post-PCI ischemic event occurrence, including stent thrombosis (ST) [2].

Platelets are activated by multiple pathways, and thrombotic event occurrence is influenced by multiple factors in addition to platelet activation and aggregation. Therefore, a single antiplatelet treatment strategy directed against a specific receptor cannot be expected to overcome all thrombotic event occurrences. Therefore, clinical treatment failure (occurrence of an ischemic event) during clopidogrel treatment is not synonymous with clopidogrel resistance. The optimal definition of resistance or nonresponsiveness (a PD property) to any antiplatelet agent should be the failure of the antiplatelet agent to inhibit the target of its action [3]. The identification of resistance should therefore utilize a laboratory technique that detects the activity of the target receptor before and after administration of the specific antiplatelet agent. For example, the absence of a change in platelet response to ADP from baseline to after clopidogrel administration is an indicator of clopidogrel resistance [3].

Antiplatelet Therapy in Cardiovascular Disease, First Edition. Edited by Ron Waksman, Paul A. Gurbel, and Michael A. Gaglia, Jr.
© 2014 John Wiley & Sons, Ltd. Published 2014 by John Wiley & Sons, Ltd.

The unpredictable antiplatelet response to clopidogrel was reported nearly a decade ago using conventional platelet aggregometry and flow cytometry in patients undergoing PCI who had received a 300 mg loading dose followed by 75 mg daily maintenance dose. In this study, there was a negligible (≤10% absolute change from baseline) or no antiplatelet effect in a significant percentage of patients. The latter phenomenon was defined as clopidogrel "resistance" or "nonresponsiveness" to clopidogrel therapy [4]. Similar observations have been made in numerous subsequent studies utilizing various laboratory methods to assess platelet reactivity to ADP such as turbidimetric aggregation, flow cytometry to measure platelet surface P-selectin and activated GPIIb/IIIa expression and vasodilator-stimulated phosphoprotein phosphorylation levels, and point-of-care methods (VerifyNow P2Y12 assay, platelet mapping with thrombelastography, and Multiplate analyzer). It was also demonstrated that clopidogrel resistance was dependent on the dose and timing of *ex vivo* platelet function measurements in relation to dose administration and performance of the stent procedure [2].

Given the interindividual variability in baseline ADP-induced platelet aggregation, the measurement of clopidogrel responsiveness (absolute or relative changes in platelet aggregation from baseline) may overestimate ischemic risk in nonresponders with low pretreatment reactivity as well as underestimate risk in responders who remain with high platelet reactivity (HPR) after treatment [3]. Therefore, the absolute level of platelet reactivity during treatment (i.e., on-treatment platelet reactivity) has been proposed as a better measure of thrombotic risk than responsiveness to clopidogrel.

Evidence for a threshold of posttreatment platelet reactivity (high on-treatment platelet reactivity) associated with long-term ischemic events

In the earliest study linking on-treatment platelet reactivity to ADP and the occurrence of postdischarge ischemic events following stenting, a threshold of approximately 50% periprocedural platelet aggregation in response to 20 μM ADP was associated with a 6-month ischemic event occurrence [5]. Subsequent translational research studies conducted worldwide involving thousands of patients utilizing multiple laboratory tests have reached the identical conclusion: patients treated with PCI who have high on-treatment platelet reactivity (HPR) are at increased risk for both short-term and long-term post-PCI ischemic event occurrences, including ST [2]. These studies have primarily used a single measurement of reactivity determined either immediately before PCI or at the time of hospital discharge. A recent consensus statement proposed HPR cutoff values based on receiver operating characteristic curve analysis for different platelet function assays (Table 34.1) [6, 7, 8, 9].

Table 34.1 Studies linking high on-treatment platelet reactivity (HPR) to adenosine diphosphate (ADP) to ischemic events based on a receiver operating characteristic curve with a specific cutoff value.

Study	Assay	Cutoff value
Price et al. [6] Stone et al. [11]	VerifyNow assay	>208 PRU
Sibbing et al. [7]	Multiplate analyzer	>468 AU*min
Gurbel et al. [8]	LTA	>46% 5 μM ADP
		>59% 20 μM ADP
Bonello et al. [9]	VASP-PRI	>50% PRI

ADP, adenosine diphosphate; AU, aggregation units; LTA, light transmittance aggregometry; MACE, major adverse clinical events; MI, myocardial infarction; NA, not addressed: PCI, percutaneous coronary intervention; PRU, P2Y12 reaction units; VASP-PRI, vasodilatorstimulated phosphoprotein – platelet reactivity index.

In a time-covariate Cox regression analysis of on-treatment platelet reactivity in the Gauging Responsiveness with A VerifyNow Assay – Impact on Thrombosis And Safety (GRAVITAS) study, HPR to ADP defined as a P2Y12 reaction units (PRU) greater than 208 was an independent predictor of event-free survival at 60 days (hazard ratio (HR) [95% CI] = 0.23 [0.05–0.98], $p = 0.047$) and strongly trended to be an independent predictor at 6 months (HR [95% CI] = 0.54 [0.28–1.04], $p = 0.06$) [6,10]. In the recently presented Assessment of Dual Antiplatelet Therapy With Drug-Eluting Stents (ADAPT-DES) trial that included higher-risk population (~50% had ACS), those patients with greater than 208 PRU (42.5%) had a 3-fold adjusted hazard (95% CI = 1.39, 6.49, $p = 0.005$) for 30-day ST and a 2.49 adjusted hazard for 1-year ST (95% CI = 1.43, 4.31, $p = 0.001$) [11]. Finally, in a recent meta-analysis of 20 observational studies comprising a total number of 9187 PCI patients, HPR (>208) was demonstrated to be a strong predictor of myocardial infarction (MI), ST, and the composite end point of reported ischemic events (HR [95% CI] = 3.00 [2.26–3.99], 4.14 [2.74–6.25], and 4.95 [3.34–7.34], respectively, $P < 0.00001$ for all cases). Furthermore, the predicted risk for CV death, MI, or ST was not heterogeneous (I^2, 0%, 0%, and 12%, respectively; $p =$ not significant for all cases) despite large differences in the methodology and in the definition of HPR between studies [12].

In medically managed unstable angina or NSTEMI patients who were randomly assigned to treatment with either clopidogrel or prasugrel in the TRILOGY-PFS [13], platelet reactivity and HPR (>208 PRU) significantly correlated with a higher risk of ischemic event occurrence, but this relationship did not persist after multivariable adjustment. The prevalence of HPR (>208) during clopidogrel therapy was about 50% during the 30-month treatment period. Since on-treatment PRU values were not strongly associated with ischemic outcomes in this study, the mechanism of recurrent thrombotic event occurrence in medically managed ACS patients may differ from PCI-treated patients where the recurrent ischemic event occurrences are strongly influenced by intensified P2Y$_{12}$ inhibition.

Mechanisms responsible for clopidogrel nonresponsiveness

Multiple lines of evidence strongly suggest that variable and insufficient active metabolite generation is the primary explanations for clopidogrel response variability and nonresponsiveness, respectively [14]. Variable levels of active metabolite generation following clopidogrel administration could be explained by (i) variable or limited intestinal absorption that may be influenced by *ABCB1* gene polymorphism and (ii) functional variability in P450 isoenzyme activity that is influenced by drug–drug interactions (DDI) and single nucleotide polymorphisms (SNPs) in genes encoding CYP450 isoenzymes [14].

Numerous studies have evaluated the influence of SNPs of the gene encoding CY2C19 as well as SNPs of the P-glycoprotein transporter (ABCB1) gene on clopidogrel response variability and clinical outcomes. The most widely analyzed and most frequent SNPs are *CYP2C19*2 (loss-of-function or LoF allele)* associated with complete absence of enzyme activity and **17 (gain-of-function or GoF allele)* associated with increased expression and enzymatic activity [15, 16]. Less plasma clopidogrel active metabolite exposure (34% relative reduction, $p < 0.001$) and less platelet inhibition (9% absolute reduction from baseline, $p < 0.001$) were demonstrated in healthy carriers of at least one *CY2C19 LoF* allele compared to noncarriers [15]. It was reported that, although both **2* and **17* allele carriage influence ADP-induced platelet aggregation, the influence of **2* is more pronounced in patients undergoing stenting during maintenance therapy [17]. In the first genome-wide association study, conducted in healthy Amish subjects, *CYP2C19*2* was the only SNP associated with clopidogrel response variability and accounted for only 12% of the variation in platelet aggregation to ADP after clopidogrel treatment. In a replication study of PCI patients, carriers of the *CYP2C19*2* allele had a approximately 2.4× higher cardiovascular event rate compared with noncarriers [15]. In a collaborative meta-analysis of various clinical trials involving primarily patients who underwent PCI (91%), there was an increased risk of the composite end point occurrence of CV death, MI, or stroke among carriers of 1 *LoF* allele (1.6×) and also carriers of 2 *LoF* alleles (1.8×) as compared with noncarriers. A significantly increased risk of ST in both carriers of 1 *LoF* allele (2.7×) and 2 *LoF* alleles (4×) as compared with noncarriers was also observed [18].

Subsequent retrospective analyses of trials involving non-PCI patients failed to demonstrate a significant association between *CYP2C19 LoF* allele carriage and adverse clinical outcomes. The relation of the GoF allele (*CYP2C19*17*) carrier status and *ABCB1* genotype to antiplatelet response and clinical outcomes in clopidogrel-treated patients is inconclusive at this time [19, 20]. Taken together, *LoF* allele carrier status is an important independent predictor of the PD response to clopidogrel and the outcomes of high-risk clopidogrel-treated patients who have undergone PCI. In 2009, the FDA noted that healthcare professionals should be aware that tests are available to determine genotype and that the antiplatelet response in poor metabolizers is increased by high-dose clopidogrel. The FDA also recommended the use of other antiplatelet medications or alternative dosing strategies for clopidogrel in poor metabolizers [21].

Finally, it should be noted that the CYP2C19 isoenzyme is not the only factor determining the antiplatelet response to clopidogrel, as even in poor metabolizers, some degree of platelet inhibition has been observed where no enzyme activity is expected [16]. The stimulation of CYP3A4 activity by rifampin and St. John's wort (SJW) and CYP1A2 activity by tobacco smoking has been shown to enhance platelet inhibition induced by clopidogrel [22]. The effect of smoking on the antiplatelet effect of clopidogrel has been associated with clinical outcomes and may, in part, explain the "smoker's paradox" [22]. Conversely, agents that compete with clopidogrel for CYP and/or inhibit CYP attenuate the antiplatelet effect of clopidogrel. A diminished PD response to clopidogrel has been observed with the coadministration of proton pump inhibitors (PPIs) such as omeprazole, lipophilic statins, and calcium channel blockers (CCB) that are metabolized by the CYP2C19 and CYP3A4 isoenzymes [22]. Although a diminished level of platelet inhibition induced by clopidogrel has been demonstrated in some ex vivo studies following the coadministration of these agents, the consequence of these interactions with respect to the risk for ischemic event occurrence remains controversial. In addition to the aforementioned mechanisms explaining clopidogrel PD variability, old age, increased body mass index (BMI), renal insufficiency, diabetes mellitus, and ACS have also been associated with a diminished antiplatelet response to clopidogrel [23]. Finally, noncompliance is an obvious factor that must be excluded in the diagnosis of clopidogrel nonresponsiveness. When attempting to define causality for HPR related to the occurrence of clinical events in patients receiving clopidogrel, all of the aforementioned mechanisms should be considered (Figure 34.1) [23].

Conclusions

Currently, clopidogrel response variability and nonresponsiveness are widely accepted phenomena, and HPR during clopidogrel therapy is an established risk factor in high-risk PCI patients for recurrent ischemic event occurrence. It was clearly demonstrated that treatment with high-dose clopidogrel (600 mg loading dose plus 150 mg maintenance dose) is not an optimal strategy to overcome HPR and to reduce recurrent ischemic event occurrence. Treatment with more potent $P2Y_{12}$ receptor

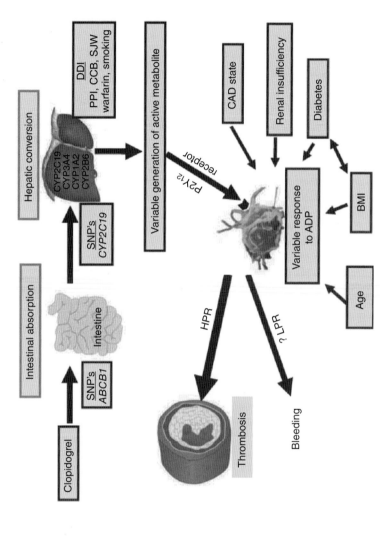

Figure 34.1 Various factors influencing platelet reactivity and clinical outcome during clopidogrel therapy. BMI, body mass index; CAD, coronary artery disease; CCB, calcium channel blocker; DDI, drug–drug interactions; HPR, high platelet reactivity; LPR, low platelet reactivity; PPIs, proton pump inhibitors; SJW, St. John's wort; SNP, single nucleotide polymorphism. (Source: Gurbel PA et al., 2012 [23]. Reproduced with permission of Oxford University Press.)

blockers, such as prasugrel and ticagrelor, is associated with faster and greater platelet inhibition than clopidogrel therapy and is a credible alternative strategy to overcome HPR during clopidogrel therapy. However, recent data indicate that prasugrel therapy is also associated with nonresponsiveness (although <10%). Finally, the demonstration of clopidogrel response variability was the foundation for personalized antiplatelet therapy based on objective platelet function testing and genetic analyses.

References

1 Gurbel, P.A. and Tantry, U.S. (2010) Combination antithrombotic therapies. *Circulation*, **121**, 569–583.

2 Bonello, L., Tantry, U.S., Marcucci, R. *et al.* (2010) Consensus and future directions on the definition of high on treatment platelet reactivity to adenosine diphosphate. *Journal of the American College of Cardiology*, **56**, 919–933.

3 Gurbel, P.A., Becker, R.C., Mann, K.G., Steinhubl, S.R., and Michelson, A.D. (2007) Platelet function monitoring in patients with coronary artery disease. *Journal of the American College of Cardiology*, **50**, 1822–1834.

4 Gurbel, P.A., Bliden, K.P., Hiatt, B.L., and O'Connor, C.M. (2003) Clopidogrel for coronary stenting: response variability, drug resistance, and the effect of pretreatment platelet reactivity. *Circulation*, **107**, 2908–2913.

5 Gurbel, P.A., Bliden, K.P., Guyer, K. *et al.* (2005) Platelet reactivity in patients and recurrent events post-stenting: results of the PREPARE POSTSTENTING Study. *Journal of the American College of Cardiology*, **46**, 1820–1826.

6 Price, M.J., Endemann, S., Gollapudi, R.R. *et al.* (2008) Prognostic significance of post-clopidogrel platelet reactivity assessed by a point-of-care assay on thrombotic events after drug-eluting stent implantation. *European Heart Journal*, **29**, 992–1000.

7 Sibbing, D., Morath, T., Braun, S. *et al.* (2010) Clopidogrel response status assessed with Multiplate point-of-care analysis and the incidence and timing of stent thrombosis over six months following coronary stenting. *Thrombosis and Haemostasis*, **103**, 151–159.

8 Gurbel, P.A., Antonino, M.J., Bliden, K.P. *et al.* (2008) Platelet reactivity to adenosine diphosphate and long-term ischemic event occurrence following percutaneous coronary intervention: a potential antiplatelet therapeutic target. *Platelets*, **19**, 595–604.

9 Bonello, L., Paganelli, F., Arpin-Bornet, M. *et al.* (2007) Vasodilator-stimulated phosphoprotein phosphorylation analysis prior to percutaneous coronary intervention for exclusion of postprocedural major adverse cardiovascular events. *Journal of Thrombosis and Haemostasis*, **5**, 1630–1636.

10 Price, M.J., Berger, P.B., Teirstein P.S. et al. (2011) GRAVITAS Investigators. Standard- vs high-dose clopidogrel based on platelet function testing after percutaneous coronary intervention: the GRAVITAS randomized trial. *Journal of American Medical Association*, **305**, 1097–1105.

11 Stone G.W., Witzenbichler B., Weisz G. *et al.* (2013) ADAPT-DES Investigators. Platelet reactivity and clinical outcomes after coronary artery implantation of drug-eluting stents (ADAPT-DES): a prospective multicentre registry study. *Lancet*, **382**, 614–623.

12 Aradi, D., Komócsi, A., Vorobcsuk, A. *et al.* (2010) Prognostic significance of high on-clopidogrel platelet reactivity after percutaneous coronary intervention: systematic review and meta-analysis. *American Heart Journal*, **160**, 543–551.

13 Gurbel, P.A., Erlinge, D., Ohman, E.M. *et al.* (2012) Platelet function during extended prasugrel and clopidogrel therapy for patients with ACS treated without revascularization: The TRILOGY ACS Platelet Function Substudy. *JAMA*, **308**, 1785–1794.

14 Gurbel, P.A. and Tantry, U.S. (2012) Do platelet function testing and genotyping improve outcome in patients treated with antithrombotic agents? Platelet function testing and genotyping improve outcome in patients treated with antithrombotic agents. *Circulation*, **125**, 1276–1287.

15 Mega, J.L., Close, S.L., Wiviott, S.D. *et al.* (2009) Cytochrome p-450 polymorphisms and response to clopidogrel. *The New England Journal of Medicine*, **360**, 354–362.

16 Shuldiner, A.R., O'Connell, J.R., Bliden, K.P. *et al.* (2009) Association of cytochrome P450 2C19 genotype with the antiplatelet effect and clinical efficacy of clopidogrel therapy. *JAMA*, **302**, 849–857.

17 Gurbel, P.A., Shuldiner, A.R., Bliden, K.P., Ryan, K., Pakyz, R.E. and Tantry, U.S. (2011) The relation between CYP2C19 genotype and phenotype in stented patients on maintenance dual antiplatelet therapy. *American Heart Journal*, **161**, 598–604.

18 Simon, T., Verstuyft, C., Mary-Krause, M. *et al.* (2009) Genetic determinants of response to clopidogrel and cardiovascular events. *The New England Journal of Medicine*, **360**, 363–375.

19 Pare, G., Mehta, S.R., Yusuf, S. *et al.* (2010) Effects of CYP2C19 genotype on outcomes of clopidogrel treatment. *The New England Journal of Medicine*, **363**, 1704–1714.

20 Wallentin, L., James, S., Storey, R.F. *et al.* (2010) Effect of CYP2C19and ABCB1 single nucleotide polymorphisms on outcomes of treatment with ticagrelor versus clopidogrel for acute coronary syndromes: a genetic substudy of the plato trial. *Lancet*, **376**, 1320–1328.

21 Plavix package insert. www.Plavix.Com. http://products.sanofi.us/plavix/plavix.html [accessed January 28, 2011]

22 Price, M.J., Tantry, U.S., and Gurbel, P.A. (2011) The influence of CYP2C19 polymorphisms on the pharmacokinetics, pharmacodynamics, and clinical effectiveness of P2Y(12)inhibitors. *Reviews in Cardiovascular Medicine*, **12**, 1–12.

23 Gurbel, P.A., Ohman, E.M., Jeong, Y.H., and Tantry, U.S. (2012) Toward a therapeutic window for antiplatelet therapy in the elderly. *European Heart Journal*, **33**, 1187–1189.

35 Genetics of Clopidogrel Poor Response

Pierre Fontana[1,2] and Jean-Luc Reny[1,2,3]
[1] Geneva Platelet Group, University of Geneva, Geneva, Switzerland
[2] Trois-Chêne Hospital, Geneva, Switzerland
[3] Geneva University Hospitals and Faculty of Medicine (Geneva Platelet Group), Geneva, Switzerland

Introduction

At least one-third of patients treated with clopidogrel display high on-treatment platelet reactivity (HTPR) and are potentially not adequately protected from recurrent major adverse cardiovascular events (MACE) [1]. The prognostic value of HTPR is particularly important in acute coronary syndromes and becomes much less relevant as the clinical condition is more stable [2, 3]. Although some clinically meaningful cutoffs have been consensually suggested for some platelet function assays defining HTPR [4], there remain some uncertainties with regard to the universal value of such cutoffs. Moreover, uncertainties relate also to the platelet function assay to be used since they do not necessarily identify the same patients as having HTPR. A genetic approach to identify patients at risk is thus tempting since fast, cheap, and reliable genotyping is around the corner. Indeed, the important variability of the biological response to clopidogrel is hardly explained by demographic factors [5], while it is believed to be highly heritable ($h^2 = 0.73$) [6], suggesting an important genetic contribution. This has prompted a quest for genetic culprits, starting with a conventional candidate gene approach and evolving to next-generation sequencing strategies.

Candidate gene approach

The first attempt to unravel the genetic basis of clopidogrel response variability was based on the identification of associations between genetic variations within prespecified genes of interest and the biological response to clopidogrel (candidate gene approach). This approach implies thorough knowledge of genes implicated in clopidogrel metabolism including absorption, activation of the prodrug, and degradation [7]. Although

---

Antiplatelet Therapy in Cardiovascular Disease, First Edition. Edited by Ron Waksman, Paul A. Gurbel, and Michael A. Gaglia, Jr.
© 2014 John Wiley & Sons, Ltd. Published 2014 by John Wiley & Sons, Ltd.

Table 35.1 Allelic frequency of common functional alleles of the *CYP2C19* gene.

CYP2C19 variant	Impact of DNA change	Allelic frequency	
		Europeans	Asians
*2 (rs4244285)	Splicing defect	0.12–0.16	0.29
*3 (rs1057910)	Premature stop codon	<0.01	0.04–0.12
*17 (rs12248560)	Increased gene transcription	0.19–0.27	0.01

clopidogrel is on the market for about 15 years, its exact metabolism is not fully understood and represents a field of active research.

Clopidogrel absorption is mediated by the efflux transporter P-glycoprotein (P-gp) that is encoded by the *ABCB1* (*MDR1*) gene [8]. The *ABCB1* gene is highly polymorphic, and one variant (C3435T in exon 26 [rs1045642]) was evaluated in several studies. Although the initial publication clearly showed an association between this latter polymorphism and the pharmacokinetic profile of clopidogrel [8], its association with the recurrence of ischemic cardiovascular events was more mitigated with a recent meta-analysis showing no significant association with clinical events [9].

After the absorption of the prodrug, clopidogrel is exposed to carboxylesterases that hydrolyzed around 85% of the molecule into an inactive carboxyl metabolite. Recent data showed indeed the implication of carboxylesterase 1 as well as a genetic variant (G143E, rs71647871) associated with clopidogrel response [10, 11]. The remaining approximately 15% of the drug absorbed undergoes a two-step oxidation process by hepatic cytochromes P450 (CYPs) resulting in 2-oxo-clopidogrel followed by the opening of the thiophene group to the thiol metabolite. The cis-thiol metabolite inhibits covalently the platelet ADP receptor P2Y12 [12]. Various CYPs are implicated in this activation process including CYP3A4, CYP2C19, CYP2C9, and CYP2B6 [12].

CYP2C19 drew a particular attention due to its relative large contribution in the activation of clopidogrel [12], and carriers of loss-of-function genetic variants in the *CYP2C19* gene have been consistently associated with lower active clopidogrel metabolite levels and diminished platelet inhibition. Table 35.1 summarized the allelic frequency in different populations of various loss- and gain-of-function *CYP2C19* genetic variants [13]. The first description of the impact of a genetic variant of the *CYP2C19* gene on the biological response to clopidogrel was by the publication of Hulot *et al.* [14] and Fontana *et al.* [15] who evaluated the association of the loss-of-function *CYP2C19*2* allele (rs4244285) with platelet reactivity in clopidogrel-treated healthy subjects. When considering the distributions of the platelet response to clopidogrel according to the *CYP2C19*1/*2* status, a large overlap is obvious (Figure 35.1). Thus, based on a 50% VASP assay cutoff [4], a significant proportion of *CYP2C19*2* carriers have an "adequate" response to

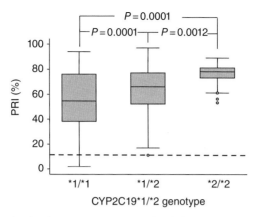

Figure 35.1 Clopidogrel responsiveness as assessed with the VASP assay according to the CYP2C19*1/*2 genotype in 538 clopidogrel-treated patients. (Source: Adapted from Fontana P *et al.*, 2011 [16]. Reproduced with permission of John Wiley & Sons Ltd.). The dotted line represents the 50% cutoff value to define clopidogrel poor responders [4].

clopidogrel, while another important proportion of *CYP2C19*2* noncarriers are clopidogrel poor responders [7, 16]. This reflects the fact that the *CYP2C19*1/*2* genotype has only a minor influence (5–12%) on the pharmacodynamic response to clopidogrel [6, 16, 17, 18, 5]. In the same line, the association between *CYP2C19*2* and the recurrence of ischemic events in clopidogrel-treated patients yielded mitigated results with recent meta-analyses showing a poor predictive value of this polymorphism, mostly related to a small study bias effect and restricted to stent thrombosis [19, 20, 21]. Thus, a strategy of routine antiplatelet drug tailoring according to CYP2C19*1/*2 would be limited to improving the rate of stent thrombosis with the risk of overlooking an important proportion of CYP2C19*2 noncarriers bearing HTPR (false-negatives of genetic testing) who are at increased risk for ischemic events.

The gain-of-function *CYP2C19*17* genetic variant (Table 35.1) is associated with an increased catalytic activity of CYP2C19 due to an increased transcription rate [22] and is thus supposed to be associated with an increased antiplatelet effect that would expose clopidogrel-treated patients to an increased rate of bleeding events. Although there are only few data regarding the biological and clinical impact of this polymorphism, two meta-analyses [21, 23] evidenced that carriers of the *CYP2C19*17* allele had a lower risk of cardiovascular events but an increased risk of bleeding [5].

PON1: Have we found the grail?

In 2011, paraoxonase-1 (PON1), an esterase synthesized in the liver and present in the serum, was reported to be strongly involved in clopidogrel bioactivation [24]. In the same publication, a PON1 genetic variant

(Q192R, rs662, A576G) was reported to account for more than 70% of the variability of clopidogrel responsiveness with the PON1-192Q allele being associated with an increased risk of recurrent ischemic events in clopidogrel-treated patients [24]. However, these associations were recently challenged by the results of several independent studies that showed no influence of the Q192R polymorphism on the biological response to clopidogrel or on the risk of ischemic events, and a meta-analysis suggested that the PON1-Q192R polymorphism had no major impact on the risk of MACE (OR = 1.28 [0.97, 1.68], $p = 0.08$) and did not alter the biological response to clopidogrel [25]. Subsequent *in vitro* studies showed that PON1 only catalyzes the formation of a minor thiol metabolite isomer [16, 26, 27]. Altogether, the PON1-Q192R variant does not account for the variability of the response to clopidogrel.

Genome-wide association studies

Genome-wide association studies (GWAS) search for associations between very large numbers of genetic variants, usually single nucleotide polymorphisms (SNPs), and specific diseases, clinical outcomes, or biological responses. In the field of clopidogrel pharmacogenetics, the first GWAS published by Shuldiner *et al.* confirmed the association of the CYP2C19*2 variant with diminished platelet response to clopidogrel treatment and did not identify in an Amish population any other polymorphism significantly associated with on-clopidogrel platelet reactivity, assessed with ADP-induced platelet aggregation [6]. GWAS have limitations that are inherent to their design. Thus, only a limited, though large, number of SNPs are included in the GWAS (500 K to 1 M arrays in Shuldiner's GWAS and up to 5 M arrays in 2013), thus leaving out most of coding or regulatory DNA regions. As an example, only 8% of the DNA coding for esterases, enzymes potentially involved in the metabolism of clopidogrel, is covered by current DNA arrays (personal communication). In addition, individual GWAS may be limited by the number of participants included, thus restricting the potential for the analysis of various associations of genetic variants through a haplotypic or epistatic approach. The combination of large databases with individual patients' data through an ongoing consortium will certainly help in improving the power of GWAS.

Perspectives and conclusion

Next-generation sequencing, including whole-exome sequencing (WES) and whole-genome sequencing (WGS), may also provide novel findings. WES is based on the capture of protein-coding DNA sequences and has so far been mostly used for the study of rare diseases in related subjects. In multigenic diseases such as cardiovascular diseases and clopidogrel pharmacogenomics, promising results have been communicated by Price *et al.* at the 2012 ACC meeting [28]. WGS has the major advantage of also covering noncoding DNA, which includes regulatory regions upstream or downstream of coding sequences. When it becomes affordable to perform WGS on large populations of patients with a pharmacodynamic evaluation, bioinformatics may help to unravel most of the unknown in the genetically determined response to clopidogrel. This effort will also encompass patients treated with newer anti-P2Y12 drugs for which the paradigm is shifted to the prediction of the bleeding risk. Indeed, patients treated with prasugrel also display a large interindividual variability in their pharmacodynamic response and are overall at greater risk of bleeding.

References

1 Combescure, C., Fontana, P., Mallouk, N. *et al.* (2010) Clinical implications of clopidogrel non-response in cardiovascular patients: a systematic review and meta-analysis. *Journal of Thrombosis and Haemostasis*, **8**, 923–933.

2 Reny, J.L., Berdague, P., Poncet, A. *et al.* (2012) Antiplatelet drug response status does not predict recurrent ischemic events in stable cardiovascular patients: results of the antiplatelet drug resistances and ischemic events study. *Circulation*, **125**, 3201–3210.

3 Cuisset, T., Quilici, J., Loosveld, M. *et al.* (2012) Comparison between initial and chronic response to clopidogrel therapy after coronary stenting for acute coronary syndrome and influence on clinical outcomes. *American Heart Journal*, **164**, 327–333.

4 Bonello, L., Tantry, U.S., Marcucci, R. *et al.* (2010) Consensus and future directions on the definition of high on-treatment platelet reactivity to adenosine diphosphate. *Journal of the American College of Cardiology*, **56**, 919–933.

5 Trenk, D., Kristensen, S.D., Hochholzer, W., and Neumann, F.J. (2013) High on-treatment platelet reactivity and P2Y12 antagonists in clinical trials. *Thrombosis and Haemostasis*, **109 (5)**, 834–845.

6 Shuldiner, A.R., O'Connell, J.R., Bliden, K.P. *et al.* (2009) Association of cytochrome P450 2C19 genotype with the antiplatelet effect and clinical efficacy of clopidogrel therapy. *JAMA*, **302**, 849–857.

7 Ancrenaz, V., Daali, Y., Fontana, P. *et al.* (2010) Impact of genetic polymorphisms and drug-drug interactions on clopidogrel and prasugrel response variability. *Current Drug Metabolism*, **11**, 667–677.

8 Taubert, D., von Beckerath, N., Grimberg, G. *et al.* (2006) Impact of P-glycoprotein on clopidogrel absorption. *Clinical Pharmacology and Therapeutics*, **80**, 486–501.

9 Luo, M., Li, J., Xu, X., Sun, X., and Sheng, W. (2012) ABCB1 C3435T polymorphism and risk of adverse clinical events in clopidogrel treated patients: a meta-analysis. *Thrombosis Research*, **129**, 754–759.

10 Lewis, J.P., Horenstein, R.B., Ryan, K. *et al.* (2013) The functional G143E variant of carboxylesterase 1 is associated with increased clopidogrel active metabolite levels and greater clopidogrel response. *Pharmacogenetics and Genomics*, **23**, 1–8.

11 Zhu, H.J., Wang, X., Gawronski, B., Brinda, B., Angiolillo, D., and Markowitz, J. (2013) Carboxylesterase 1 as a determinant of clopidogrel metabolism and activation. *Journal of Pharmacology and Experimental Therapeutics*, **344 (3)**, 665–672.

12 Kazui, M., Nishiya, Y., Ishizuka, T. *et al.* (2010) Identification of the human cytochrome P450 enzymes involved in the two oxidative steps in the bioactivation of clopidogrel to its pharmacologically active metabolite. *Drug Metabolism and Disposition*, **38**, 92–99.

13 Kurose, K., Sugiyama, E., and Saito, Y. (2012) Population differences in major functional polymorphisms of pharmacokinetics/pharmacodynamics-related genes in Eastern Asians and Europeans: implications in the clinical trials for novel drug development. *Drug Metabolism and Pharmacokinetics*, **27**, 9–54.

14 Hulot, J.S., Bura, A., Villard, E. *et al.* (2006) Cytochrome P450 2C19 loss-of-function polymorphism is a major determinant of clopidogrel responsiveness in healthy subjects. *Blood*, **108**, 2244–2247.

15 Fontana, P., Hulot, J.S., De Moerloose, P., and Gaussem, P. (2007) Influence of CYP2C19 and CYP3A4 gene polymorphisms on clopidogrel responsiveness in healthy subjects. *Journal of Thrombosis and Haemostasis*, **5**, 2153–2155.

16 Fontana, P., James, R., Barazer, I. *et al.* (2011) Relationship between paraoxonase-1 activity, its Q192R genetic variant and clopidogrel responsiveness in the ADRIE study. *Journal of Thrombosis and Haemostasis*, **9**, 1664–1666.

17 Hochholzer, W., Trenk, D., Fromm, M.F. *et al.* (2010) Impact of cytochrome P450 2C19 loss-of-function polymorphism and of major demographic characteristics on residual platelet function after loading and maintenance treatment with clopidogrel in patients undergoing elective coronary stent placement. *Journal of the American College of Cardiology*, **55**, 2427–2434.

18 Bouman, H.J., Harmsze, A.M., van Werkum, J.W. *et al.* (2011) Variability in on-treatment platelet reactivity explained by CYP2C19*2 genotype is modest in clopidogrel pretreated patients undergoing coronary stenting. *Heart*, **97**, 1239–1244.

19 Holmes, M.V., Perel, P., Shah, T., Hingorani, A.D., and Casas, J.P. (2011) CYP2C19 genotype, clopidogrel metabolism, platelet function, and cardiovascular events: a systematic review and meta-analysis. *JAMA*, **306**, 2704–2714.

20 Bauer, T., Bouman, H.J., van Werkum, J.W., Ford, N.F., ten Berg, J.M., and Taubert, D. (2011) Impact of CYP2C19 variant genotypes on clinical efficacy of antiplatelet treatment with clopidogrel: systematic review and meta-analysis. *BMJ*, **343**, d4588.

21 Zabalza, M., Subirana, I., Sala, J. *et al.* (2012) Meta-analyses of the association between cytochrome CYP2C19 loss- and gain-of-function polymorphisms and cardiovascular outcomes in patients with coronary artery disease treated with clopidogrel. *Heart*, **98**, 100–108.

22 Sim, S.C., Risinger, C., Dahl, M.L. *et al.* (2006) A common novel CYP2C19 gene variant causes ultrarapid drug metabolism relevant for the drug response to proton pump inhibitors and antidepressants. *Clinical Pharmacology and Therapeutics*, **79**, 103–113.

23 Li, Y., Tang, H.L., Hu, Y.F., and Xie, H.G. (2012) The gain-of-function variant allele CYP2C19*17: a double-edged sword between thrombosis and bleeding in clopidogrel-treated patients. *Journal of Thrombosis and Haemostasis*, **10**, 199–206.

24 Bouman, H.J., Schomig, E., van Werkum, J.W. *et al.* (2011) Paraoxonase-1 is a major determinant of clopidogrel efficacy. *Nature Medicine*, **17**, 110–116.

25 Reny, J.L., Combescure, C., Daali, Y., and Fontana, P. (2012) Influence of the paraoxonase-1 Q192R genetic variant on clopidogrel responsiveness and

recurrent cardiovascular events: a systematic review and meta-analysis. *Journal of Thrombosis and Haemostasis*, **10**, 1242–1251.

26 Dansette, P.M., Rosi, J., Bertho, G., and Mansuy, D. (2012) Cytochromes P450 catalyze both steps of the major pathway of clopidogrel bioactivation, whereas paraoxonase catalyzes the formation of a minor thiol metabolite isomer. *Chemical Research in Toxicology*, **25**, 348–356.

27 Ancrenaz, V., Desmeules, J., James, R. *et al.* (2012) The paraoxonase-1 pathway is not a major bioactivation pathway of clopidogrel in vitro. *British Journal of Pharmacology*, **166**, 2362–2370.

28 Price, M.F., Carson, A.R., Murray, S.S. *et al.* (2012) First pharmacogenomic analysis using whole exome sequencing to identify novel Genetic determinants of clopidogrel response variability: results of the Genotype Information and Functional Testing (GIFT) exome study. *Journal of the American College of Cardiology*, **59**, E9.

36 Proton Pump Inhibitors and Clopidogrel

Michael A. Gaglia, Jr

University of Southern California Keck School of Medicine, Los Angeles, CA, USA

Introduction

Dual antiplatelet therapy (DAPT) with aspirin and a P2Y12 receptor inhibitor, often clopidogrel, is indicated for patients with an acute coronary syndrome (ACS) or undergoing percutaneous coronary intervention [1, 2]. This places such patients, however, at considerably higher risk of gastrointestinal (GI) bleeding [3, 4]. Concurrent proton pump inhibitor (PPI) therapy is thus recommended for most patients on DAPT [5], as this strategy has been shown to reduce the incidence of GI bleeding and ulcers [6, 7].

The US Food and Drug Administration (FDA), however, issued a statement in November 2009, recommending against the administration of clopidogrel with the PPIs omeprazole and esomeprazole [8]. This was largely based upon pharmacokinetic studies of clopidogrel and omeprazole, which showed that concurrent administration increased the levels of platelet reactivity when compared to clopidogrel alone [9]. This spawned considerable controversy; retrospective studies were inconclusive in regard to an increased risk of adverse cardiac events, and the randomized Clopidogrel and the Optimization of Gastrointestinal Events Trial (COGENT) showed no clinically apparent interaction [7]. This chapter reviews the pharmacokinetic, pharmacodynamic, and clinical evidence for, and against, this interaction between clopidogrel and PPIs.

Metabolism of clopidogrel and proton pump inhibitors

Clopidogrel, a thienopyridine, acts by irreversibly binding the P2Y12 adenosine diphosphate receptor on the surface of platelets, ultimately attenuating platelet activation. The majority of clopidogrel is hydrolyzed by esterases to an inactive compound, whereas the remainder requires activation by the cytochrome P450 (CYP) system in the liver.

Antiplatelet Therapy in Cardiovascular Disease, First Edition. Edited by Ron Waksman, Paul A. Gurbel, and Michael A. Gaglia, Jr.
© 2014 John Wiley & Sons, Ltd. Published 2014 by John Wiley & Sons, Ltd.

Importantly, this generation of the active metabolite involves a two-step pathway that consists of the CYP isoenzymes 3A4 and 2C19 [10, 11, 12, 13]. The latter pathway appears to be the most important, as carriers of the reduced function allele of 2C19 (the so-called poor metabolizers) generate less active metabolite and have reduced levels of platelet inhibition [14].

PPIs inhibit the H^+/K^+ ATPase of gastric parietal cells, which results in decreased production of gastric acid. PPIs are also prodrugs, but they are converted to an active sulfenamide derivative in nonenzymatic fashion [15]. The CYP system converts PPIs via 3A4 and 2C19 to inactive metabolites, with 2C19 again playing a key role. The affinity of different PPIs for CYP2C19, however, appears to vary, with omeprazole having the highest affinity [16]. The metabolism of PPIs is relevant because they are in essence competitive inhibitors of CYP2C19. Given that clopidogrel has less affinity than PPIs for CYP2C19, it is at least plausible that an interaction may occur [17]. Therefore, in the presence of a PPI that is a strong inhibitor of CYP2C19 (e.g., omeprazole), the metabolism of clopidogrel might be reduced.

Pharmacodynamic studies of clopidogrel and proton pump inhibitors

Evidence from pharmacodynamic studies generally supports the conclusion that certain PPIs reduce *ex vivo* platelet inhibition in subjects taking clopidogrel, although the studies are quite heterogeneous. A recent systematic review by Focks *et al.* counted 28 pharmacokinetic studies examining the interaction, with 18 studies demonstrating reduced platelet inhibition in at least one platelet function test in those on clopidogrel and a PPI [18].

Two recent randomized, crossover design studies, albeit in healthy volunteers, examined the effects of different PPIs upon the pharmacokinetics and pharmacodynamics of clopidogrel. Angiolillo *et al.* found that omeprazole decreased the levels of the active metabolite of clopidogrel and increased the levels of platelet aggregation, as measured by both light transmission aggregometry and vasodilator-stimulated phosphoprotein phosphorylation. Furthermore, these effects did not vary significantly when clopidogrel and omeprazole doses were separated by 12 h. Pantoprazole resulted in a less dramatic, but still significant, reduction in the active metabolite; it had inconclusive effects upon platelet aggregation [9]. Similarly, Frelinger *et al.* showed that among CYP2C19 "extensive metabolizers," omeprazole and esomeprazole increased the levels of platelet aggregation; lansoprazole and dexlansoprazole did not. All PPIs reduced the peak levels of the active metabolite of clopidogrel, but omeprazole had the most pronounced effect [19]. It thus appears that all PPIs likely have some degree of interaction with clopidogrel as measured by *ex vivo* assays, but the effect is most pronounced with omeprazole and esomeprazole.

Retrospective clinical studies and meta-analyses

The pharmacokinetic and pharmacodynamic data summarized earlier prompted numerous retrospective data analyses examining the interaction between PPIs and clopidogrel. One of the first, by Pezalla *et al.*, showed an increase of more than 300% in the relative risk of acute myocardial infarction (MI) among patients taking clopidogrel and highly adherent to PPI therapy [20]. This was a relatively small study, however, based upon claims data and with limited adjustment for comorbidities. Larger retrospective studies with multivariable adjustment therefore followed, including one by Ho *et al.* showing an increased risk of death or rehospitalization with concurrent PPI therapy [21] and another by Juurlink *et al.* showing an increased risk of recurrent MI [22].

A large number of retrospective studies were ultimately reported, with widely varying populations, follow-up, methods of multivariable adjustment, and end points. Siller-Matula *et al.* attempted to condense this muddle with a thorough meta-analysis in 2010, which included 24 retrospective studies and the randomized COGENT. The pooled risk ratio for major adverse cardiac events with PPI therapy was 1.29 (95% CI 1.15–1.44, $p < 0.001$) and for MI was 1.31 (95% CI 1.12–1.53, $p < 0.001$).

At least 33 clinical studies assessing the potential interaction between PPIs and clopidogrel were ultimately reported. According to the systematic review by Focks *et al.*, 25 of these studies reported an adjusted incidence of major adverse cardiac events, and 48% showed an increased risk with PPI therapy. Adjusted hazard ratios ranged from 1.20 to 4.58. A pooled risk ratio including only the studies with prospective data collection, however, did not show an increased risk of MACE with PPI therapy [18].

Data from randomized trials of newer P2Y12 inhibitors is also instructive. The PRINCIPLE-TIMI 44 study showed increased levels of platelet aggregation in patients on clopidogrel and a PPI as compared to prasugrel and a PPI; but in the TRITON-TIMI 38 randomized study of prasugrel versus clopidogrel, there was no association of PPIs with cardiovascular death, MI, or stroke in either group [23]. In a prespecified subgroup analysis of the PLATO randomized study of ticagrelor versus clopidogrel, there was an association between PPIs and increased cardiovascular death, MI, and stroke, but this was true for both ticagrelor and clopidogrel [24]. This suggests that PPIs may be a marker for patients at higher risk of cardiovascular events, regardless of clopidogrel therapy. Data available from retrospective studies and meta-analyses, therefore, is at best inconclusive and raises doubt about the clinical relevance of the interaction between PPIs and clopidogrel.

Randomized clinical trials

There are only two randomized trials of the effect of PPI therapy in patients on clopidogrel. The first, however, was a small study by Wu *et al.* of 665 patients with ACS and at increased risk of GI bleeding. This showed a borderline reduction in GI bleeding with pantoprazole (1.2% vs. 3.6%, $p = 0.046$), which was given for only 7 days [25]. There was no effect upon mortality or pneumonia at 30 days, although the study was not powered to assess cardiovascular events.

The randomized COGENT, however, was designed to assess both cardiovascular (death, MI, revascularization, and stroke) and GI (bleeding, ulcers, obstruction, and perforation) end points. It ultimately included only 3761 of 5000 planned subjects, due to bankruptcy of the sponsor. Nevertheless, it is the largest randomized study available, comparing omeprazole to placebo in patients on aspirin and clopidogrel. In regard to GI events, omeprazole was superior to placebo (1.1% vs. 2.9%, $p < 0.001$); there was no significant impact upon cardiovascular events (4.9% vs. 5.7%, $p = 0.96$) [7]. COGENT therefore established that PPI therapy, specifically omeprazole, reduces GI events in patients with ACS on DAPT. Also worth noting is that study patients were not necessarily at high risk for GI bleeding, so it may be that all patients on DAPT might benefit from omeprazole. From a strict statistical perspective, COGENT did not exclude the possibility of an increase in MACE with omeprazole and DAPT. But there was no signal present for a clinically important interaction between omeprazole and clopidogrel.

Conclusion

It is reasonable to conclude that the interaction between PPIs and clopidogrel is a real and measurable phenomenon as assessed by pharmacokinetic and pharmacodynamic studies. It is also logical to conclude that retrospective clinical studies of this interaction are subject to bias and uncontrolled confounders. Lastly, the data from COGENT (albeit underpowered) is the highest quality available, and a similar study is unlikely to be repeated in the future. At the very least, the FDA overstated the case for the clinical relevance of this highly publicized interaction. Perhaps the most important conclusion from the PPI and clopidogrel controversy is that patients at DAPT are at high risk of GI bleeding, and PPIs effectively reduce this risk. Reasonable clinicians should agree on this and exercise their own clinical judgment in regard to the rest.

References

1 Jneid, H., Anderson, J.L., Wright, R.S. *et al.* (2012) 2012 ACCF/AHA focused update of the guideline for the management of patients with unstable angina/non-ST-elevation myocardial infarction (updating the 2007 guideline and replacing the 2011 focused update): a report of the American College of Cardiology Foundation/American Heart Association Task Force on Practice Guidelines. *Journal of the American College of Cardiology*, **60 (7)**, 645–681.

2 O'Gara, P.T., Kushner, F.G., Ascheim, D.D. *et al.* (2013 Jan 29) 2013 ACCF/AHA guideline for the management of ST-elevation myocardial infarction: a report of the American College of Cardiology Foundation/American Heart Association Task Force on Practice Guidelines. *Journal of the American College of Cardiology*, **61 (4)**, e78–e140.

3 Hallas, J., Dall, M., Andries, A. *et al.* (2006) Use of single and combined antithrombotic therapy and risk of serious upper gastrointestinal bleeding: population based case–control study. *BMJ*, **333** (7571), 726.

4 Yusuf, S., Zhao, F., Mehta, S.R., Chrolavicius, S., Tognoni, G. and Fox, K.K. (2001 Aug 16) Effects of clopidogrel in addition to aspirin in patients with acute coronary syndromes without ST-segment elevation. *The New England Journal of Medicine*, **345** (7), 494–502.

5 Bhatt, D.L., Scheiman, J., Abraham, N.S. *et al.* (2008) ACCF/ACG/AHA 2008 expert consensus document on reducing the gastrointestinal risks of antiplatelet therapy and NSAID use: a report of the American College of Cardiology Foundation Task Force on Clinical Expert Consensus Documents. *Circulation*, **118** (18), 1894–1909.

6 Lanas, A., Garcia-Rodriguez, L.A., Arroyo, M.T. *et al.* (2007 Mar) Effect of antisecretory drugs and nitrates on the risk of ulcer bleeding associated with nonsteroidal anti-inflammatory drugs, antiplatelet agents, and anticoagulants. *The American Journal of Gastroenterology*, **102** (3), 507–515.

7 Bhatt, D.L., Cryer, B.L., Contant, C.F. *et al.* (2010 Nov 11) Clopidogrel with or without omeprazole in coronary artery disease. *The New England Journal of Medicine*, **363** (20), 1909–1917.

8 United States Food and Drug Administration. *Information for healthcare professionals: update to the labeling of clopidogrel bisulfate (marketed as Plavix) to alert healthcare professionals about a drug interaction with omeprazole (marketed as Prilosec and Prilosec OTC)*.

9 Angiolillo, D.J., Gibson, C.M., Cheng, S. *et al.* (2010) Differential effects of omeprazole and pantoprazole on the pharmacodynamics and pharmacokinetics of clopidogrel in healthy subjects: randomized, placebo-controlled, crossover comparison studies. *Clinical Pharmacology and Therapeutics*, **89 (1)**, 65–74.

10 Pereillo, J.M., Maftouh, M., Andrieu, A. *et al.* (2002) Structure and stereochemistry of the active metabolite of clopidogrel. *Drug Metabolism and Disposition*, **30 (11)**, 1288–1295.

11 Savi, P., Combalbert, J., Gaich, C. *et al.* (1994) The antiaggregating activity of clopidogrel is due to a metabolic activation by the hepatic cytochrome P450-1A. *Thrombosis and Haemostasis*, **72 (2)**, 313–317.

12 Savi, P., Pereillo, J.M., Uzabiaga, M.F. *et al.* (2000 Nov) Identification and biological activity of the active metabolite of clopidogrel. *Thrombosis and Haemostasis*, **84 (5)**, 891–896.

13 Clarke, T.A. and Waskell, L.A. (2003 Jan) The metabolism of clopidogrel is catalyzed by human cytochrome P450 3A and is inhibited by atorvastatin. *Drug Metabolism and Disposition*, **31 (1)**, 53–59.

14 Mega, J.L., Close, S.L., Wiviott, S.D. *et al.* (2009) Cytochrome p-450 polymorphisms and response to clopidogrel. *The New England Journal of Medicine*, **360 (4)**, 354–362.

15 Desta, Z., Zhao, X., Shin, J.G., and Flockhart, D.A. (2002) Clinical significance of the cytochrome P450 2C19 genetic polymorphism. *Clinical Pharmacokinetics*, **41 (12)**, 913–958.

16 Li, X.Q., Andersson, T.B., Ahlstrom, M., and Weidolf, L. (2004) Comparison of inhibitory effects of the proton pump-inhibiting drugs omeprazole, esomeprazole, lansoprazole, pantoprazole, and rabeprazole on human cytochrome P450 activities. *Drug Metabolism and Disposition*, **32 (8)**, 821–827.

17 Andersson, T. (1996) Pharmacokinetics metabolism and interactions of acid pump inhibitors. Focus on omeprazole, lansoprazole and pantoprazole. *Clinical Pharmacokinetics*, **31** (1), 9–28.

18 Focks, J.J., Brouwer, M.A., van Oijen, M.G., Lanas, A., Bhatt, D.L., and Verheugt, F.W. (2013) Concomitant use of clopidogrel and proton pump inhibitors: impact on platelet function and clinical outcome – a systematic review. *Heart*, **99 (8)**, 520–527.

19 Frelinger, A.L., 3rd, Lee, R.D., Mulford, D.J. *et al.* (2012) A randomized, 2-period, crossover design study to assess the effects of dexlansoprazole, lansoprazole, esomeprazole, and omeprazole on the steady-state pharmacokinetics and pharmacodynamics of clopidogrel in healthy volunteers. *Journal of the American College of Cardiology*, **59 (14)**, 1304–1311.

20 Pezalla, E., Day, D. and Pulliadath, I. (2008) Initial assessment of clinical impact of a drug interaction between clopidogrel and proton pump inhibitors. *Journal of the American College of Cardiology*, **52 (12)**, 1038–1039 author reply 1039.

21 Ho, P.M., Maddox, T.M., Wang, L. *et al.* (2009) Risk of adverse outcomes associated with concomitant use of clopidogrel and proton pump inhibitors following acute coronary syndrome. *JAMA*, **301 (9)**, 937–944.

22 Juurlink, D.N., Gomes, T., Ko, D.T. *et al.* (2009) A population-based study of the drug interaction between proton pump inhibitors and clopidogrel. *CMAJ*, **180 (7)**, 713–718.

23 O'Donoghue, M.L., Braunwald, E., Antman, E.M. *et al.* (2009) Pharmacodynamic effect and clinical efficacy of clopidogrel and prasugrel with or without a proton-pump inhibitor: an analysis of two randomised trials. *Lancet*, **374** (9694), 989–997.

24 Goodman, S.G., Clare, R., Pieper, K.S. *et al.* (2012) Association of proton pump inhibitor use on cardiovascular outcomes with clopidogrel and ticagrelor: insights from the platelet inhibition and patient outcomes trial. *Circulation*, **125 (8)**, 978–986.

25 Wu, H., Jing, Q., Wang, J., and Guo, X. (2011) Pantoprazole for the prevention of gastrointestinal bleeding in high-risk patients with acute coronary syndromes. *Journal of Critical Care*, **26 (4)**, 434.e1–434.e6.

37 Other Drug Interactions with Clopidogrel

Eric R. Bates

University of Michigan, Ann Arbor, MI, USA

Introduction

Clopidogrel, atorvastatin, omeprazole, and many other drugs require hepatic cytochrome P450 (CYP) metabolism. Because many of these drugs are concomitantly administered to patients with coronary artery disease, the clinical implications of possible pharmacodynamic interactions have raised concern [1]. The proton pump inhibitor interaction with clopidogrel is reviewed in Chapter 36. The purpose of this chapter is to summarize the pharmacodynamic and clinical evidence regarding the other clopidogrel–drug interactions.

Drug metabolism

Clopidogrel bisulfate, an inactive thienopyridine prodrug, is 85% hydrolyzed *in vivo* by esterases to an inactive carboxylic acid derivative (Figure 37.1). The remaining drug undergoes oxidative biotransformation to its active thiol metabolite by a two-step, CYP-dependent process where CYP3A4/5 and CYP2C19 have the greatest roles, with lesser involvement from CYP2B6, CYP1A2, and CYP2C9. The active metabolite then irreversibly inhibits the platelet $P2Y_{12}$ adenosine diphosphate (ADP) receptor. This blocks ADP from binding to the receptor and stimulating platelet activation and aggregation. Genetic, cellular, and clinical factors that induce, inhibit, or compete for CYP activity can modulate biotransformation of clopidogrel to its active metabolite and result in interindividual variability of clopidogrel responsiveness. Drug–drug interactions are also important.

Antiplatelet Therapy in Cardiovascular Disease, First Edition. Edited by Ron Waksman, Paul A. Gurbel, and Michael A. Gaglia, Jr.
© 2014 John Wiley & Sons, Ltd. Published 2014 by John Wiley & Sons, Ltd.

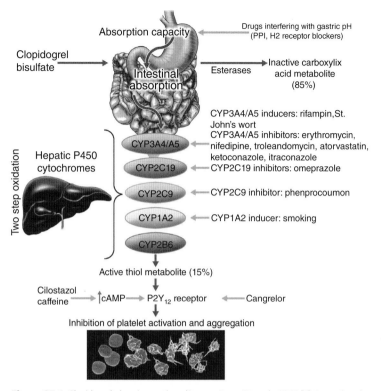

Figure 37.1 Clopidogrel–drug interactions (Source: Bates ER et al., 2011 [1]. Reproduced with permission of Elsevier.)

The clopidogrel–atorvastatin interaction

Atorvastatin was the first drug noted to interact with clopidogrel, establishing that clopidogrel is metabolized by CYP3A4 in humans [2]. However, other pharmacodynamic studies have shown no impact with clopidogrel and atorvastatin coadministration for various reasons, especially when a higher clopidogrel loading dose (600 mg) was tested, when measurements were made several weeks later, or when atorvastatin was added to clopidogrel [1].

Registry, administrative database, and *post hoc* randomized clinical trial reports have evaluated the potential clinical interaction. Increased risk was seen in two studies [3, 4], but not in three studies [5, 6, 7], two of which used a high clopidogrel loading dose [6, 7]. In other studies, there was an insignificant trend for worse outcomes with atorvastatin compared with pravastatin or no statin [8, 9, 10, 11] and with CYP-metabolized statins compared with non-CYP-metabolized statins [10, 11, 12], but no consistent signal for increased cardiovascular risk with drug coadministration.

Other clopidogrel–drug interactions

CYP3A4 inhibitors (erythromycin, troleandomycin, ketoconazole) decrease and CYP3A4 inducers (rifampin) increase the antiplatelet activity of clopidogrel [2, 13]. Several other clopidogrel–drug interactions have also been described (Figure 37.1).

CYP inhibitors

Ketoconazole is a potent inhibitor of both CYP3A4 and CYP3A5. Healthy subjects given loading and maintenance doses of clopidogrel had decreased production of active metabolite and significantly reduced platelet inhibition on ketoconazole compared with control [14]. Similarly, the CYP3A inhibitor itraconazole significantly decreased the ability of clopidogrel to inhibit platelet aggregation [15].

Dihydropyridine calcium channel blockers (nifedipine, amlodipine) also inhibit CYP3A4. In *ex vivo* platelet function studies, they have been shown to decrease clopidogrel responsiveness [16, 17, 18], but no impact on the clinical efficacy of clopidogrel has been demonstrated [19, 20, 21].

Phenprocoumon, an oral anticoagulant used in Europe, is a coumarin derivative metabolized by CYP3A4 and CYP2C9. Concomitant treatment with clopidogrel attenuated the antiplatelet effect of clopidogrel and increased the number of nonresponders [22].

Cangrelor, an ATP analog, is a parenteral reversible $P2Y_{12}$ receptor inhibitor with a short half-life that results in the normalization of platelet aggregation approximately 30 minutes after discontinuation of the infusion. When clopidogrel was given simultaneously with cangrelor and cangrelor was continued for 2 hours, there was no inhibition of the $P2Y_{12}$ receptor by clopidogrel after the infusion was stopped because the clopidogrel active metabolite was unavailable for binding due to its short half-life [23]. When clopidogrel was started at the time the cangrelor infusion was discontinued, there was inhibition of the $P2Y_{12}$ receptor.

CYP inducers

Clopidogrel responsiveness can be increased by coadministration with rifampin, a CYP3A4 and CYP2C19 inducer, and nonresponders can become responsive [2, 13]. Judge *et al.* [24] have proven that this response is due to increased production of the clopidogrel active metabolite and increased $P2Y_{12}$ receptor blockade.

By inhibiting the platelet $P2Y_{12}$ receptor, clopidogrel increases intracellular cyclic adenosine monophosphate (cAMP), a key signaling molecule in inhibiting platelet aggregation. Caffeine also increases cAMP levels and has been shown to enhance platelet inhibition by clopidogrel [25]. Other methylxanthines (theophylline) and phosphodiesterase inhibitors (cilostazol) also increase platelet cAMP levels [26].

Smoking is a known CYP1A2 inducer, and several studies have demonstrated increased platelet inhibition [27, 28], fewer ischemic events [29, 30], and increased bleeding risk [30] in smokers following clopidogrel administration. Other studies have found no impact on clinical events [31, 32].

Omega-3 polyunsaturated fatty acids (PUFA) were shown in one small prospective randomized trial to increase clopidogrel responsiveness, but the mechanism is unclear [33].

St. John's wort (*Hypericum perforatum*) is an herbal product used to treat depression. It also induces CYP3A4 activity. In healthy volunteers who were nonresponders to clopidogrel, St. John's wort 300 mg thrice daily for 14 days improved the platelet inhibitory activity of clopidogrel by increasing CYP3A4 metabolic activity [34].

Confounding variables in the drug interaction debate

There are many confounding variables contributing to the discordant results regarding potential clopidogrel–drug interactions [1]. First, drug interactions can be dose dependent. Second, suboptimal production of active metabolite following a clopidogrel loading dose could eventually be overcome as active metabolite eventually accumulates from maintenance dosing and binds to initially unblocked platelet receptors. Moreover, only 10–15% of the platelet pool is regenerated daily, and platelet reactivity decreases with time after the initiating event, making it unlikely that a sustained reduction in inhibition of platelet aggregation could be maintained by a drug interaction. Third, drug interactions may only be important in patients with borderline platelet inhibition, where small reductions in platelet inhibition might result in posttreatment platelet reactivity above therapeutic thresholds. Additionally, alternative CYP isoenzyme pathways may become more active in patients with concomitant treatment of competing agents. Fourth, there may be offsetting clinical effects. Atorvastatin has a number of beneficial pleiotropic effects (LDL reduction, decreased inflammation, plaque stabilization, fibrinolysis stimulation, improved endothelial function), including platelet inhibition, associated with decreased MI and death rates that could offset the negative clinical effect of any potential reduction in platelet inhibition with clopidogrel.

Research challenges in the drug interaction debate

There are many research challenges in scientifically measuring the clinical importance of drug–drug interactions. First, study design is critical. Treatment in observational studies is based on clinical need or physician preference, creating selection bias, so these studies can only suggest association, not conclude causality. Claims-based studies are particularly limited by missing or misclassified data. Outcome events in randomized trials are often adjudicated, but multivariable or propensity score analyses in *post hoc* studies cannot completely adjust for differences in unknown or unmeasured confounders. Only a randomized clinical trial could confirm the importance of a drug–drug interaction at the population level, although the generalizability of the results would be modified by inclusion and exclusion criteria and the potential cost of such a trial would probably be prohibitive. Second, published studies have not been appropriately powered to address clopidogrel–drug interactions. The absolute reduction in major adverse cardiac events at 30 days when clopidogrel is added to aspirin compared with aspirin monotherapy is only 1% [35], making it possible that studies demonstrating no clopidogrel–drug interactions were insufficiently powered to detect a small, but clinically meaningful, difference in event rates when millions of patients are prescribed these drugs. Third, composite end points that include variables that are not platelet mediated may obscure a potential drug interaction. Fourth, drug–drug interactions in subgroups of patients may not be recognized in population analyses. Moreover, the small reduction in platelet aggregation (10–15%) with clopidogrel–drug interactions may not be clinically significant in many subgroups. Fifth, patient compliance with coadministration of both medications during the study period needs to be proven.

Conclusions

There are many pharmacodynamic clopidogrel–drug interactions, but there is no consistent evidence that these interactions have clinical significance. The therapeutic benefit of coadministering these medications to appropriate patients should greatly exceed any theoretical harm from clopidogrel–drug interactions that appear to be dose dependent, time limited, and mild compared with the larger challenges of medication adherence and interindividual variability in clopidogrel responsiveness.

References

1 Bates, E.R., Lau, W.C. & Angiolillo, D.J. (2011) Clopidogrel-drug interactions. *Journal of the American College of Cardiology*, **57**, 1251–1263.

2 Lau, W.C., Waskell, L.A., Watkins, P.B. *et al.* (2003) Atorvastatin reduces the ability of clopidogrel to inhibit platelet aggregation: a new drug-drug interaction. *Circulation*, **107**, 32–37.

3 Gulec, S., Ozdol, C., Rahimov, U., Atmaca, Y., Kumbasar, D. & Erol, C. (2005) Myonecrosis after elective percutaneous coronary intervention: effect of clopidogrel-statin interaction. *The Journal of Invasive Cardiology*, **17**, 589–593.

4 Brophy, J.M., Babapulle, M.N., Costa, V. & Rinfret, S. (2006) A pharmacoepidemiology study of the interaction between atorvastatin and

clopidogrel after percutaneous coronary intervention. *American Heart Journal*, **152**, 263–269.

5 Mukherjee, D., Kline-Rogers, E., Fang, J., Munir, K. & Eagle, K.A. (2005) Lack of clopidogrel-CYP3A4 statin interaction in patients with acute coronary syndrome. *Heart*, **91**, 23–26.

6 Trenk, D., Hochholzer, W., Frundi, D. *et al.* (2008) Impact of cytochrome P450 3A4-metabolized statins on the antiplatelet effect of a 600-mg loading dose clopidogrel and on clinical outcome in patients undergoing elective coronary stent placement. *Thrombosis and Haemostasis*, **99**, 174–181.

7 Geisler, T., Zürn, C., Paterok, M. *et al.* (2008) Statins do not adversely affect post-interventional residual platelet aggregation and outcomes in patients undergoing coronary stenting treated by dual antiplatelet therapy. *European Heart Journal*, **29**, 1635–1643.

8 Wienbergen, H.A., Gitt, A.K., Schiele, R. *et al.* (2003) Comparison of clinical benefits of clopidogrel therapy in patients with acute coronary syndromes taking atorvastatin versus other statin therapies. *The American Journal of Cardiology*, **92**, 285–288.

9 Wahab, N.N. & Cox, J.L. (2003) Does the use of atorvastatin with clopidogrel increase clinical adverse events after percutaneous coronary intervention? *The Canadian Journal of Cardiology*, **19** (Suppl A), 231A–232A abst.

10 Saw, J., Steinhubl, S.R., Berger, P.B. *et al.* (2003) Lack of adverse clopidogrel-atorvastatin clinical interaction from secondary analysis of a randomized, placebo-controlled clopidogrel trial. *Circulation*, **108**, 921–924.

11 Saw, J., Brennan, D.M., Steinhubl, S.R. *et al.* (2007) Lack of evidence of a clopidogrel-statin interaction in the CHARISMA trial. *Journal of the American College of Cardiology*, **50**, 291–295.

12 Blagojevic, A., Delaney, J.A.C., Levesque, L.E., Dendukuri, N., Boivin, N.F. & Brophy, J.M. (2009) Investigation of an interaction between statins and clopidogrel after percutaneous coronary intervention: a cohort study. *Pharmacoepidemiology and Drug Safety*, **18**, 362–369.

13 Lau, W.C., Gurbel, P.A., Watkins, P.B. *et al.* (2004) The contribution of hepatic cytochrome P450 3A4 metabolic activity to the phenomenon of clopidogrel resistance. *Circulation*, **109**, 166–171.

14 Farid, N.A., Payne, C.D., Small, D.S. *et al.* (2007) Cytochrome P450 3A inhibition by ketoconazole affects prasugrel and clopidogrel pharmacokinetics and pharmacodynamics differently. *Clinical Pharmacology and Therapeutics*, **81**, 735–741.

15 Suh, J.W., Koo, B.K., Zhang, S.Y. *et al.* (2006) Increased risk of atherothrombotic events associated with cytochrome P450 3A5 polymorphism in patients taking clopidogrel. *CMAJ*, **174**, 1715–1722.

16 Siller-Matula, J.M., Lang, I., Christ, G. & Jilma, B. (2008) Calcium-channel blockers reduce the antiplatelet effect of clopidogrel. *Journal of the American College of Cardiology*, **52**, 1557–1563.

17 Gremmel, T., Steiner, S., Seidinger, D., Koppensteiner, R., Panzer, S. & Kopp, C.W. (2010) Calcium-channel blockers decrease clopidogrel-mediated platelet inhibition. *Heart*, **96**, 186–189.

18 Harmsze, A.M., Robijns, K., van Werkum, J.W. *et al.* (2010) The use of amlodipine, but not of P-glycoprotein inhibiting calcium channel blockers is associated with clopidogrel poor-response. *Thrombosis and Haemostasis*, **103**, 920–925.

19 Olesen, J.B., Gislason, G.H., Charlot, M.G. *et al.* (2011) Calcium-channel blockers do not alter the clinical efficacy of clopidogrel after myocardial infarction. *Journal of the American College of Cardiology*, **57**, 409–417.

20 Sarafoff, N., Neumann, L., Morath, T. *et al.* (2011) Lack of impact of calcium-channel blockers on the pharmacodynamic effect and the clinical efficacy of clopidogrel after drug-eluting stenting. *American Heart Journal*, **161**, 605–610.

21 Good, C.W., Steinhubl, S.R., Brennan, D.M., Lincoff, A.M., Topol, E.J. & Berger, P.B. (2012) Is there a clinically significant interaction between calcium channel antagonists and clopidogrel? *Circulation. Cardiovascular Interventions*, **5**, 77–81.

22 Sibbing, D., von Beckerath, N., Morath, T. *et al.* (2010) Oral anticoagulation with coumarin derivatives and antiplatelet effects of clopidogrel. *European Heart Journal*, **31**, 1205–1211.

23 Steinhubl, S.R., Oh, J.J., Oestreich, J.H., Ferraris, S., Charnigo, R. & Akers, W.S. (2008) Transitioning patients from cangrelor to clopidogrel: pharmacodynamic evidence of a competitive effect. *Thrombosis Research*, **121**, 527–534.

24 Judge, H.M., Patil, S.B., Buckland, R.J., Jakubowski, J.A. & Storey, R.F. (2010) Potentiation of clopidogrel active metabolite formation by rifampicin leads to greater P2Y12 receptor blockade and inhibition of platelet aggregation following clopidogrel. *Journal of Thrombosis and Haemostasis*, **8**, 1820–1827.

25 Lev EI, Arikan ME, Vaduganathan M, et al. Effect of caffeine on platelet inhibition by clopidogrel in healthy subjects and patients with coronary artery disease. *American Heart Journal* 2007;**154**:694.e1-694.e7

26 Angiolillo, D.J., Capranzano, P., Goto, S. *et al.* (2008) A randomized study assessing the impact of cilostazol on platelet function profiles in patients with diabetes mellitus and coronary artery disease on dual antiplatelet therapy: results of the OPTIMUS-2 study. *European Heart Journal*, **29**, 2202–2211.

27 Bliden, K.P., DiChiara, J., Lawal, L. *et al.* (2008) The association of cigarette smoking with enhanced platelet inhibition by clopidogrel. *Journal of the American College of Cardiology*, **52**, 531–533.

28 Park, K.W., Kang, S.-H., Kang, J. *et al.* (2012) Enhanced clopidogrel response in smokers is reversed after discontinuation as assessed by VerifyNow assay: additional evidence for the concept of 'smokers' paradox'. *Heart*, **98**, 1000–1006.

29 Desai, N.R., Mega, J.L., Jiang, S., Cannon, C.P. & Sabatine, M.S. (2009) Interaction between cigarette smoking and clinical benefit of clopidogrel. *Journal of the American College of Cardiology*, **53**, 1273–1278.

30 Berger, J.S., Bhatt, D.L., Steinhubl, S.R. *et al.* (2009) Smoking, clopidogrel, and mortality in patients with established cardiovascular disease. *Circulation*, **120**, 2337–2344.

31 Hochholzer, W., Trenk, D., Mega, J.L. *et al.* (2011) Impact of smoking on antiplatelet effect of clopidogrel and prasugrel after loading dose and on maintenance therapy. *American Heart Journal*, **162**, 518–526.

32 Cornel JH, Becker RC, Goodman SG, et al. Prior smoking status, clinical outcomes, and the comparison of ticagrelor with clopidogrel in acute coronary syndromes – Insights from the PLATelet inhibition and patient Outcomes (PLATO) trial. *American Heart Journal* 2012;**164**:334.e1–342.e1

33 Gajos, G., Rostoff, P., Undas, A. & Piwowarska, W. (2010) Effects of polyunsaturated omega-3 fatty acids on responsiveness to dual antiplatelet

therapy in patients undergoing percutaneous coronary intervention. *Journal of the American College of Cardiology*, **55**, 1671–1678.

34 Lau, W.C., Welch, T.D., Shields, T., Rubenfire, M., Tantry, U.S. & Gurbel, P.A. (2011) The effect of St. John's wort on the pharmacodynamic response of clopidogrel in hyporesponsive volunteers and patients: increased platelet inhibition by enhancement of CYP 3A4 metabolic activity. *Journal of Cardiovascular Pharmacology*, **57**, 86–93.

35 The CURE Trial Investigators (2001) Effects of clopidogrel in addition to aspirin in patients with acute coronary syndromes without ST-segment elevation. *The New England Journal of Medicine*, **345**, 494–502.

Index

Antiplatelet Therapy in Cardiovascular Disease, First Edition. Edited by Ron Waksman,
Paul A. Gurbel and Michael A. Gaglia, Jr.
© 2014 John Wiley & Sons, Ltd. Published 2014 by John Wiley & Sons, Ltd.